Vol. 3

INTERNATIONAL

COLLATION

OF

TRADITIONAL

AND

FOLK MEDICINE

NORTHEAST ASIA

Part III

International Collation of Traditional and Folk Medicine

Vol. 3

A project of UNESCO

INTERNATIONAL

COLLATION

OF

TRADITIONAL

AND

FOLK MEDICINE

Editor-in-Chief

Chung Ki Sung
Chonnam National University

Editors

Takeatsu Kimura
Daiichi College of Pharmaceutical Sciences

Paul P. H. But
The Chinese University of Hong Kong

Ji-Xian Guo
Shanghai Medical University

NORTHEAST ASIA

Part III

World Scientific
Singapore • New Jersey • London • Hong Kong

Published by

World Scientific Publishing Co. Pte. Ltd.

P O Box 128, Farrer Road, Singapore 912805

USA office: Suite 1B, 1060 Main Street, River Edge, NJ 07661

UK office: 57 Shelton Street, Covent Garden, London WC2H 9HE

Library of Congress Cataloging-in-Publication Data
Northeast Asia / editor-in-chief, Paul P. H. But; editors, Takeatsu Kimura, Ji-Xian Guo, Chung Ki Sung.
    p.   cm. -- (International collation of traditional and folk medicine : vol. 3)
  "A project of UNESCO."
  Includes bibliographical references and index.
  ISBN 9810236395
  1. Materia medica, Vegetable -- East Asia.   2. Medicinal plants -- East Asia.
  3. Traditional medicine -- East Asia.   I. Kimura, Takeatsu.   II. UNESCO.
  III. Series.
    [DNLM: 1. Medicine, Herbal.   2. Plants, Medicinal -- chemistry.
  3. Plant Extracts -- therapeutic use.   4. Drug Design.
  5. International Cooperation.   WB 925 N874 1996]
  RS180.E18N67   1997
  615'.321'095--dc20
  DNLM/DLC   96-4659
  for Library of Congress   CIP

British Library Cataloguing-in-Publication Data
A catalogue record for this book is available from the British Library.

Printed in Singapore by Uto-Print

FOREWORD

The plant floras and animal faunas in China, Hong Kong, Japan, and Korea – located nearly in the same temperature zone – share much similarity with the result that traditional folk medical experiences in this region are comparable in nature. Nonetheless, since folk medical experience in different countries have been developed rather independently each with a long history, both similarities and differences coexist in traditional folk medical knowledge from different countries.

Folk medical knowledge may be regarded as clinical experience obtained naturally. However, part of the experience might be mythical reflecting regional differences in culture. The task of separating fact from myth and isolating placebo-effects from objective bio-activity in folk and traditional medicine is a difficult one. We believe that when folk medical experiences derived from the same source are collated comparatively the real medical effects associated with bio-activity of the drug will emerge. From this perspective, an international collation of folk medical knowledge should help in establishing objective and reliable medical experience.

The search for bio-active components from natural materials as a source of lead compounds in drug development, is a major endeavor in natural product chemical research. This book is aimed at assisting natural product chemists to identify the natural products which most likely contain bio-active components of interest and which may warrant further investigation.

The folk medical knowledge of each entry in the book includes the scientific and local names of the drug, special processing involved, method used for administration, apparent folk medical efficacy in each country, contraindications and side effects. Also included is the information concerning modern scientific data relating to the associated chemistry and pharmacology as well as references to the available literature.

This third volume continues to cover the outcome generated by the "international collation project" propelled by the Regional Network for the Chemistry of Natural Products in Southeast Asia, operated by the United Nations Educational, Scientific and Cultural Organization(UNESCO). The Ministry of Education, Republic of Korea has kindly provided financial support for this ongoing project. On behalf of the Managing Board, I am most grateful to Professor Chung Ki Sung, the *Editor-in-Chief* of volume III, and other members of the editorial board who undertook the painstaking job of making a literature survey, as well as writing and editing this volume. My sincere gratitude is also extended to the UNESCO Office, Jakarta(ROSTSEA) and the Korea National Commission for UNESCO for their valuable help in the planning and organizing this project.

Byung Hoon Han, Prof., PhD.
Chairman, Managing Board

CONTENTS

x

xi

EXPLANATIONS AND ABBREVIATIONS

Plant and Animal Name
One hundred ninety eight important medicinal plants and two animals are presented in this volume. The sequence of the plant families follows the classification and arrangement of plant families of Engler's system and the sequence of the individual species in a family follows the alphabetical order of their scientific names. Synonyms are shown as (=). Each representative vernacular name is shown in Roman script followed by an abbreviation of a country/region name. Chinese characters of the herb and plant names are shown in the "Chinese Character Index." Related plants are shown in similar manner. Animals are arranged at the end of plants in an alphabetical order of their scientific names.

Part
Pharmacopoeias which adopt a particular drug are shown in abbreviations. Local drug names are the standard or representative vernacular names for that particular drug.

Processing
Procedures for processing the crude drug.

Method of Administration
Routes of administration and preparation methods.

Folk Medicinal Use
Names of diseases or symptoms treated with the drug, followed by an abbreviation of the country which uses the drug for that purpose.

Contra-indications and Side Effects
Warnings for conditions to be avoided in the application of a particular drug and adverse reactions that may be induced by the drug.

Scientific Research
Chemical components and pharmacology reported before 1998 are summarized.

Literature
Format of the literature citation is as follows: First author, *journal title or book title*(in italics), **year**(boldface), volume, and first page.

401.   *Codium fragile* Hariot   (Codiaceae)

Ci-hai-song(C), Miru(J), Cheong-gak-chae(K)

Whole plant
Local Drug Name: Ci-hai-song(C), Suisho(J), Su-song(K),
Processing: Dry under the sun(C, K)
Method of Administration: Oral(decoction, C, K)
Folk Medicinal Uses:
        1) Ascariasis(C, K)
        2) Astonishment(K)

Scientific Research:
Chemistry
  1) Carbohydrates: 1-Glycerophosphoryl-2-hydroxy-3-(5'-dimethyl-arsinoyl-β-ribofuranosyl-oxy)
    propane, 1'-(1,2-dihydroxy-propyl)-5'-deoxy-5'-dimethyl-arsinoyl β-ribofuranoside[1]
  2) Amines: Trimethyl amine, trimethyl amine N-oxide[2], taurine[3]
  3) N-Heterocycles: Chlorophyll a, b[4]
  4) Miscellaneous: Dimethyl arsinic acid[1]
Phamacology
  1) Cytotoxic activity[5]
  2) Plant growth inhibition[5]
  3) Phytohemagglutinin[6]

Literature:
[1] Jin, K. *et al.*: *Appl. Organometallic Chem.* **1988**, 2(4), 365.
[2] Fujiwara-Arasaki, T. and Mino, N.: *Proc. Int. Seaweed Symp. 7ᵗʰ 1971* **1972**, 506.
[3] Kataoka, H. and Ohnishi, N.: *Agr. Biol chem.* **1986**, 50(7), 1887.
[4] Zeng, C. K. *et al.*: *Hai Yang Yu Hu Chao* **1980**, 11(2), 134.
[5] Chenieux, J. C. *et al.*: *Planta Med. Suppl.* **1980**, 40, 152.
[6] Blunden, G. *et al.*: *Lloydia* **1975**, 38, 162.

                                                    [C. K. Sung]

402.   *Laminaria japonica* Aresch.   (Laminariaceae)

Hai-dai (C), Hoi-dai (H), Makonbu (J), Da-si-ma (K)

Related Plant: *Ecklonia kurome* Okam.: Kum-bu (C), Gam-tae (K).

Thalline (CP)
Local Drug Name: Kun-bu (C), Hoi-dai (H), Konbu (J), Gon-po (K).
Processing: Eliminate foreign matter, rinse, briefly dry in the air, cut into wide slivers, and dry in the sun (C, K).
Method of Administration: Oral (decoction: C, H, K).
Folk Medicinal Uses:
        1) Goiter (C, H, J, K).
        2) Edema (C, H, J, K).
        3) Swelling and pain of the testis (C, H).
        4) Scrofula (C, H).
        5) Hematemesis (K).
        6) Hypoaciditic (K).
Contraindication: Incompatible with Radix Glycyrrhizae (C).

Scientific Research:
Chemistry
1) Carbohydrates: alginate [1-3], laminarin (laminariose), mannitol, galactan [1], arsenic-containing ribofuranoside [4], uronofucan [5].
2) Amino acids: laminine, glutamic acid, aspartic acid, proline, methionine, histidine, gysteine,trypotophan, alanine, glycine, valine, arginine [6-8].
3) Trace elements: I_2, Ca, Fe, Na, K, Mg, Al, Mn, Cu, Co, Ti, F, Pb, Zn, As, Cr, Ni, Mo, Sn, Cd, Ag, Au, Si, Li, V, Bi, Se, Y [2-4, 6,8,9].
4) Organic acids [10]: nicotinic acid [11].
5) Vitamins: vitamin B_1, vitamin B_2, vitamin C [11].
6) Essential oils: cubenol, (E,Z)-2,6-nonodienal, (E)-2-nonenal, (Z,Z)-3,6-nonadienal, (E,Z)-2,6-nonadienol, (E)-2-noneol, myristic acid, w-hexadecenoic acid [12].
7) Pigments: carotene [11], chlorophylls [13].
Pharmacology
1) Effect on thyroid.
2) Chlolesterol lowering effect [14,15].
3) Antihypertensive effect [15-19].
4) Relieving asthma and cough [16].
5) Styptic effect [18,19].
6) Antitumor effect [18,19].
7) Anticoagulant effect [20,21].
8) Radioprotective effect (polysaccharides) [22].
9) Antiviral effect (polysaccharides) [23].
10) Antioxidative effect [24].
11) Immunomodulating effect (polysaccharides) [25-27].
12) Analgesic effect [28].
13) Heterogenous antimutagenic activity [29].

Literature:
[1] Ji, M. H. *et al.*: *Hydrobigologia* **1984,** 116, 554.
[2] Evtushenko. Z.S.: *Okeanologiya* **1986,** 26(6), 933.
[3] Fan, X. *et al.*: *Haiyang Yu Huzhao* **1988,** 19(1), 64.
[4] Shibata, Y. *et al.*: *Agric. Biol. Chem.* **1987,** 51(2), 391.
[5] Shaposhnikova, G. M. *et al.*: *Dokl. Akad. Nauk* **1992,** 324(4), 881.
[6] Yoshimura, A. *et al.*: *Nippon Suisan Gakkaishi* **1973,** 39(3), 317.
[7] Takagi, S.: *Nara Igaku Zsshi* **1973,** 24(5), 575.
[8] Gryzhankova, L. N. *et al.*: *Izv. Akad. Nauk SSSR, Ser. Biol.* **1975,** (1), 76.
[9] Saenko, G. . *et al.*: *Okeanologiya* **1988,** 28(2), 322.
[10] Kaneniwa, M. *et al.*: *Nippon Suisan Gakkaishi* **1987,** 53(5), 861.
[11] *"Shiwu Chengfenbiao"* **1977,** 164.
[12] Kajiwra, T. *et al.*: *J. Food Sci.* **1988,** 53(2), 960.
[13] Sasaki, K. *et al.*: *Jpn. Kokai Tokkyo Koho JP* 06,113,872 [94,113,872] (cl. c12P17/18), 26 Apr. **1994,** APPL. 92/287,096 02 Oct. **1991.**
[14] *Arch. Pathol.* **1955,** 59, 717.
[15] Ren. D. *et al.*: *Fish Sci.* **1994,** 60(1), 83.
[16] *"Zhongyao Dacidian"* **1977,** Vol.1, 1351.
[17] Funayama, S. *et al.*: *Planta Med.* **1981,** 41(1), 29.
[18] *Guowai Yaoxue (Zhiwuyao Fence)* **1981,** (5), 22.
[19] *Guowai Yaoxee (Z hiwuyao Fence)* **1982,** (2), 36.
[20] Han, Q. Q. *et al.*: *Zhonghua Xinxueguanbing Zazhi* **1980,** (8), 218.
[21] Yu, B. Q.: *Zhonghua Xinxueguanbing Zazhi* **1981,** (3), 212.
[22] Deng, H. C. *et al.*: *Zhonghua Fangshe Yixue Yu Fanghu Zazhi* **1987,** 7(1), 49.
[23] Muto, S. *et al.*: *Eur. Pat. Appl. Ep.* 295,956 21 Dec JP, APPL. **1988** 87/152,086, 18 Jun **1987.**
[24] Nishibori, S. *et al.*: *Kaseigaku Zasshi* **1985,** 36(11), 845.

[25] Fa, M.F. *et al.*: *Zhongguo Yaoke Daxue Xuebao* **1988,** 19(1), 30.
[26] Inagwa, H. *et al.*: *Chem. Pharm. Bull.* **1992,** 40(4), 994.
[27] Wang, W. T. *et al.*: *Zhongguo Yaolixue Yu Dulixue Zazhi* **1994,** 8(3), 199.
[28] Soma, G. *et al.*: *Eur. Pat. APPL. EP* 472,467 (cl. A61k37/20), 26 Feb **1992,** JP APPL. 90/218, 599, 29 Aug **1990.**
[29] Okai, Y. *et al.*: *Mutat. Res.* **1993,** 303(2), 63.

[J.X. Guo]

403   *Laminaria ochotensis* **Miyabe**   (Laminariaceae)

Rishiri-konbu(J), Da-si-ma(K)

Related plants: *L. japonica* Areschoug, *L. japonica* var. *ochotensis*: Konbu(J)

Whole plant
  Local Drug Name: Konbu(J), Hae-dae(K)
  Processing: Dry under the sun(K)
  Method of Administration: Oral(decoction, K)
  Folk Medicinal Uses:
           1) Scrofula(J)
           2) Edema(J)
           3) Stegnotic(K)
           4) Hematemesis(K)
           5) Hypoaciditic(K)
           6) Leukorrhea(K)

Scientific Research:
  Chemistry
   1) Laminarins[1]
  Phamacology
   1) Inhibition of Sarcoma-180 cell[2]

Literature:
[1] Elyakova, L. A. and Zvyagintseva, T. N.: *Carbohyd. Res.* **1974,** 34(2), 241.
[2] Yamamoto, I. *et al.*: *Cancer Lett.* **1986,** 30(2), 125.

[C. K. Sung]

404.   *Undaria pinnatifida* **Suring**   (Laminariaceae)

Qun-dai-cai(C), Wakame(J), Mi-yeok(K)

Whole plant
  Local Drug Name: Kun-bu(C), Kuntaisai(J), Gon-po(K)
  Processing: Dry under the sun(C, K) or use in fresh(C)
  Method of Administration: Oral(decoction, C, K)
  Folk Medicinal Uses:
           1) Weakness after child birth(J, K)
           2) Constipation(J, K)
           3) Thyroid enlargement(C)
           4) Chronic bronchitis(C)
           5) Scrofula(C)

6) Ancylostomiasis(K)
  7) Dysentery(K)
  8) Neuralgia(K)
  9) Acute gastritis(K)
  10) Alcohol poisoning(K)

Scientific Research:
Chemistry
  1) Carbohydrates: Alginic acid[1], polysaccharide[2]
  2) Lipids: Digalactosyldiacyl glycerol[3]
  3) Terpenes: (-)-Loliolide[4]
  4) Amines: Trimethyl amine, trimethyl amine N-oxide[5]
  5) Benzenoids: Phenyl acetic acid, p-hydroxy phenyl acetic acid[6]
  6) Carotenoids: β-Carotene[7]
Phamacology
  1) Cardiotonic activity[8]
  2) Antibacterial activity[9]
  3) Repellant activity(animal)[9]
  4) Antimutagenic activity[10, 15]
  5) Antitumor activity[11, 13, 14, 16]
  6) Cytotoxic activity[11]
  7) Macrophage cytotoxicity enhancement[11]
  8) Antioxidant activity[12]
  9) Antitumor-promoting activity[15, 18]
  10) Uterine stimulant effect[17]

Literature:
[1] Ji, M. H. *et al.*: *Hydrobiologia* **1984**, 1984, 116,7.
[2] Fujikawa, T. *et al.*: *Nippon Nogei Kagaku Kaishi* **1975**, 49, 667.
[3] Sakata, K. and Ina, K.: *Agr. Biol. Chem.* **1983**, 47(12), 2957.
[4] Pettit, G. R. *et al.*: *J. Nat. Prod.* **1980**, 43, 752.
[5] Fujiwara-Arasaki, T. and Mino, N.: *Proc. Int. Seaweed Symp. 7th 1971* **1972**, 506.
[6] Abe, H. *et al.*: *Agr. Biol. Chem.* **1974**, 38, 897.
[7] Okuda, H. and Ukegawa, K.: *Hiroshima Jogakuin Daigaku Ronshu* **1981**, 24, 63.
[8] Searl, P. B. *et al.*: *Proc. West Pharmacol. Soc.* **1981**, 24, 63.
[9] Keiichi, O.: *Proc. Int. Seaweed Symp. 1977* **1979**, 1979, 401.
[10] Okai, Y. *et al.*: *Mutat. Res.* **1993**, 303(2), 63.
[11] Ogawa, T. *et al.*: *Phytochemisty* **1990**, 29(1), 303.
[12] Le Tutour, B.: *Phytochemisty* **1990**, 29(12), 3759.
[13] Furusawa, E. and Furusawa, S.: *Cancer Lett.* **1990**, 50(1), 71.
[14] Furusawa, E. *et al.*: *Cancer Lett.* **1991**, 56(3), 197.
[15] Okai, Y. *et al.*: *Chem. Lett.* **1994**, 87(1), 25.
[16] Furusawa, E. and Furusawa, S.: *Fed. Proc.* **1985**, 44(4), 4260.
[17] Huh, K. *et al.*: *Korean J. Pharmacog.* **1992**, 23(3), 146.
[18] Ohigashi, H. *et al.*: *Biosci. Biotech. Biochem.* **1992**, 56(6), 994

[C. K. Sung]

405.   *Porphyra tenera* **Kjellim**   (Bangiaceae)

Asakusanori(J), Gim(K)

Whole plant
  Local Drug Name: Hae-tae(K)

4

Processing: Dry under the sun(K)
Method of Administration: Oral(decoction, K)
Folk Medicinal Uses:
        1) Burn(K)
        2) Haemorroid(K)
        3) Abortion(K)
        4) Erysipelas(K)
        5) Hemeralopia(K)
        6) As foodstuff(J)

Scientific Research:
Chemistry
1) Alkanes: n-nonadecane, n-octadecane, pentadecan-1-al, pentadecan-1-ol, n-pentadecane, n-tetradecane, tetradecan-1-al, tetradecan-1-ol, n-tridecane, tridecan-1-al[1]
2) Alkenes: Deca-trans-2-cis-4-dien-1-al, deca-trans-2-trans-4-dien-1-al, heptadec-cis-8-1-al, heptadeca-cis-8-cis-11-dien-1-al, n-heptadecane, hexadec-cis-7-en-1-al, hexadeca-cis-7-cis-10-dien-1-al, n-hexadecan, n-icosane, nona-trans-2-cis-6-dien-1-al, n-nonadecane, octa-trans-2-trans-4-dien-al[1]
3) Lipids: Decanoic acid, lauric acid, myristic acid, nonanoic acid, oleic acid, palmitic acid, pentadecanoic acid[1]
4) Monoterpenes: Limonene, α-terpineol[1]
5) Sesquiterpenes: Dihydroactinidiolide, α-cadinol, cubenol, α-, β-ionone[1]
6) Diterpenes: 6,10,14-Trimethylpentadecan-2-one, phytol[1]
7) Benzenoids: Benzyl alcohol[1]
8) Amines: Trimethylamine, trimethylamine N-oxide[2]
9) Sulfur compounds: Benzothiazole, dimethyl β-propiothetin[1], methyl sulfide[3]
Phamacology
1) Hypocholesterolemic acivity[4]
2) Antitumor activity[5, 6]
3) Immunostimutant activity[7]

Literature:
[1] Kajiwara, T. *et al.*: *Phytochemistry* **1990**, 29(7), 2193.
[2] Hujiwara-Arasaki, T. and Mino, N.: *Proc. 7th Int. Seaweed Symp.* **1971**(Ed: Nisizawa, K.), Wiley, New York, NY, p. 506.
[3] Noda, A. and Horiguchi, Y.: *Nippon Suisan Gakkaishi* **1975**, 41, 481.
[4] Abe, S. and Kaneda T.: *Nippon Suisan Gakkaishi* **1967**, 33(4), 361.
[5] Yamamoto, I. *et al.*: *Cancer Lett.* **1987**, 35(2), 109.
[6] Okai, T. *et al.*: *Chem. Lett.* **1994**, 87(1), 25.
[7] Cho, K. J. *et al.*: *Hanguk Susan Hakhaechi* **1990**, 23(5), 345.

[C. K. Sung]

406   *Shiraia bambusicola* **P. Henn.**   (Hypocreaceae)

Zhu-huang (C), Juk-wong (H)

Stroma
Local Drug Name: Zhu-huang (C), Juk-wong (H)
Processing: Dry under the sun (C).
Method of Administration: Oral (decoction: C, H; tincture: C)
Folk Medicinal Uses:
        1) Cough and sputum (C, H).
        2) Bronchitis (C, H).

3) Arthritis (C, H).
4) Whooping cough (C).
5) Stomachache (C).
6) Infantile epilepsy (C).
7) Toothache (C).
8) Stroke (C).
Side effects: Occasionally causing photosensitive response and sinus bradycardia [1].

Scientific Research:
  Chemistry
  1) Mannitol, stearic acid, hypocrellines A and B [2].
  Pharmacology
  1) Analgesic effect [3].
  2) Anti-inflammatory effect [3].
  3) Local anesthetic effect [4].
  4) Inhibitory effect on the heart [5].
  5) Hypotensive effect [5].
  6) LD_{50}: 6.471 g/kg i.v. [5].

Literature:
  [1] Lin, X. Y.: *Zhongguo Zhongyao Zashi* **1993**, 18, 755.
  [2] Wang, J. X. *et al.*: *Zhongcaoyao* **1990**, 21, 292.
  [3] Zhu, L. Q. *et al.*: *Zhongcaoyao* **1990**, 21, 22.
  [4] Xiong, D. S.: *Zhongcaoyao* **1985**, 16, 552.
  [5] Wan, F. C.: *Zhongyao Tongbao* **1982**, 7(5), 31.

[P.P.H. But]

407.   *Macrolepiota procera* **(Fr.) Sing**   (Agaricaceae)
                        [= *Lepiota procera*]

                        Gat-beo-seot(K)

Fruiting body
  Local Drug Name: Gat-beo-seot(K)
  Processing: Dry under the sun(K)
  Method of Administration: Oral(decoction, K)
  Folk Medicinal Uses:
                1) Mouth being sore(K)
                2) Pain of lip(K)

Scientific Research:
  Chemistry
  1) Alkaloids[1]
  Phamacology
  1) Platelet aggregation inhibition[2]
  2) Cytotoxic activity[3]
  3) DNA synthesis inhibition[3]

Literature:
  [1] Kim, B. K. *et al.*: *Korean J. Pharmacog.* **1971**, 2, 31.
  [2] Pinto, A. *et al.*: *J. Ethnopharmacol.* **1988**, 22(1), 91.
  [3] Dornberger, K. *et al.*: *Z. Allg. Mikrobiol.* **1978**, 18, 647.

[C. K. Sung]

408. *Auricularia auricula* **(L. ex Hook.) Underw.**   (Auriculariaceae)

Mu-er (C), Muk-yee (H), Kikurage (J)

Related plants: *Auricularia auricula-judae* (Fr.) Quel.

Fruiting body
  Local Drug Name: Mu-er (C), Muk-yee (H), Mokuji (J).
  Processing: Dry under the sun (H, J).
  Method of Administration: Oral (decoction and food: C, H, J).
  Folk Medicinal Uses:
                 1) General weakness (C, H, J).
                 2) Anemia (C, H).
                 3) Cough (C, H).
                 4) Hemoptysis (C, H).
                 5) Hematemesis (C, H).
                 6) Epistaxis (C, H).
                 7) Uterine bleeding (C, H).
                 8) Hypertension (C, H).
                 9) Constipation (C, H).
                 10) Limbs convulsion (C).

Scientific Research:
  Chemistry
    1) Polysaccharides [1, 21].
    2) Copper [23].
  Pharmacology
    1) Antitumor effect [1].
    2) Antifertility effect [2].
    3) Anticoagulant effect [3-4, 25].
    4) Antiaging effect [5].
    5) Antidiabetic effect [6, 18].
    6) Immunostimulatory effect [7].
    7) Antiradical effect [7].
    8) Antileukocytopenic effect [7].
    9) Antiinflammatory effect [7].
    10) Hepatoprotective effect [8].
    11) Antimutation effect [8].
    12) Antilepemic effect [9].
    13) Stimulatory effect on lymphocyte proliferation [10] .
    14) Macrophage-activating effect [19-20].
    15) Antiviral effect [19].
    16) Cholesterol-lowering effect [20].
    17) Analgesic effect [21].

Literature:
  [1] Qi, D. S. *et al.*: *Huazhong Nongye Daxue Xuebao* **1994,** 13, 160.
  [2] He, B. F. *et al.*: *Zhongguo Yaoke Daxue Xuebao* **1991,** 22, 48.
  [3] Shen, J. H. *et al.*: *Zhongguo Yaoke Daxue Xuebao* **1990,** 21, 39.
  [4] Shen, J. H. *et al.*: *Zhongguo Yaoke Daxue Xuebao* **1987,** 18, 137.
  [5] Zhou, H. P. *et al.*: *Zhongguo Yaoke Daxue Xuebao* **1989,** 20, 303.
  [6] Xue, W. J. *et al.*: *Zhongguo Yaoke Daxue Xuebao* **1989,** 20, 181.
  [7] Xia, E. N. *et al.*: *Zhongguo Yaoke Daxue Xuebao* **1989,** 20, 227.
  [8] Zhou, H. P. *et al.*: *Zhongguo Yaoke Daxue Xuebao* **1989,** 20, 51.
  [9] Shen, J. H. *et al.*: *Zhongguo Yaoke Daxue Xuebao* **1989,** 20, 344.

[10] Xia, E. N. *et al.*: *Zhongguo Yaoke Daxue Xuebao* **1987,** 18, 141 .

[11] Teaumroong, N. *et al.*: *Microb. Util. Renewable. Resour.* **1989,** 6, 126.

[12] Xia, E. N. *et al.*: *Shengwu Huaxue Yu Shengwu Wuli Xuebao* **1988,** 20, 614.

[13] Ho, H. K. *et al.*: *Mem. Coll. Agr., Natl. Taiwan Univ.* **1956,** 4(3), 101.

[14] Ho, H. K. *et al.*: *Formosan Sci.* **1952,** 6, 1.

[15] Su, C. C. *et al.*: *Chung Kuo Nung Yeh Hua Hsueh Hui Chih* **1963,** (1-2), 35.

[16] Zhang, L. N. *et al.*: *Gaodeng Xuexiao Huaxue Xuebao* **1993,** 14, 1320.

[17] Zhang, L. N. *et al.*: *Gaodeng Xuexiao Huaxue Xuebao* **1994,** 15, 1231.

[18] Soma, G. *et al.*: *Eur. Pat. Appl. Ep 462,022,* 18 Dec **1991,** JP Appl. 90/155,428, 15 Jun 1990; 34pp.

[19] Soma, G. *et al.*: *Eur. Pat. Appl. Ep 462,020,* 18 Dec **1991,** JP Appl. 90/155,426, 15 Jun 1990; 36pp.

[20] Soma, G. *et al.*: *Eur. Pat. Appl. Ep 462,021,* 18 Dec **1991,** JP Appl. 90/155,428, 15 Jun 1990; 36pp.

[21] Soma, G. *et al.*: *Eur. Pat. Appl. Ep 472,467,* 26 Feb **1992,** JP Appl. 90/218,599, 20 Aug 1990; 48pp.

[22] Yokokawa, H. *et al.*: *Tachikawa Tandai Kiyo* **1994,** 27, 29.

[23] Zhang, W. D.: *Shipin Kexue* **1991,** 141, 49.

[24] Bukhalo, A. S. *et al.*: *Mikrobiol. Zh. (Kiev)* **1971,** 33, 663.

[25] Agarwal, K. C. *et al.*: *Thrombosis & Haemostasis* **1982,** 48, 162.

[P.P.H. But]

409. *Omphalia lapidescens* Schroet. (Polyporaceae)

Lei-wan (C), Lui-yuan (H), Raigan (J)

Sclerotium (CP)
Local Drug Name: Lei-wan (C), Lui-yuan (H), Raigan (J).
Processing: Wash clean, dry in the sun and break to pieces. Do not boil or bake at a high temperature (C).
Method of Administration: Oral (powder: C, H, J).
Folk Medicinal Uses:
1) Intestinal parasitosis with abdominal pain or with infantile malnutrition (C, H, J).
2) Taeniasis (C, H, J).
3) Ancylostomiasis (C, H).
4) Ascariasis (C, H).

Scientific Research:
Chemistry
1) Proteinase [1,2].
2) Trace elements: Ca, Al, Mg [3].
3) Sugars [4]: water-insol. polysaccharide [5,6], OL-2-I, OL-2-II, OL-2-III, OL-2 [7,8], water-sol. polysaccharide, D-glucose, 2-acetamido-2-deoxy-D-glucose, D-glucurenic acid [9].
Pharmacology
1) Antitumor activity [1,7,8,10,11].
2) Taenifugal effect [12,13].
3) Antiscolic effect on ascaris [13].
4) Anti-trichomonas vaginalic [14].

Literature:
[1] Qiu, X. B. *et al.*: *Weishengwuxue Tongbao* **1986,** 13(2), 68.

[2] Du, C. X. *et al.*: *Zhongcaoyao* **1987,** 18(3), 114.

[3] *"Quanguo Zhongcaoyao Huibian"* **1975,** Vol.1, 867.

[4] *"Zhongyao Zhi"* **1994,** Vol.5, 815.
[5] Miyazaki, T. *et al.*: *Chem. Pharm. Bull.* **1980,** 28(10), 3118.
[6] Saito, K. *et al.*: *Chem. Pharm. Bull.* **1990,** 38(6), 1745.
[7] Saito, K. *et al.*: *Chem. Pharm. Bull.* **1992,** 40(1), 261.
[8] Ohno, N. *et al.*: *Chem. Pharm. Bull.* **1992,** 40(8), 2215.
[9] Miyazaki, T. *et al.*: *Carbohydr. Res.* **1981,** 96(1), 105.
[10] Miyazaki, T. *et al.*: *Shinkin to Shinkinsho* **1983,** 24(2), 95.
[11] Yao, Y.H. *et al.*: *Ningxia Yixueyuan Xuebao* **1979,** (1), 50.
[12] Jing, H.D. *et al.*: *Zhonghua Xinyixuebao* **1951,** 2(10), 753.
[13] Wu, Y.R. *et al.*: *Zhonghua Yixue Zazhi* **1948,** 34(10), 347.
[14] Dept. of Pharmacology: *Henan Yixueyuan Xuebao* **1960,** (7), 23.

[J.X. Guo]

410.   *Hericium erinaceus* **(Bull. ex Fr.) Pers.**   (Hydnaceae)

Hou-tou (C), Hau-tau-gwoo (H)

Fruiting body
Local Drug Name: Hou-tou (C), Hau-tau-gwoo (H)
Processing: Dry under the sun (C, H)
Method of Administration: Oral (eat as vegetable or soup: C, H)
Folk Medicinal Uses:
         1) Chronic gastritis and stomach cancer (C, H).
         2) Tumor (C, H).
         3) Stomach and duodenal ulcer (C).
         4) Indigestion (C).

Scientific Research:
Chemistry
   1) Saponins: oleanolic acid saponins [1].
   2) Herierins III and IV, 4-chloro-3,5-dimethoxybenzoic-0-arabitol ester, 4-chloro-3,5-dimethoxy-
      benzoic methyl ester, 4-chloro-3,5-dimethoxybenzoic acid, palmic acid, stearic acid, behenic
      acid, tetracosanic acid, 5α-ergostan-3-one, 5α-stigmasten-22-en-3-one, 5α-stigmastan-3-one
      [2].
   3) Polysaccharides [4–5].
   4) Sialic acid-binding lectin [7].
Pharmacology
   1) Therapeutic effect on atrophic gastritis [3].
   2) Immunomodulatory effect [4].
   3) Anitumor effect [5–6].

Literature:
[1] Qian, F.G. *et al.*: *Chin. Trad. Herbal Drugs* **1988,** 19, 290.
[2] Qian, F.G. *et al.*: *Yaoxue Xuebao* **1990,** 25, 522.
[3] Xu, C.P. *et al.*: *Chin. Med. J.* **1985,** 98, 455.
[4] Xu, H.M.. *et al.*: *Zhongguo Zhongxiyi Jiehe Zazhi.* **1994,** 14, 427.
[5] Mizuno, T. *et al.*: *Biosc., Biotech. Biochem.* **1992,** 56, 347.
[6] Chen, Z.Y. *et al.*: *Zhonghua Zhongliu Zazhi* **1987,** 9, 109.
[7] Kawagishi, H. *et al.*: *FEBS Lett.* **1994,** 340, 56.

[P.P.H. But]

411. *Pleurotus ostreatus* **(Jacq. ex Fr.) Kumm.** (Tricholomataceae)

Zhai-er (C), Bau-yue-gwoo (H)

Stroma
Local Drug Name: Zhai-er (C), Bau-yue-gwoo (H)
Processing: Use when fresh or dry under the sun (C).
Method of Administration: Oral (eat as vegetable or soup: C, H)
Folk Medicinal Uses:
               1) Weakness (C, H).
Remarks: Avoid eating raw [1].

Scientific Research:
Chemistry
  1) Mannitol, sesquiterpenoids [2–3].
  2) Polysaccharides [4, 14].
  3) Vitamins, sterols, amino acids, peptides [20].
Pharmacology
  1) Hypocholesterolaemic effect [5–11, 15–16, 22].
  2) Antioxidant and lipid peroxidation effect [12, 19].
  3) Immunomodulatory effect [13, 17–18].
  4) Antitumor effect [21, 23].
  5) LD_{50}: 3 g/kg i.g., 3 g/kg i.p. [1].

Literature:
[1] Al-Deen, I.H. *et al.*: *J. Ethnopharm.* 21, 297.
[2] Gallois, A. *et al.*: *Mycological Research* **1990,** 94, 494.
[3] Dijkstra, F.Y.: *Zeitschrift fur Lebensmittel-Unterschung und -Forschung* 160, 401.
[4] Yoshioka, Y. *et al.*: *Carbohydrate Res.* **1975,** 43, 305.
[5] Bobek, P. *et al.*: *Nutrition* **1991,** 7, 105.
[6] Bobek, P. *et al.*: *Physiol. Res.* **1991,** 40, 327.
[7] Bobek, P. *et al.*: *Zeitschrift fur Ernahrungswissenschaft* **1994,** 33, 44.
[8] Bobek, P. *et al.*: *Physiol. Res.* **1994,** 43, 205.
[9] Bobek, P. *et al.*: *Nahrung* **1995,** 39, 98.
[10] Bobek, P. *et al.*: *Physiol. Res.* **1994,** 44, 287.
[11] Bobek, P. *et al.*: *Nahrung* **1996,** 40, 222.
[12] Bobek, P. *et al.*: *Pharmazie* **1995,** 50, 441.
[13] Paulik, S. *et al.*: *Zentralblatt Fur Veterinarmedizin - Reihe B* **1996,** 43, 129.
[14] Gutierrez, A. *et al.*: *Carbohydrate Res.* **1996,** 281, 143.
[15] Chang, R. *et al.*: *Nutrition Reviews* **1996,** 54, 891.
[16] Bobek, P. *et al.*: *Zeitschrift fur Ernahrungswissenschaft* **1996,** 35, 249.
[17] Wang, W.S. *et al.*: *Comp. Immun. Microbio. Infect. Dis.* **1997,** 20, 261.
[18] Paulik, S. *et al.*: *Veterinarni Medicina* **1992,** 37, 675.
[19] Filipek, J.: *Pharmazie* **1992,** 47, 393.
[20] Opletal, L.: *Ceskoslovenska Farmacie* **1993,** 42, 160.
[21] Kurashige, S. *et al.*: *Immunopharm. Immunotox.* **1997,** 19, 175.
[22] Bobek, P. *et al.*: *Casopis Lekaru Ceskych.* **1997,** 136, 186.
[23] Zusman, J. *et al.*: *Anticancer Res.* **1997,** 17, 2105.

[P.P.H. But]

412. *Tricholoma matsutake* **(S. Ito et Imai) Sing** (Tricholomataceae)

Song-moa(C), Matsutake(J), Song-i-beo-seot(K)

Fruiting body
  Local Drug Name: Song-moa(C), Song-i(K)
  Processing: Dry under the sun(K) (C)
  Method of Administration: Oral(decoction, K)
  Folk Medicinal Uses:
  1) Lumbago(C)
  2) Constipation(C)
  3) Food stuff(J)
  4) Apepsia(K)
  5) Boil(K)
  6) Tonsillitis(K)
  7) Fever(K)
  8) Acute gastritis(K)
  9) Infant astonishment(K)

Scientific Research:
  Chemistry
  1) Benzoids: Acetophenone, benzaldehyde, benzyl acetate, phenylacetaldehyde [1]
  2) Monoterpenes: Borneol acetate, butan-1-ol 3-methyl, cymene para, limonene, linalool oxide cis,linalool oxide trans, pinene alpha, terpineol alpha [1]
  3) Sesquiterpenes: Cadinene delta[1]
  4) Penylpropanoids: Cinnamaldehyde, cinnamic acid ethyl ester, cinnamic acid cis methyl ester, cinnamic acid trans methylester [1]
  5) Courmarins: Courmarin [1]
  6) Lipids: Deca-2-4-dienolic acid methyl ether, oct-2-enoic acid methyl ester, palmitic acid ethyl ester [1]
  7) Oxygen heterocycles: Furan 2-hexyl, furan 2-pentyl [1]
  8) Alkanes: Heptane-2-one, hexane-1-al, hexane-1-ol, hexanoic acid methyl ester, hexyl acetate, octan-1-ol, octan-3-one, pentane-1-ol, non-2-en-1-al, nona-trans-2-trans-4-dien-1-al, oct-1-en-3-ol, oct-1-en-3-one, oct-2-en-1-al, oct-3-en-1-ol, oct-cis-2-en-1-ol [1]
  9) Polycyclics: Naphthalene [1]
  10) Proteids: Alanine, alanine phenyl, arginine, aspartic acid, butyric acid alpha-amino, gllutaamic acid, glycine, histidine, leucine, leucine iso,leucine iso: allo, lysine, ornithine, proline, serine, threonine, tryptophan, tyrosine, valine [2]
  11) Alkaloids: Cystine, ethalolamine [2]
  12) Antibiotics: Emitanin A, B, C, D [3]
  13) Structure unknown: Emitanin M-A[4]

Literature:
  [1]Yajima, I. *et al.: Agr. biol. Chem.* **1981**, 45, 373.
  [2] Park, W. H.: *Korean J. Pharmacog.***1982**, 13, 43.
  [3]Sakakida, K., Ikegawa, T.: *Patent-Japan Kokai Tokkyo Koho-80* **1980**, 68, 4.
  [4] Sakakida, K., Ikegawa, T.: *Patent-Ger-2*, 809, 092 **1978**

[C. K. Sung]

413. *Volvariella volvacea* **(Bull. ex Fr.) Sing.** (Pluteaceae)

Cao-gu (C), Cho-gwoo (H)

Fruiting body
  Local Drug Name: Cao-gu (C), Cho-gwoo (H)
  Processing: Use when fresh or dry under the sun (C, H)
  Method of Administration: Oral (eat as mushroom: C, H)

Folk Medicinal Uses:

    1) Weakness (C, H).

    2) Febrile diseases (C).

Side effects: Avoid eating raw as it contains a cardiotoxic and hemolytic protein [1, 2].

Scientific Research:

Chemistry

  1) Protein: Volvatoxin [1–2], Fip-vvo [3], lectin [4].

  2) Glucan [5].

Pharmacology

  1) Immunomodulatory effect [3].

  2) Antitumor effect [5–6].

  3) Free radical scavenging effect [7].

  4) LD_{50} of lectin: 17.5 mg/kg [4].

Literature:

[1] Lin, J.Y. et al.: Nature **1973,** 246, 524.

[2] Lin, J.Y. et al.: Proteins **1996,** 24, 141.

[3] Hsu, H.C. et al.: Biochem. J. **1997,** 323, 557.

[4] Lin, J.Y. et al.: J. Biochem. **1984,** 96, 35.

[5] Kishida, E. et al.: Carbohydrate Res. **1989,** 193, 227.

[6] Kishida, E. et al.: Biosc. Biotech. Biochem. **1992,** 56, 1308.

[7] Liu, F. et al.: Life Sc. **1997,** 60, 763.

[P.P.H. But]

414.   *Dictyophora indusiata* **(Vent. ex Pers.) Fischer**   (Phallaceae)

Zhu-sun (C), Juk-suan {Juk-sunk} (H)

Fruiting body

Local Drug Name: Zhu-sun (C), Juk-suan {Juk-sunk} (H)

Processing: Dry under the sun (C, H)

Method of Administration: Oral (eat as vegetable or soup: C, H)

Folk Medicinal Uses:

    1) Weakness (C, H).

    2) Diarrhea (C).

Scientific Research:

Chemistry

  1) Polysaccharides [1–3].

  2) Sesquiterpenes: dictyophorines A and B [4].

Pharmacology

  1) Anti-inflammatory effect [1].

  2) Antitumor effect [2].

  3) Mitogenic and colony-stimulating effects [3].

  4) Promoting nerve growth factor synthesis by astroglial cells [4].

Literature:

[1] Hara, C. et al.: Carbohydrate Res. **1982,** 110, 77.

[2] Ukai, S. et al.: Chem. Pharm. Bull. **1983,** 31, 741.

[3] Hara, C. et al.: Chem. Pharm. Bull. **1991,** 39, 1615.

[4] Kawagishi, H. et al.: Phytochem. **1997,** 45, 1203.

[P.P.H. But]

415.   *Cladonia rangiferina* **Webb**   (Cladoniaceae)

Shi-rui(C), Ggot-i-ggi(K)

Whole plant
Local Drug Name: Shi-rui(C), Seok-ye-cho(K)
Processing: Dry under the sun(C, K)
Method of Administration: Oral(decoction: C, K), topical(powder: C)
Folk Medicinal Uses:

          1) Headache(C, K)
          2) Rheumatalgia(C)
          3) Hemoptysis(C)
          4) Hemorrhage(K)
          5) Hematemesis(K)
          6) Jaundice(K)

Scientific Research:
Chemistry
  1) Depsides: Atranorin[1]
  2) Carotenoids: β-Carotene, α-cryptoxanthin, violaxanthin[2], astaxanthin, zeaxanthin[2, 3], mutatochrome, neoxanthin, rhodoxanthin[3]
  3) Oxygen heterocycles: Usnic acid[1], α-Tocopherol[4]
Phamacology
  1) Plant root growth inhibition[5]

Literature:
[1] Nourish, R. and Oliver, R. W. A.: Biol. *J. Linn. Soc.* **1974**, 6, 259.
[2] Czeczuga, B.: *Biochem. Syst. Ecol.* **1985**, 13(2), 83.
[3] Czeczuga, B. and Alstrup, V.: *Biochem. Syst. Ecol.* **1987**, 15(3), 297.
[4] Dasilva, E. J. and Englund, B.: *Lichenologist* **1974**, 6, 96.
[5] Oswiecimska, M. *et al.*: *Herba Pol.* **1979**, 25, 317.

[C. K. Sung]

416.   *Lycopodium japonicum* **Thunb.** (Lycopodiaceae)

Shi-song (C), Sun-gun-cho(H),

Related plant: *L. claratum* L.: Hikagenokazura(J), Seok-song (K).

Herb (CP)
Local Drug Name: Shen-jin-cao (C), Sun-gun-cho(H), Sekisho(J), Sin-geun-cho (K).
Processing: Eliminate foreign matter, wash clean, cut into sections, and dry (C, H, J, K), or use in
          fresh (H).
Method of Administration: Oral (decoction: C, H, J, K); Topical (decoction or powder: H).
Folk Medicinal Uses:

          1) Arthralgia with limited mobility of the joints (C, H, K).
          2) Articular pain (H, J, K).
          3) Rheumatalgia (C, H).
          4) Acute hepatitis (C).
          5) Sprain (C).
          6) Conjunctival congetion (C).
          7) Weakness (J).

8) Traumatic injury (H).
9) Eye diseases (K).

Spore
Local Drug Name: Sekishoshi (J), Seok-song-ja (K).
Processing: Dry under the sun (J, K).
Method of Administration: Powder (J, K).
Folk Medicinal Uses:
                1) Diarrhea (J, K).
                2) Edema (J).

Scientific Research:
Chemistry
1) Alkaloids: Lycopodine, clavatine [1-3], clavolonine, fawcettiine, fawcettimine, deacetylfawcettiine, dihydrolycopodine [4].
2) Triterpene alcohols: Serraten-3β-ol-2l-one, α−onocerin (onocerol), serratenediol, 2l-episerratenediol, diepiserratenediol, 16-oxodiepiserratenediol, 16-oxo-2l-episerratenediol, 16-oxoserratenediol, 2l-episerratriol, lycoclavanol, diepiserratriol, 16-oxolyclavanol, clavatol, lyclaninol, lycoclavanin, diepilycocryptol, lyclanitin, 16-oxolyclanitin [5-9].
3) Organic acids: Vanillic acid, ferulic acid, azelaic acid [10].
4) Flavonoid glycosides: Apigenin-4'-O-(2",6"-di-O-p-coumaroyl-β−D-glucopyranoside) [11].
5) Anthraquinones: Physcion [12].
Pharmacology
1) Antibacterial effect [13].
2) Antipyretic effect (alkaloids) [14].
3) Effect on blood pressure and heart (alkaloids) [15].
4) Effect on smooth muscles (alkaloids) [15,16].
5) Causing muscular incoordination and paralysis [15,16].
6) Estrogenic activity [17].

Literature:
[1] Achmatowicz, O. *et al.*: *Roczniki Chem.* **1938,** 18, 88.
[2] Achmatowicz, O. *et al.*: *Bull. Acad. Polon. Sci., Ser. Sci. Chim.* **1964,** 12(5), 311.
[3] Podewald, W.J. *et al.*: *Bull. Acad. Pol. Sci. Ser., Ser. Sci. Chim.* **1967,** 15(12), 579.
[4] Burnell, R.H. *et al.*: *Can. J. Chem.* **1961,** 39, 1090.
[5] Inubushi, Y. *et al.*: *Yakugaku Zasshi* **1962,** 82, 1083, 1537.
[6] Tsuda, Y. *et al.*: *J. Chem. Soc. (D)* **1969,** 1040, 1042.
[7] Sano, T. *et al.*: *J. Chem. Soc. (D)* **1970,** 1274.
[8] Tsuda, Y. *et al. J. Chem. Soc. (D)* **1979,** 260.
[9] Tsuda, Y. *et al.*: *Yakugaku Zasshi* **1974,** 94, 970.
[10] Achmatowicz, O. *et al.*: *Roczniki Chem.* **1958,** 32, 1127.
[11] Ansari, F.R. *et al.*: *Planta Med.* **1979,** 36(3), 196.
[12] Cai, X. *et al.*: *Shanghai Yike Daxue Xuebao* **1991,** 18(5), 383.
[13] *"Quanguo Zhongcaoyao Huibian"* **1975,** Vol.1, 460.
[14] Maksym, N.: *Acta Polon. Pharm.* **1939,** 3, 23.
[15] Henry, M.L. *et al.*: *J. Am. Pharm. Assoc.* **1945,** 34, 197.
[16] Guy, M. *et al.*: *Can. J. Research 26E* **1948,** 174.
[17] Watt, J.M.: *Medicinal and Poisonous: Plant of Southern and Eastern Africa 2Ed,* **1962,** 1137.

[J.X. Guo]

417.　　　　*Equisetum arvense* **L. var.** *boreale*　(Equisetaceae)

Sugina(J), Soe-ddeu-gi(K)

Related plants: *Equisetum arvense* L.

Herb
　Local Drug Name: Monkei(J), Mun-hyung(K)
　Processing: Dry under the sun(J, K)
　Method of Administration: Oral(decoction, J, K)
　Folk Medicinal Uses:
　　　　　　1) Edema(J, K)
　　　　　　2) Poisoned dermatitis with lacquer(K)
　　　　　　3) Urticaria(K)
　　　　　　4) Gonorrhoea(K)
　　　　　　5) Anti-cancer(K)
　　　　　　6) Edema(K)

Scientific Research:
　Chemistry
　1) Inorganic salts: Mg[1]
　Pharmacology
　1) Uterine stimulant effect[2, 3]
　2) Antibacterial activity[4]
　3) Spontaneous activity stimulation[4]

Literature:
　[1] Mino, Y. *et al.*: *Obihiro Chikusan Daigaku Gakujutsu Kenkyu Hokoku, Dai-1-Bu* **1981**, 12(2), 139
　[2] Lee, E. B.: *Korean J. Pharmacog.* **1982**, 13, 99.
　[3] Lee, E. B.: *Annu. Rept. Nat. Prod. Res. Inst. Seoul Natl. Univ.* **1981**, 20, 1.
　[4] Woo, W. S. *et al.*: **Arch. Pharm. Res**. 1979, 2, 127.

[C. K. Sung]

418.　　　　*Pseudodrynaria coronans* **(Wall.) Ching**　(Polypodiaceae)

Ya-jiang (C), Ngie-keung (H)

Rhizome
　Local Drug Name: Ya-jiang (C), Ngie-keung (H).
　Processing: Wash, remove fone hair, slice and dry under sun (C, H).
　Method of Administration: Oral (decoction: C, H); Topical (macerated fresh rhizome: C, H)
　Folk Medicinal Uses:
　　　　　　1) Rheumatic arthritis (C, H)
　　　　　　2) Traumatic injury, fractures (C, H)
　　　　　　3) Otitis media (C, H)

Scientific Research:
　Chemistry
　1) Triterpenoids: tetracyclictriterpenoid acetate, neohop-13(18)-ene, fern-9(11)-ene, hop-22(29)-ene [1]

Literature:
[1] Tanaka, Y. et al.: *Shoyakugaku Zasshi* **1978,** 32, 260.

[P.P.H. But]

419.   *Pyrrosia lingua* **(Thunb.) Farwell**   (Polypodiaceae)

Shi-wei (C), Sak-wai (H), Hitotsuba (J), Seok-wi (K)

Related Plants: *P. sheareri* (Bak.) Ching: Lu-shan-shi-wei (C); *P. petiolosa* (Christ) Ching: You-bing-shi-wei(C), Ae-gi-seok-wi (K).

Leaf (CP)
  Local Drug Name: Shi-wei (C), Sak-wai (H), Sekii (J), Seok-wi (K).
  Processing: Eliminate foreign matter, wash clean, cut into sections, dry in the sun and sift (C, K).
  Method of Administration: Oral (decoction: C, H, K).
  Folk Medicinal Uses:
      1) Urinary infection and urolithiasis with difficult painful urination (C, H, J, K).
      2) Cough and asthma due to heat in the lung (C, H, J, K).
      3) Spitting of blood, epistaxis, hematuria, abnomal uterne bleeding (C, H, K).
      4) Acute and chronic nephritis (C, H).
      5) Urinary tract stones (C, H).
      6) Leucopenia (C, H).
      7) Chronic bronchitis (C, H).

Scientific Research:
  Chemistry
    1) Tannins [1].
    2) Sugars: Sucrose [1,2].
    3) Organic acids: Fumaric acid, caffeic acid [1], chlorogenic acid [2].
    4) Steroids: β–Sitosterol [1,2].
    5) Flavonoids: Mangiferin, isomagiferin [1], kaempferol, quercetin, isoquercetin, trifolin [2], astragalin, liquiritin [3].
  Pharmacology
    1) Antitussive effect and eliminate sputum [4].

Literature:
[1] *"Zhongyao Zhi"* **1988,** Vol.4, 221.
[2] Mizuno, M. et al.: *Zhiwu Xuebao* **1986,** 28(3), 339.
[3] Do, J.C. et al.: *Seengyak Hakhoechi* **1992,** 23(4), 276.
[4] Shanghai First Medical College, et al.: *Yiyao Gongye* **1973,** 6, 1.

[J.X. Guo]

420.   *Nephrolepis cordifolia* **(L.) Presl.**   (Davalliaceae)

Shen-jue (C), Sun-kuit (H)

Tubers or Whole Plant
  Local Drug Name: Shen-jue (C), Sun-kuit (H).
  Processing: Remove scales, wash, use in fresh or dry under the sun (C, H).
  Method of Administration: Oral (decoction: C, H); Topical (macerated fresh herb or tuber: C).
  Folk Medicinal Uses:

1) Colds (C, H).
2) Fever (C, H).
3) Pulmonary tuberculosis and hemoptysis (C, H).
4) Enteritis (C, H).
5) Urinary tract infection (C, H).
6) Dysentery (C, H).
7) Infantile malabsorption and malnutrition (C, H).
8) Mastitis (C, H).
9) Cough (C).
10) Lymphnoditis (C).
11) Orchitis (H).
12) Diarrhea (H).

Scientific Research:
Chemistry
1) Thioredoxin, NADP-thioresoxin reductase [1].
2) Sucrose phosphatase [2].
3) 3,4-dihydroxycinnamic acid [3].
Pharmacology
1) Inhibitory effects on the activities of murine retroviral reverse transcriptase and human DNA polymerases [4].

Literature:
[1] Cao, R.Q. *et al.*: *Zhiwu Shengli Xuebao* **1989,** 15, 205.
[2] Hawker, J.S. *et al.*: *Phytoochemistry* **1984,** 23, 245.
[3] Murata, K. *et al.*: *J. Nutr. Sci. Vitaminol.* **1974,** 20, 351.
[4] Ono, K. *et al.*: *Chem. Pharm. Bull.* **1989,** 37, 1810.

[P.P.H. But]

421. *Pseudolarix kaempferi* **Gord.** (Pinaceae)

Jin-qian-song (C)

Root bark or stem bark near the root (CP)
Local Drug Name: Tu-jing-pi (C), Toh-ging-pay (H).
Processing: Wash clean, slightly soften, cut into slivers and dry in the sun (C).
Method of Administration: Topical (tincture or paste: C, H).
Folk Medicinal Uses:
1) Scabies (C, H).
2) Tinea (C, H).

Scientific Research:
Chemistry
1) Diterpenoids: Pseudolaric acid A, B, C and C_2 [1], pseudolaric acid A-β–D-glucoside, pseudolaric acid B-β–D-glucoside [2], pseudolaric acid D, E [3].
2) Triterpenoids: Pseudolarifuroic acid, betulinic acid [4].
3) Steroids: β-sitosterol, β-sitosterol-β–D-glucoside [4].
4) Tannins [5].
5) Phlegms [5].
Pharmacology
1) Antifungal effect [1,6-8].
2) Antifertility effect [9-11].
3) Toxicity [10,11].
4) Styptic effect [12].

17

Literature:

[1] Li, Z.L. *et al.*: *Shanghai Til I Hsueh Yuan Hsueh Pao* **1980,** 7(5), 386.
[2] Li, Z.L. *et al.*: *Huaxue Xuebao* **1985,** 43(8), 786.
[3] Li, Z.L.: *Huaxue Xuebao* **1989,** 47(3), 258.
[4] Chen, K.: *Huaxue Xuebao* **1990,** 48(6), 591.
[5] *"Zhongyao Zhi"* **1994,** Vol.5, 344.
[6] Zhou, B.N. *et al.*: *Planta Med.* **1983,** 47(1), 35.
[7] Li, E.G. *et al.*: *J. Nat. Prod.* **1995,** 58(1), 56.
[8] Wu, S.X. *et al.*: *Zhonghua Pifuke Zazhi* **1960,** 8(1), 18.
[9] Xie, J.X. *et al.*: *Zhongcaoyao* **1986,** 17, 226.
[10] Wang, W.C.: *Zhongguo Yaoli Xuebao* **1988,** 9(5), 445.
[11] Wang W.C. *et al.*: *Shengzhi Yu Biyun* **1989,** 9(1), 34.
[12] *"Zhongyao Da Cidian"* **1975,** 89.

[J.X. Guo]

422.   *Thuja orientalis* **L.**   (Cupressaceae)
                         [= *Biota orientalis* (L.) Endl.]

                  Bin-park(H), Konotegashiwa(J), Cheuk-baek-na-mu(K)

Leaf
Local Drug Name: Bin-park(H), Sokuhakuyo(J), Cheuk-baek-yeop(K)
Processing: Dry under the sun(K)
Method of Administration: Oral(decoction, H, K)
Folk Medicinal Uses:
                    1) Hemostasis(H, J, K)
                    2) Hematemesis(H, J, K)
                    3) Hemoptysis(H, K)
                    4) Rheumatism(H)
                    5) Diarrhea(J)
                    6) Hemostatic(K)
                    7) Epistaxis(K)
                    8) Uterine hemostatic(K)
                    9) Leucorrhea(K)

Seed
Local Drug Name: Hakushinin(J), Baek-ja-in(K)
Processing: Dry under the sun(K)
Method of Administration: Oral(decoction, J, K)
Folk Medicinal Uses:
                    1) Weakness(J, K)
                    2) Liver disease(K)

Scientific Research:
Chemistry
  1) Diterpene: Abietatriene, ferruginol, 6-dehydroferruginol[1], totarol[1, 7], pinusolide [7],
     pinusolide, pimaric acid [8], 15-hydroxy pinusolidic acid, sandaracopimaric acid, trans-
     communic acid, isopimaric acid [8, 9], 12ε,13(RS)-dihydroxy communic acid, 13-oxo-15,16-
     bis-nor-labd-8(17)-en-19-oic acid, 14,15,16-tris-nor labd-8(17)-ene-13-19-dioic acid, 13-oxo-
     15,16-bis-nor-labda-8(17)-trans-11-dien-19-oic acid[9]
  2) Steroid: β-Sitosterol [1]
  3) Flavonoid: Mono-O-methyl amentoflavone, apigenin, hinokiflavone mono-methyl ether,

18

myricitrin, quercetin-7-O-rhamnoside [2], amentoflavone, cupressuflavone[2, 3], quercetin [2, 10, 14], quercitrin [2, 15, 17, 18], populnin [2, 10], myricetin[2, 14], 4'-monomethyl amentoflavone[3], hinokiflavone [2, 3, 14], (+)-catechin, (-)-epicatechin, procyanidin B-1, procyanin B-3 [5], flavone 5-hydroxy-4',7-dimethoxy [7, 8], luteolin [10]

4) Monoterpenes: Car-3-ene, β-phellandrene, α-pinene, α-thujene, thujopsene[4], β-thujaplicin, γ-thujaplicin[6], platidiol, α-thujone[8]

5) Sesquiterpenes: Cedrol [4, 6,7], α-cedrol [8], thujapsene[4, 6]

6) Essential oils[6]

7) Alkanes: N-Dotriacontane[7], nonacosan-1-ol [15]

8) Steroids: β-Sitosterol [8], daucosterol, ikshusterol [10]

9) Phenylpropanoids: *p*-Coumaric acid, ferulic acid, 16-feruloyl-oxy palmitic acid, quinic acid 5-O-*p*-coumaroyl methyl ester [10]

10) Lipids: Eicosa-5-11-14-17-tetraenoic acid [11], fatty acid (18:1) (9C), fatty acid (18:2) (9C, 12C), fatty acid (18:3) (9C, 12C, 15C), fatty acid (20:0), fatty acid (20:1) (11C), fatty acid (20:2) (11C,14C), fatty acid (20:2) (5C, 11C), fatty acid (20:3) (11C, 14C, 17C), fatty acid (20:3) (5C, 11C, 14C), fatty acid (20:4) (5C, 11C, 14C, 17C), palmitic acid, stearic acid [12]

11) Inorganic: Fluoride[13]

12) Lignans: Deoxy podophyllotoxin [16]

Pharmacology

1) PAF inhibition effect [20, 22, 6]

2) Antibacterial effect [21, 23, 26, 41]

3) Serotonin secretion inhibition effect [22]

4) Colony formation inhibition effect [16]

5) Cytotoxic activity [24]

6) Hemostatic activity [15, 25]

7) Plaque formation suppressant effect [27]

8) Antifungal effect [28, 30]

9) Dentifrice effect [29]

10) Hair stimulant effect [31]

11) Unsfecified antimicrobial activity [32]

12) Antitumor activity, cytotoxic efect [33]

13) Antiinflammatory activity [34]

14) Antiamnesic effect, barbiturate potentiation effect, conditioned avoidance response decreased effect [35]

15) Cholecystokinin receptor binding effect, HMG-CoA reductase inhibition [36]

16) Learning enhancement effect [37]

17) Platelet aggregation inhibition effect [39]

18) Immunosuppressant effect [40]

19) Antioxytocic effect [41, 42]

Literature:

[1] Ohgaku, A. *et al.*: *Agr. Biol. Chem.* **1984**, 48, 2523

[2] Khabir, M. *et al.*: *Curr. SCI.* **1985**, 54, 1180

[3] Gadek, P. A., Quinn, C. J.: *Phytochemistry.* **1985**, 24, 267

[4] Chen, Y. *et al.*: *Lincaan Hua. Hsueh. Yu. Gong. Yi.* **1984**, 4, 1

[5] Sakar, M. K., Engelshowe, K.: *Istanbul Univ. Eczacilik Fak. Mecm.* **1985**, 21, 80

[6] Hirose, Y., Nakatsuka, T..: *Mokuzaki Gakkaishi.* **1958**, 4, 26

[7] Yang, H. O. *et al.*: *Planta. Med.* **1995**, 61, 37

[8] Kuo, Y. H., Chen, W.C..: *Heterocycle.* **1984**, 48, 2523

[9] Inoue, M. *et al.* : *Phytochemistry.* **1985**, 24, 1602.

[10] Ohmoto, T., Yamaguchi, K. : *Chem. Phar. Bull.* **1988**, 36, 807.

[11] Kikuji, H., Izu, S. : *Patent-Japan Kokai. Yokkyo Koho-04 100.* **1992**, 898, 9.

[12] Jie, Jsflk. *et al.* : *J. Chromatogr.* **1991**, 543, 257.

[13] Sakai, T. *et al.* : *Shoyakugaku Zasshi.* **1985**, 39, 165.

[14] Natarajan, S. *et al.* : *Phytochemistry.* **1970**, 9, 575.

[15] Xu, Z. W. *et al.* : *Chung. Yao. T'ung Pao.* **1983**, 8, 30.
[16] Kosuge, T. *et al.* : *Chem. Pharm. Bull.* **1985**, 33, 5565.
[17] Sun, W. J. *et al.* : *Yao. Hsueh. Pao.* **1987**, 22, 385.
[18] Kosuge, T. et al. : *Chem. Pharm. Bull.* **1985**, 33, 206.
[19] Pinto-Scognamiglio, W. : *Boll. Chim. Farm.* **1967**, 106, 292.
[20] Han, B. H. *et al.* : *Yakhak. Hoe. Chi.* **1994**, 38, 462.
[21] Chen, C. P. *et al.* : *J. Ethnopharmacol.* **1989**, 27, 285.
[22] Son, K. H. *et al.* : *Korean J. Pharmacog.* **1994**, 25, 167.
[23] Chen, C. P. *et al.* : *Shoyakugaku Zasshi.* **1987**, 41, 215.
[24] Sato, A. : *Yakugaku. Zasshi.* **1989**, 109, 407.
[25] Kosuge, T. *et al.* : *Yakugaku. Zasshi.* **1981**, 101, 501.
[26] Sharma, S. *et al.* : *Fitoterapia.* **1990**, 61, 453.
[27] Namba, T. *et al.* : *Shoyakugaku Zasshi.* **1984**, 38, 253.
[28] Singh, J. *et al.* : *Int. J. Pharmacog.* **1994**, 32, 314.
[29] Zhang, S. : *Patent-Faming Zhuanli Shenquing Gongkai Shuomingshu-1, 039.* **1990**, 535, 9.
[30] Deshmukh, S. K. *et al.* : *Fitoterapia.* **1986**, 58, 295.
[31] Haung, M. F. *et al.* : *Patent-Faming Zhuanli Shenquing Shuomingshu-1, 043.* **1990**, 624, 6.
[32] Dornberger, K., Lich, H. : *Pharmazie.* **1982**, 37, 215.
[33] Kosuge, T. *et al.* : *Yakugaku. Zasshi.* **1985**, 105, 791.
[34] Han, B. H. *et al.* : *Korean. J. Pharmacog.* **1972**, 4, 205.
[35] Nishyama, N. *et al.* : *Shoyakugaku Zasshi.* **1992**, 46, 62.
[36] Han, G. Q. *et al.* : *Int. J. Chinese Med.* **1991**, 16, 1.
[37] Nishiyama, N. *et al.* : *Phytother. Res.* **1992**, 6, 289.
[38] Woo, W. S. *et al.* : *Arch. Pharm. Res.* **1979**, 2, 127.
[39] Yun-Choi, H. S. *et al.* : *Korean. J. Pharmacog.* **1986**, 17, 19.
[40] Lai, L. T. Y. *et al.* : *Clin. Immunol. Immunopathol.* **1994**, 71, 293.
[41] Lee, E. B. : *Korean. J. Pharmacog.* **1982**, 13, 99.
[42] Lee, E. B. : *Annu. Rept. Nat. Prod. Res. Inst. Seoul natl. Univ.* **1981**, 20, 1.

[C. K. Sung]

423.　　　　　　　*Torreya nucifera* Sieb. et Zucc.　　(Taxaceae)

Kaya(J), Bi-ja-na-mu(K)

Leaf
 Local Drug Name: Bi-ja-yeop(K)
 Processing: Dry under the sun(K)
 Method of Administration: Oral(decoction, K)
 Folk Medicinal Uses:
　　　　　　　1) Ancylostomiasis(K)
　　　　　　　2) Tapeworm(K)
　　　　　　　3) Gingivitis(K)
　　　　　　　4) Enuresis(K)
　　　　　　　5) Ascariasis(K)
　　　　　　　6) Peritonitis(K)

Fruit
 Local Drug Name: Hijitsu(J), Bi-ja(K),
 Processing: Dry under the sun(K)
 Method of Administration: Oral(decoction, J, K)
 Folk Medicinal Uses:
　　　　　　　1) Ascariasis(J, K)

Scientific Research:

Chemistry

1) Lipids: Behnic acid, fixed oil, linoleic acid, oleic acid, palmitic acid[1]

2) Steroids: Campesterol, cholesterol [1], campesterol[1, 2], β-sitosterol, stigmasterol[2], β-ecdysone [4]

3) Diterpenes: Communic acid, ferruginol, 18-hydroxy ferruginol, 18-oxo-ferruginol, hinokiol, kayadiol, isopimaric acid[3]

4) Oxygen heterocycles: δ-Tocopherol [3]

5) Sesquiterpenes: trans-2, trans-6-Fanesol [3]

6) Flavonoids: Kayaflavone[5, 6], vitexin[7]

Phamacology

1) Spasmogenic activity ,uterine stimulant effect(methanol extract) [8]

2) Uterine stimulant effect(alkaloid fraction)[9]

3) Antihelmintic activity[10, 12]

4) Aldose reductase inhibition activity[11]

Literature:

[1] Lott, G. and Izzo, R.: *Agr. Ital.(Pisa)* **1974**, 74: 163.

[2] Chung, B. S. and Ko, Y. S.: *Yakhak Hoe Chi* **1978**, 22 : 87.

[3] Harrison, L. J. and Asakawa, Y.: *Phytochemistry* **1987**, 26, 4: 1211.

[4] Jones, C. G. and Firn, R. D.: *J. Chem. Ecol.* **1978**, 4 : 117.

[5] Kozuka, M. *et al.*: *Patent-Japan Kokai Tokkyo Koho* **1989**, 01 221, 314, 5pp.

[6] Kozuka, M. *et al.*: *Patent-Japan Kokai Tokkyo Koho* **1989**, 01 221, 314, 5pp

[7] Lebreton, P. *et al.*: *C. R. Acad. SCI Ser. D*. **1978**, 287: 1255.

[8] Lee, E. B. and Lee, Y. S.: *Korean J. Pharmacog.* **1991**, 22,(4), 246.

[9] Kobayashi, K.: *Sei-I-Kwai Med. J.* **1931**, 50, 6.

[10] Kim, N. D.: *Yakhak Hoe Chi* **1974**, 19, 87.

[11] Shin, K. H. *et al.*: *Fitoterapia* **1993**, 64(2), 30.

[12] Kim, N. D. *et al.*: *Korean J. Pharmacog.* **1977**, 8, 121.

[C. K. Sung]

424.   *Juglans regia* **L.**   (Juglandaceae)

[= *J. sinensis* Dode]

Hu-tao (C), Hup-toh (H), Kurumi (J), Ho-du-na-mu (K)

Seed (CP)

Local Drug Name: He-tao-ren (C), Hup-top (H), Kotonin (J), Ho-do-in (K).

Processing: Eliminate the fleshy pericarp, dry in the sun, then remove the nut-shell (C, K).

Method of Administration: Oral (decoction: C, H, K).

Folk Medicinal Uses:

                  1) Aching and weakness of the loins and kness (C, H, J, K).

                  2) Asthma and cough of deficiency-cold type (C, H).

                  3) Seminal emission (C, H).

                  4) Impotence (C, H).

                  5) Arteriosclerosis (J).

                  6) Ancylostomiasis (K).

                  7) Cough (K).

                  8) Tympanitis (K).

Scientific Research:

Chemistry

1) Fatty oils: glyceride of linoleic acid, oleic acid, linolenic acid [1].

2) Proteins [2].
3) Carbohydrates [2].
4) Trace elements: Ca, P, Fe [2].
5) Pigments: carotene [2].
6) Vitamins: vitamin B_2 [2], α-and γ-ritamin E [3].

Literature:

[1] *"Zhongguo Jingji Zhiwuzhi"* **1961,** 704.
[2] *"Shiwu Chengfenbiao"* **1957,** 72.
[3] Lambertsen, G. *et al.: J. Sci. Food Agr.* **1962,** 13, 617.

[J.X. Guo]

425.   *Castanea crenata* **Sieb. et Zucc.**   (Fagaceae)

Kuri (J), Bam-na-mu (K)

Leaf
　Local Drug Name: Ritsu-yo (J), Yul-yeop (K).
　Processing: Use in fresh or dry under the sun (J, K).
　Method of Administration: Oral (decoction; K). Decoction for external application (J).
　Folk Medicinal Uses:
　　　　　　1) Irritation of the skin caused by fresh natural lacquer (J).
　　　　　　2) Allergy (K).
　　　　　　3) Cough (K).

Flower
　Local Drug Name: Ritsu-ka (J), Yul-hwa (K).
　Processing: Dry under the sun (J, K).
　Method of Administration: Decoction (J, K).
　Folk Medicinal Uses:
　　　　　　1) Scrofula (J).
　　　　　　2) Poisoning dermatitis with lacquer (K).
　　　　　　3) Sea-sickness (K).
　　　　　　4) dyscrasia (K).
　　　　　　5) Centiped bite (K).

Bark
　Local Drug Name: Yul-su-pi (K).
　Processing: Dry under the sun (J, K).
　Method of Administration: Decoction (external) (J, K).
　Folk Medicinal Uses:
　　　　　　1) Irritation of the skin caused by lacquer (J, K).
　　　　　　2) Poisones wound (J).
　　　　　　3) Tinapedis (K).
　　　　　　4) Eczema (K).
　　　　　　5) Hydrocele (K).

Fruit
　Local Drug Name: Bam (K).
　Processing: Use in fresh (K).
　Method of Administration: Fresh (K).
　Folk Medicinal Uses:
　　　　　　1) Common cold (K).

2) Cough (K).
3) Snake bite (K).
4) Poisoned dermatitis by lacquer (K).
5) Gonorrhoea (K).
6) Weakness (K).

Scientific Research:
Chemistry
1) Tannins: 5-O-Galloyl hamamelofuranose, 1,2'-di-O-galloyl hamamelofuranose, 1,2',5-tri-O-galloyl hamamelofuranose, 1,2',3,5-tetra-O-galloyl hamamelofuranose, 3-O-galloyl hamamelitannin[6], kurigalin [7], acutissimin A and B [8], castacrenin A, B and C[9], castalagin, vescalagin in the woods [1], C-glycosidic ellag-tannins metabolite in the heartwood [2].
2) Phenolics: 4-Hydroxybenzoic acid, scopoletin, 3,4-dihydroxybenzoic acid, 4-hydroxy-3-methoxybenzoic acid, quercetin, 6,7-dihydroxy-2H-1-benzopyran-2-one, 3-(3,4-dihydroxyphenyl)-2-propenoic acid, gentisic acid, syringic acid, sinapic acid, ferulic acid, 3-(4-hydroxyphenyl)-2-propenoic acid [4], hyperin [10].
3) Organic acids [3].
4) Lipids: Fatty acids, glyceride, glycolipids and phospholipids [5].

Literature:
[1] Tanaka, T. et al.: Tennen Yuki Kagobutsu Toronkai Koen Yoshishu, 37th, 1995, 452.
[2] Tanaka, T. et al.: Chem. Pharm. Bull., 1996, 44(12), 2236.
[3] Manabe, T. : Nippon Shokuhin Kogyo Gakkai-Shi, 1969, 16(2), 81.
[4] Cortizo, M. et al.: An. Edafol. Agrobiol. 1981, 40(7-8), 1253.
[5] Rhee, C.-O. et al.: Hanguk Nonghwa Hakhoe Chi, 1982, 25(4), 239; 1983, 26(1), 19.
[6] Nonaka, G. et al.: Chem. Pharm. Bull. 1984, 32(2), 483.
[7] Ozawa, T. et al.: Agric. Biol. Chem. 1984, 48(6), 1411.
[8] Ishimaru, K. et al.: Chem. Pharm. Bull., 1987, 35(2), 602.
[9] Tanaka, T. et al.: Tennen Yuki Kagobutsu Toronkai Koen Yoshishu, 1995, 37th, 457.
[10] Nakaoki, T. et al.: Yakugaku Zasshi 1960, 80, 1473.

[T. Kimura]

426.   *Quercus salicina* **Blume**   (Fagaceae)
[= *Q. stenophylla* Makino]

Urajirogashi (J), Cham-ga-si-na-mu (K)

Leaf
Local Drug Name: Urajirogashi (J), Cham-ga-si-na-mu-yeop (K).
Processing: Dry under the sun (J, K).
Method of Administration: Decoction (J, K).
Folk Medicinal Uses:
1) Urinary calculus (J, K).
2) Calculus of kidney (J, K).

Scientific Research:
Chemistry
1) Tannins: Gallic acid, ellagic acid, (+)-catechin, procyanidin B-1, B-2, salidroside 6"-O-gallate, salidroside 3"-O-gallate, salidoside 4',6"-di-O-gallate, salidroside 4",6"-di-O-gallate, salidroside 3",4",6"-tri-O-gallate, 3',4'-dihydroxyphenethyl alcohol 1-O-β-D-(6"-O-galloyl)-glucopyrano-side and 2,4,6,-trimethoxyphenol 1-O-β-D- (6"-O-galloyl)-glucopyranoside [1].

2",3",4",6"-tetra-*O*-galloyl salidroside, 2",3"-di-*O*-galloyl-4",6"-(*S*)-hexahydroxydiphenoyl salidroside and 3"-*O*-galloyl-4",6"-(*S*)-hexahydroxydiphenyl salidroside. Protoquercitol 4,5-di-*O*-gallate, 3,4,5-tri-*O*-gallate, 2,4,5-tri-*O*-gallate, 1,4,5-tri-*O*-gallate, 1,3,5-tri-*O*-gallate, 1,3,4,5-tetra-*O*-gallate, 1,2,4,5-tetra-*O*-gallate, 1,2,3,4,5-penta-*O*-gallate, 1,5-di-*O*-galloyl-3,4-(*S*)-hexahy-droxydiphenoyl proto-quercitol and 5-*O*-galloyl-3,4-(*S*)-hexahydroxydiphenoyl proto-quercitol[2], stenophynin A and B [3], acutissimin A and B [4].

Pharmacology
   1) Biliary and urinary calculi removal (extract) [5].
   2) Hyaluronidase-inhibiting, antiallergic and atopic dermatitis treatment agent (extract) [6].

Literature:
[1] Nonaka, G. *et al.*: *Chem. Pharm. Bull.* **1982**, 30(6), 2061.
[2] Nishimura, H. *et al.*: *Chem. Pharm. Bull.* **1984**, 32(5), 1735; 1741; 1750.
[3] Nishimura, H. *et al.*: *Chem. Pharm. Bull.* **1986**, 34(8), 3223.
[4] Ishimaru, K. *et al.*: *Chem. Pharm. Bull.* **1987**, 35(2), 602.
[5] Tsuji, T. *et al.*: *Japan Kokai Tokkyo Koho* JP 7358113, 730815, Appl. Japan JP 7194994, 711126.
[6] Sayama, Y.: *Japan Kokai Tokkyo Koho* JP 94239757 A2 730815, JP 06239757 940830.

[T. Kimura]

427.   *Cudrania tricuspidata* **Bureau**   (Moraceae)
               [= *Maclura tricuspidata* Carr.]

             Zhe-shu(C), Ggu-ji-bbong-na-mu(K)

Stem and Leaf
  Local Drug Name: Zhe-shu-keung-yip(C), Ja-su-yeop(K)
  Processing: Dry under the sun(K)
  Method of Administration: Oral(decoction, K)
  Folk Medicinal Uses:
          1) Mumps(C, K)
          2) Tuberculosis(C, K)
          3) Eczema(K)
          4) Cancer(K)

Fruit
  Local Drug Name: Ja-su-gwa-sil(K)
  Processing: dry under the sun(K)
  Method of Administration: oral(decoction, K)
  Folk Medicinal Uses:
          1) Hypertension(K)
          2) Contusion(K)

Scientific Research:
  Chemistry
    1) Flavonoids: Morin, kaempferol-7-glucoside, gericudranins A-C[1]
    2) Benzylated dihydroflavonols: Gericudranins D, E[2]
    3) Amino acids: Proline, glutamic acid, arginine, asparagic acid[2]
  Phamacology
    1) Cytotoxic activity(gericudranins)[1](gericudranins)[2]

Literature:
[1] Lee, I. K. *et al.*: *Phytochemistry* **1996**, 41(1), 213.
[2] Lee, I. K. *et al.*: *J. Nat. Prod.* **1995**, 58(10), 1614.

[C. K. Sung]

428.   *Viscum articulatum* **Burm f.**   (Loranthaceae)

Bian-zhi-hu-ji-sheng (C), Hook-gay-sung (H)

Related plants: *Viscum album* L. var. *coloratum* (Komar.) Ohwi: Yadorigi (J).

Whole Plant
  Local Drug Name: Feng-ji-sheng (C), Hook-gay-sung (H), Sokisei (J).
  Processing: Dry under the sun (C, H).
  Method of Administration: Oral (decoction: C, H); Topical (powder or decoction: H).
  Folk Medicinal Uses:
                   1) Rheumatic arthritis (C, H).
                   2) Urinary tract infection (C, H).
                   3) Leucorrhea (C, H).
                   4) Epistaxis (C, H).
                   5) Lumbar muscle strain (C).
                   6) Low back pain (H).
                   7) Bacillary dysentery (H).
                   8) Uterine bleeding (H).
                   9) Pyodermas (decoction for washing: H).
                   10) Psoriasis (powder mixed with raw egg to apply as poultice: H).
                   11) Weakness (J).
                   12) Lactation deficiency (J).

Scientific Research:
  Chemistry
    1) Triterpenes: Betulin, oleanolic acid, lupeol stearate, lupeol palmitate, lupeol acetate, α-amyrin, lupeol, betulinic acid [1, 2].
    2) Steroids: β-Sitosterol[1, 2]
    3) Flavonoids: Viscumneosides I and V, homoeridioctyol-7-O-β-D-glucoside, eriodictyol-7-O-β-D-glucoside, homoeridictyol-7-O-β-glucoside-4'-O-β-D-(5'''-cinnamoyl) apioside, pinocembrin-7-β-D-apiosyl (1→2)-β-D-glucoside, pinocembrin-7-β-D-apiosyl (1→5)-β-D-apiosyl(1→2)-β-D-glucoside [3–4].

Literature:
  [1] Wang, X.L. *et al.*: *Huaxi Yaoxue Zazhi* **1995**, 10, 1.
  [2] Ray, S. *et al.*: *J. Indian Chem. Soc.* **1984**, 61, 727.
  [3] Wang, X.L. *et al.*: *Huaxi Yaoxue Zazhi* **1990**, 5, 63.
  [4] Wang, X.L. *et al.*: *Huaxi Yaoxue Zazhi* **1992**, 7, 71.

[P.P.H. But]

429.   *Polygonum bistorta* **L.**   (Polygonaceae)

Quan-shen (C), Kuan-sum (H), Ibuki-toranoo (J)

Related plant: *Bistorta vulgaris* Hill.: Beom-ggo-ri (K).

Rhizome (CP)
  Local Drug Name: Quan-shen (C), Kuan-sum (H), Kenjin (J), Gweon-sam (K).
  Processing: Eliminate foreign matter, wash clean, soak briefly, soften thoroughly, cut into thin slices
                and dry (C, K).
  Method of Administration: Oral (decoction: C, H); Topical (decoction: C, H).

Folk Medicinal Uses:
  1) Diarrhea in acute gastroenteritis (C, H, J, K).
  2) Ulcers in the mouth and on the tougue (C, H, J).
  3) Acute respiratory infection with cough (C, H, J).
  4) Carbuncles (C, H, J).
  5) Scrofula (C, H, J).
  6) Dysentery with bloody stools (C, H).
  7) Spitting of blood (C, H).
  8) Epistaxis (C, H).
  9) Hemorrhoidal bleeding (C)
  10) Venomous snake bite (C).

Scientific Research:
Chemistry
  1) Steroids: β–Sitosterol [1].
  2) Sugars: Glucose, starch, pectin, gum, mucilage [1].
  3) Resins [1].
  4) Tannins: Hydrolysable tannins, condensed tannins, gallic acid, ellagic acid, D-catechol, L-epicatechol, glucogallin, protocatechuic acid [1-4].
  5) Phenolic acids: *cis/trans*-Ferulic acid, vanillic acid, *cis/trans*-sinapic acid, syringic acid, melilotic acid, gentisic acid, *cis/trans*-p-coumaric acid, p-hydroxybenzonic acid, *cis/trans*-caffeic acid, p-hydroxyphenylacetic acid, clorogenic acid, salicylic acid [4].
  6) Flavonoids: Proanthocyanidins [5], kojie acid [6].
  7) Trace elements [7].
Pharmacology
  1) Antibacterial effect [1].
  2) Skin lubrication [7].
  3) Styptic and anti-inflammatory effects [1,8].

Literature:
[1] *"Zhongyao Zhi"* **1982,** Vol.2, 177.
[2] Zhu, Y.Q. *et al.: Shanghai Yike Daxue Xuebao* **1994,** 21(2), 129.
[3] Halas, J. *et al.: Przegl. Skorzany* **1994,** 46(3), 63.
[4] Swiatek, L. *et al.: Farm. Pd.* **1987,** 43(7-8), 420.
[5] Liang, X.Z. *et al.: Zhongcaoyao* **1989,** 20(6), 256.
[6] Watanabe, C.: *Jpn. Kokai Tokkyo Koho* JP 03,193,712, [91, 193, 712] (cl, A61k7/00), 23 Aug **1991,** Appl. 89/33, 838, 22 Dec **1989.**
[7] Popov, A.I.: *Farm. Zhongcaoyao. (Kiev)* **1993,** (2), 59.
[8] Duwiejua, M. *et al.: J. Pharm. Pharmacol.* **1994,** 46(4), 286.

[J.X. Guo]

430. *Polygonum perfoliatum* **L.** (Polygonaceae)

Huan-ye-liao (C), Gong-barn-gwai (H), Ishimikawa (J), Myeo-neu-ri-bae-ggop (K)

Whole Plant
  Local Drug Name: Gang-ban-gui (C), Gong-barn-gwai (H), Kobanki (J), Gang-pan-gwi (K).
  Processing: Use in fresh or dry under the sun (C, H, K).
  Method of Administration: Oral (decoction: C, H, J, K); Topical (mashed fresh herb or decoction: H).
  Folk Medicinal Uses:
    1) Dysentery (C, H, J, K).
    2) Edema (C, H, J, K).

3) Nephritis (C, H, K).
4) Eczema (C, H, J).
5) Acute tonsillitis (C, H).
6) Enteritis (C, H).
7) Upper respiratory tract infection (C, H).
8) Snake bites (C, H).
9) Bronchitis (C, H).
10) Herpes zoster (C, H).
11) Pertussis (C, H).
12) Boils and pyodermas (C, H).
13) Parotitis (H).
14) Otitis media (H).

Scientific Research:
Chemistry
1) Flavonoids: Kaempferol, quercetin, quercetin-3-β-D-glucuronide methyl ester[1]
2) Phenylpropanoids: Caffeic acid methyl ester, caffeic acid, *p*-coumaric acid, ferulic acid[1]
3) Terpenoids: Betulin, betulic acid, ursolic acid[1]
4) Steroids: Sterol fatty esters, phytosteryl-β-D-glucoside [1]
5) Tannins: 3,3',4,4'-tetramethylellagic acid, 3,3'-dimethylellagic acid,[1]
6) Sugars: Fructose, glucose [2–3]
7) Protein[2]
8) Fatty acids: Long-chain fatty acids esters, alcohols., fatty acids,
9) Inorganics: Ash, K_2O, Na, Ca and Mg [2].
10) Miscellaneous: Protocatechuic acid vanillic acid, di-methyl tartrate[1]
Pharmacology
1) Antihypertensive effect on the renal hypertensive rats [1].

Literature:
[1] Lin, Y.L. *et al.*: *Kuo Li Chung-kuo I Yao Yen Chiu So Yen Chiu Pao Kao* **1983**, (7), 103.
[2] Bajracharya, D.: *Z. Lebensm. -Unters. Forsch.* **1980**, 71, 363.
[3] Maskey, K. *et al.*: *J. Nepal Chem. Soc.* **1982**, 2, 23.

[P.P.H. But]

431.　　　　　*Tetragonia tetragonioides* **O. Kuntze**　　(Aizoaceae)

Fan-xing (C), Tsuruna (J), Beon-haeng-cho (K)

Whole herb
Local Drug Name: Fan-xing (C), Bankyo, Hamajisha (J), Beon-haeng (K)
Processing: Whole herb with flowers. Dry under the sun (J, K).
Method of Administration: Decoction (J, K). Plaster of　fresh leaf with salt and steamed rice (J).
Folk Medicinal Uses:
　　　　　1) Enteritis (C).
　　　　　2) Stomach ache (J).
　　　　　3) Scorbutus (K).
　　　　　4) Enteritis (K).

Scientific Research:
Chemistry
1) Tetragonin, vitamine A and B [1].
Pharmacology
1) Antibacterial activity (tetragonin) [2].

Literature:
[1] McLaughlin, L.: *C. A.* **1930**, 24, 1890; *J. Nutrition*, **1929**, 2,197.
[2] Schiffer, A. P. *et al.*: *Nature* **1959**, 183, 988.

[T. Kimura]

432. *Dianthus superbus* **L. var.** *longicalycinus*   (Caryophyllaceae)

Qu-mai(C), Gui-muk(H), Kawara-nadeshiko(J), Sul-pae-raeng-i-ggot(K)

Related plant: *Dianthus superbus* L.

Herb(CP)
Local Drug Name: Qu-mai(C), Gui-muk(H), Kubaku(J), Gu-maek(K)
Processing: Dry under the sun(C, K)
Method of Administration: Oral(decoction, C, H, K)
Folk Medicinal Uses:
        1) Amenorrhea(C, H)
        2) Edema(H, J)
        3) Urinary infection and urolithiasis with difficult painful urination or
          hematuria(C)
        4) Conjunctivitis(H)
Contraindications: Contraindicated in pregnancy(C)

Seed
Local Drug Name: Kubakushi(J)
Processing: Dry under the sun(J)
Method of Administration: Oral(decoction, J)
Folk Medicinnal Uses:
        1) Edema(J)
        2) Menstrual disorder(J)

Scientific Research:
Chemistry
  1) Pyrans: pyran I, pyran I 4-O-β-D-glucoside[1]
  2) Saponins: dianoside A, B[2], C, D, E, F[3], G, H, I[4], azukisaponin IV[5]
  3) Flavonoids[6]
Pharmacology
  1) Analgesic activity[2]
  2) Antihepatotoxic activity[7]

Literature:
[1] Shimizu, M. *et al.*: *Phytochemistry* **1982**, 21(1), 245.
[2] Oshima, Y. *et al.*: *Planta Med.* **1984**, 50(1), 40.
[3] Oshima, Y. *et al.*: *Planta Med.* **1984**, 50(1), 43.
[4] Oshima, Y. *et al.*: *Planta Med.* **1984**, 50(3), 254.
[5] Hikino, H. *et al.*: *Planta Med.* **1984**, 50(4), 353.
[6] Chi, H. J. *et al.*: *Ann. Rep. Nat. Prod. Res. Inst. Seoul Nat'l Univ.* **1982**, 21, 46.
[7] Hikino, H.: *Yakugaku Zasshi* **1985**, 105(2), 109.

[C. K. Sung]

433.   *Pseudostellaria heterophylla* (Miq.) Rax ex Pax et Hoffem.
                        (Caryophyllaceae)

Hai-er-shen (C), Tai-gee-sum (H), Wadaso (J), Gae-byul-ggot (K)

Related plants: *P. palibiniani*: Keun-gae-byul-ggot (K); *P. coreana*: Cham-gae-byul-ggot (K).

Root (CP)
Local Drug Name: Tai-zi-shen (C), Tai-gee-sum (H), Tae-ja-sam (K).
Processing: Wash clean, treat with boiling water for a moment, then dry in the sun, or dry in the sun
           directly (C, K).
Method of Administration: Oral (decoction: C, H, K).
Folk medicinal Uses:
           1) Hypofunction of the spleen lassitude and anorexia (C, H).
           2) Debility and deficiency of qi and yin marked by spontaneous sweating and thirst
              during convolescence dry cough due to dryness of the lung (C, H).
           3) Weakness (K).

Scientific Research:
Chemistry
    1) Amino acids [1]: L-arginine [2].
    2) Saponins [3].
    3) Sugars: maltose, sucrose [2], fructose, starch [3], polysaccharides [4].
    4) Trace elements: Cu, Zn, Mn, Fe, Mg, Ca [5,6].
    5) Lipids: glycerol 1-monolinolate, 3-furfuryl-pyrrole-2-carboxylate [7].
    6) Organic acids: palmitic acid, linoleic acid [7], behenic acid, 2-minaline [8].
    7) Phytosterols: β-sitosterol [8].
    8) Cyclopeptides: heterophyllin A, B [9], C [10], pseudostellarin A, B, C [11], D, E, F [12], G [13],
       H [14].
Pharmacology
    1) Antitumor activity [15].
    2) Immunomodulatory activity [16].

Literature:
[1] *"Zhongyao Zhi"* **1982,** Vol.2, 266.
[2] Yoneda, K. *et al.*: *Shoyakugaku Zasshi* **1984,** 38(1), 7.
[3] Nanjing College of Pharmacy: *"Zhongcaoyao Xue"* **1976,** Vol. 2, 202.
[4] Liu, X.H. *et al.*: *Zhongcaoyao* **1993,** 24(3), 119.
[5] Liu, Q.Y.: *Zhongcaoyao Yanjiu* **1986,** (1), 32.
[6] Xi, Y.Y. *et al.*: *Shanxi Daxue Xuebao, Ziran Kexuebao* **1990**13(3), 334.
[7] Reinecke, M.G. et al.: *J. Nat. Prod.* **1988,** 15(6), 1236.
[8] Tan, N.H. *et al.*: *Yunan Zhiwu Yanjiu* **1991,** 13(4), 440.
[9] Tan, N.H. *et al.*: *Chin. Chem. Lett.* **1992,** 3(8), 629.
[10]Tan, N.H. *et al.*: *Yunan Zhiwu Yanjiu* **1995,** 17(1), 60.
[11]Morita, H. *et al.*: *Tetrahedron* **1994,** 50(23), 6797.
[12]Morita, H. *et al.*: *Tetrahedron* **1994,** 50(33), 9975.
[13]Morita, H. *et al.*: *Tetrahedron Lett.* **1994,** 35(21), 3563.
[14]Morita, H. *et al.*: *J. Nat. Prod.* **1995,** 58(6), 943.
[15]Wong, C.K. *et al.*: *Int. J. Immunopharmacol.* **1992,** 14(8), 1315.
[16]Wong, C.K. *et al.*: *Immunopharmacology* **1994,** 28(1), 47.

[J.X. Guo]

Chenopodium album L.   (Chenopodiaceae)

Ligh(H), Shiroza(J), Hin-myeong-a-ju(K)

Related plants: *C. album* L. var. *centrorubrum* Makino: Akaza(J).

Whole plant
Local Drug Name: Ligh(H), Yeo(K)
Processing: Dry under the sun(K)
Method of Administration: Oral(decoction, H, J, K), external(leaf juice, J)
Folk Medicinal Uses:
> 1) Dysentery(H, K)
> 2) Skin irritation(H)
> 3) Insect bite(J)
> 4) Eczema(K)
> 5) Frost bite(K)

Side effect: Allergic dermatitis(curable by vitamin B_{12})

Scientific Research:
Chemistry
1) Hydrocarbons: Octadec-1-ene, n-octatetraconane, n-pentatriacont-1-ene, n-pentatriacontane, n-tetracos-1-ene[1], triacontan-1-ol[10]
2) Phenylpropanoids: Ferulic acid[2], cinnamic acid[11]
3) Terpenes: Lupeol[1], cryptomeridiol, 8α-acetoxycryptomeridiol[3]
4) Steroids: β-Ecdysone[4, 5], 24(28)-Dehydromakisterone A[5], polypodine B[5], 24-demethyl campesterol, β-sitosterol, 24-demethyl stigmasterol, stigmasterol[10]
5) Alkaloids: Betanin, iso-betanin, celosianin[6], N-trans-feruloyl-4-O-methyldopamine[7]
6) Qunoids: Phylloquinone[8]
7) Flavonoids: Quercitrin[9]
8) Coumarins: Xanthotoxin, imperatorin, scopoletin[10]
9) Benzenoids: Vanillic acid[2], *p*-hydroxy benzaldehyde[11]
10) N-Heterocycles: Amaranthin, iso-amaranthin[6, 12]
11) Vitamins: Vitamin K[9], ascorbic acid[13, 14], vitamin A[14]
12) Proteids: Chenopodine[15], chenopodium album virus inhibitor[16], ferredoxin B[18], topoisomerase I[19], trigonelline[20]
13) Inorganics: Ca, Fe, Mn, Mg, N, P, K[17]
14) Lipids: 13-Oxo-trideca-9-trans-11-trans-dien-1-oic acid, 13-oxo-trideca-cis-9-trans-11-dien-1-oic acid[11]

Phamacology
1) Estrogenic effect[21, 22]
2) Nephrotoxic activity[22]
3) Mutagenic activity[23]
4) Hypothermic activity[24]
5) Allergenic activity[25]
6) Antiviral activity[26]
7) Antifungal activity, antiyeast activity[27]
8) Protein synthesis inhibition[28]
9) Plant germination inhibition[29]
10) Diuretic activity[30]

Literature:
[1] Bera, B. *et al.*: *Fitoterapia* **1992**, 63(4), 364.
[2] Massart, L. and Janssens, A.: *Arch. Int. Physiol. Biochim.* **1957**, 65, 163.
[3] Bera, B. *et al.*: *Fitoterpia* **1991**, 62(2), 178.
[4] Dinan, H.: *Phytochem. Anal.* **1992**, 3(3), 132.

[5] Toth, I. *et al.: Fitoterapia* **1981**, 52, 77.

[6] Piattelli, M. and Minale, L.: *Phytochemistry* **1964**, 3(5), 547.

[7] Horio, T. *et al.: Phytochemisty* **1993**, 33(4), 807.

[8] Jansson, O.: *Physiol. Plant.* **1974**, 31, 323.

[9] Ganju, K. and Puri, B.: *Indian U. Med. Res.* **1959**, 47, 563.

[10] Mukherjee, K. K. *et al.: Fitoterapia* **1985**, 56(3), 172.

[11] Tahara, S. *et al.: Experientia* **1994**, 50(2), 137.

[12] Baier, H. and Guenther, G.: *Wiss Z. Paedagog Hochsch "Karl Liebknecht" Potsdam* **1979**, 23, 159.

[13] Iwata, H. and Chiba, S.: *J. Agr. Chem. Soc. Japan* **1942**, 18, 1058.

[14] Zennie, T. M. and Ogzewalla, C. D.: *Econ. Bot.* **1977**, 31, 76.

[15] Willaman, J. J. and Schubert, B. G.: *ARS, USDA, Tech. Bull 1234, Supt Cocuments, Gont. Print Off, Washington DC* **1961**.

[16] Grasso, S. and Sherherd, R. J.: *Phytopathology* **1978**, 68, 199.

[17] Shahi, H. N.: *Plant Soil* **1977**, 46, 271.

[18] Nalbandyan, R. M.: *Biokhimiya(Moscow)* **1976**, 41, 188.

[19] Meibner, K. *et al.: Biochem. Int.* **1992**, 27(6), 1119.

[20] Willaman, J. J. and Li, H. L.: *Lloydia* **1970**, 33S, 1.

[21] Kurmukov, A. G. *et al.: Rast Resur.* **1976**, 12, 515-525.

[22] Bergeron, J. M. and Gouler, M.: *Can. J. Zool* **1980**, 58, 1575.

[23] Alkofahi, A. and Al-Khalil, S.: *Int. J. Pharmacog.* 1995, 33(1), 61.

[24] Bhakuni, O. S. *et al.: Indian J. Exp. Biol.* **1969**, 7, 250.

[25] Batabyal, S. K. *et al.: Sci. Cult.* **1985**, 51(6), 198.

[26] Sako, N.: *Saga Daigaku Nogaku Iho* **1976**, 40, 45.

[27] Saksaena, N. and Tripathi, H. H. S.: *Fitoterapia* **1985**, 56(4), 243.

[28] Gasperi-Campani, A. *et al.: J. Nat. Prod.* 1985, 48(3), 446.

[29] Watanabe, Y.: *Zasso Kenkyu* **1970**, 10, 24.

[30] Kim, T. H. *et al.: Korean J. Pharmacog.* **1985**, 16(3), 165.

[C. K. Sung]

435.   ***Kochia scoparia* (L.) Schrad.**   (Chenopodiaceae)
[= *Chenopodium scoparia* L.]

Di-fu (C), Day-foo-gee (H), Houkigi (J), Daep-ssa-ri (K)

Fruit (CP)
Local Drug Name: Di-fu-zi (C), Day-foo-gee (H), Jifushi (J), Ji-bu-ja (K).
Processing : Eliminate foreign matter, and dry in the sun (C, K).
Method of Administration: Oral (decoction: C, K); Topical (decoction: C, H).
Folk medicinal Uses:

1) Painful and difficult urination (C, H, J, K).
2) Pruritus vulvae with leukorrhea (C, H).
3) Cutaneous pruritus (C, H).
4) Eczema (C, H).
5) Rubela (C).
6) Beriberi (J).
7) Diarrhea (J).
8) Scabies (J).
9) Cystodynia (K).
10) Bed-wetting (K).
11) Panaritium (K).
12) Jaudice (K).

Scientific Research:
Chemistry
  1) Fatty oils [1].
  2) Triterpenoids [2]: oleanolic acid [3].
  3) Alkanes: triacontane [3].
  4) Flavonoids [4].
  5) Alkaloids [4]: the aerial part contains choline, harman, harmine, tetrahydro-β-carboline deriv. [5].
  6) Ecdysteroids: 20-hydroxyecdysome, 5,20-dihydroxyecdysome, 20-hydroxy-24-methyleneecdysome, 20-hydroxy-24-methylecdysome [6].
  7) Amino acids [7]: lysine, histidine, phenylalanine [8].
  8) Trace elements: Ca, Mg, Na, K, Fe, Zn, Mn, Cu, P [9].
Pharmacology
  1) Bacteriostatic effect [10, 11].

Literature:

[1] *"Zhongguo Gaodeng Zhiwu Tujian"* **1972,** Vol.1, 586.
[2] *"Zhongcaoyao Youxiaochengfen De Yanjiu"* **1972,**   Vol.2, 438.
[3] Wen, Y. *et al.: Zhongcaoyao* **1993,** 24(1), 5.
[4] *"Zhongyao Zhi"* **1984,** Vol.3, 326.
[5] Drost-karbowska, K.: *Acta Pol. Pharm.* **1978,** 35(4), 497.
[6] Bathory, M. *et al.: Herba Hung* **1984,** 23(1-2), 131.
[7] Sugahara, T. *et al.: Joshi Eiyo Daigaku Kiyo* **1989,** 20, 77.
[8] Khamdamov, I. K.: *Dokl. Akad. Nauk Uzb. SSR* **1976,** (1), 40.
[9] Sugahara, T. *et al.: Joshi Eiyo Daigaku Kiyo* **1988,** 19, 131.
[10] Cao, R. L. *et al.: Zhongguo Pifuke Zazhi* **1957,** 5(4), 286.
[11] Nanjing College of Pharmacy: *"Zhongcaoyao Xue"* **1976,** Vol.2, 180.

[J.X. Guo]

436.   *Hylocereus undatus* **(Haw.) Britt. et Rose**   (Cactaceae)

Liang-tian-chi (C), Leung-tin-chak (H)

Flower
  Local Drug Name: Liang-tian-chi (C), Leung-tin-chak (H).
  Processing: Use in fresh or dry under the sun (C, H).
  Method of Administration: Oral (decoction: C, H).
  Folk Medicinal Uses:
                1) Bronchitis (C, H).
                2) Tuberculous lymphadenitis (C, H).
                3) Pulmonary tuberculosis (C, H).

Stem
  Local Drug Name: Liang-tian-chi (C), Leung-tin-chak (H).
  Processing: Use fresh with the skin and thorns removed (H).
  Method of Administration: Topical (C, H).
  Folk Medicinal Uses:
                1) Fractures (C, H).
                2) Boils (C, H).
                3) Parotitis (C, H).

Scientific Research:
  Chemistry

1) Sterols: 24α-ethylcholest-5-en-3β-ol, 24ξ--methylcholest-5-en-3β-ol, 24α-ethylcholesta-5,22E-dien-3β-ol[1], β-sitoosterol [2].
2) Lipid: hentriacontane [2].

Literature:
[1] Salt, T.A. *et al.*: *Phytochemistry* **1987,** 26, 731.
[2] Sen, A.B. *et al.*: *J. Indian Chem. Soc.* **1968**, 45, 745.

[P.P.H. But]

437.   *Illicium difengpi* **K.I.B. et K.I.M.**   (Magnoliaceae)

Di-feng-pi (C)

Bark (CP)
Local Drug Name: Di-feng-pi (C).
Processing: Eliminate foreign matter, wash clean, break to pieces, and dry in the sun (C).
Method of Administration: Oral (decoction: C).
Folk Medicinal Uses:
           1) Rheumatic arthralgia (C).
           2) Lumbar muscle strain (C).

Scientific Research:
Chemistry
  1) Essential oils: α-pinene, β-pinene, camphene, 1,8-cineol, linalool, camphor, safrole, terpinyl acetate, eugenol, β-elenene, methyleugenol, β-selinene, nerdiol, δ-cadimol, myrcene, *p*-cymene, terpinene-4-ol, α-terpineol, γ-muurolene, trans-caryophyllene, 1,6-dimethyl-4-isoprophylnaphthalene, bornyl acetate, cupressin [1,2].
  2) Flavonoids: quercitrin [2].

Literature:
[1] Rui, H.K. *et al.*: *Zhongcaoyao* **1981,** 12(5), 17.
[2] *"Zhongyao Zhi"* **1994,** Vol.5, 380.

[J.X. Guo]

438.   *Illicium verum* **Hook. f.**   (Magnoliaceae)

Ba-jiao-hui-xiang (C), Bart-gock-hwui-heung (H), Daiuikyo (J), Keun-hoi-hyang (K)

Fruit (CP)
Local Drug Name: Ba-jiao-hui-xiang (C), Bart-gock (H), Daiuikyo (J), Pal-gak-hoi-hyang (K).
Processing: Dry after heating with boiling water for a moment or dry directly (C, K).
Method of Administration: Oral (decoction: C, H, K).
Folk Medicinal Uses:
           1) Abdominal colic (C, H).
           2) Lumbago due to dificiency in the kidney (C, H).
           3) Vomiting and epigastric pain due to cold in the stomach (C, H, J, K).

Volatile oil (CP, JP)
Local Drug Name: Ba-jiao-hui-xiang-you (C), Uikyoyu (J), Pal-gak-hoi-hyang-yu (K).
Method of Administration: Oral (C).

Folk Medicinal Uses:
        1) Stomachic (C, J, K).
        2) Aromatic (C).
        3) Flavouring (C).

Scientific Research:
Chemistry
  1) Fatty oils [1].
  2) Proteins [1].
  3) Essential oils [1]: anethole [2], methyl chavicol, anisaldehyde, anisylacetone, α-pinene, *l*-phellandrene, safrole [2-4], 3,3-dimethylallyl, *p*-propenyl phenyl ether [5], transanethole, feniculine, estragole, α-limonene, α-bergamotene, *p*-methoxyphenyl propanone-2, linalool [6], *p*-methoxyl cinnamaldehyde [7], 1,8-cineole [8].
  4) Others: gum, resin [1], shikimic acid [9].
Pharmacology
  1) Stimulation and eliminate sputum [3].
  2) Effect on plant budding [7].
  3) Photostabilization [8].
  4) Nevose corrosiveness [9].
  5) Bacteriostasis [3,10].

Literature:
[1] *"Zhongyao Jianbie Shouce"* **1979,** Vol.2, 1.
[2] Lin, Q. S.: *Zhongcaoyao Chengfen Huaxue* **1975,** 586.
[3] Nanjing College of Pharmacy: *"Zhongcaoyao Xue"* **1976,** Vol.2, 308.
[4] Small, J.: *Food* **1943,** 12, 97.
[5] Okely, H. M. *et al.*: *J. Chem. Soc. D.* **1971,** (19), 1157.
[6] Chen, Y. Z. *et al.*: *Fenxi Huaxue* **1986,** 11, 583.
[7] Wolf, R. B. *et al.*: *J. Nat. Prod.* **1986,** 49, 156.
[8] Palamand, S. R. *et al.*: *Can.* **1986,** C.A. 1, 199, 517.
[9]Yamada, T.: *Nihon Tokkyo Koho* **1987,** JP6245, 508.
[10]Patel, R. N.: *Indian J. Pharm.* **1968,** 30(2), 43.

                                        [J.X. Guo]

---

439.   *Magnolia biondii* **Pamp.**   (Magnoliaceae)

Wang-chen-hua (C)

Related Plants: *M. denudata* Desr.: Yu-lan (C), Baek-mok-ryun (K); *M. sprengeri* Pamp.: Wu-dang-yu-lan (C).

Flower bud (CP)
Local Drug Name: Xin-yi (C), Sun-yee (H), Sin-i (K).
Processing: Eliminate branchlet, and dry in the shade (C, K).
Method of Administration: Oral (decoction: C, H, K); Topical (decoction: C).
Folk Medicinal Uses:
        1) Headache and nasal obstruction in colds (C, H, K).
        2) Sinusitis with purulent discharge (C, H).
        3) Allergic rhinnitis (H, K).

Scientific Research:
Chemistry
  1) Essential oils: 1,8-cineole, camphor, β-pinene, α-terpineol [1], sabinene, α-pinene, myrcene, α-

limonene, terpinen-4-ol [2], terpinyl acetate, muurolene [3].
2) Lignans: pinoresinol dimethyl ether, lirioresinol, magnolin, fargesin [4], aschantin, demethoxyaschantin, lirioresinol-B dimethyl ether [5], biondinin A [6].
3) Alkaloids: *d*-coclurine, *d*-reticuline, yuzirine, L-N-methylcoclurine [7], magnoflorine [8].
4) Esters: ethyl-E-*p*-hydroxycinnamate [8], biondinin C, biondinin D [9].
5) Falvonoids: biondnoid I [8], biondnoid A [10].

Pharmacology
1) Antagonistic activity against platelet activating factor [5].
2) Effect on central nervous system [7].
3) Antihypertensive effect [11,12].
4) Effect on uterus [12].
5) Effect on striated muscle [13].
6) Antihistaminic effect [14].
7) Local apocrustic effect [15].
8) Antifungal effect [16].
9) Local anesthetic effect [17].

Literature:
[1] Liu, Y. A. *et al.*: *Zhongcaoyao* **1984,** (4), 23.
[2] Zhang, J. *et al.*: *Fenxi Huaxue* **1986,** 4(5), 325.
[3] Chen, Y. D. *et al.*: *Linchan Huaxue Yu Gongye* **1994,** 14(4), 46.
[4] Kakisawa, H. *et al.*: *Phytochem.* **1972,** 11, 2289.
[5] Pan, J. X. *et al.*: *Phytochem.* **1987,** 26(5), 1377.
[6] Ma, Y. L. *et al.*: *Chin. Chem. Lett.* **1992,** 3(2), 121.
[7] Kimura, I. *et al.*: *Planta Med.* **1983,** 48(1), 43.
[8] Chen, Y. Y. *et al.*: *Yaoxue Xuebao* **1994,** 29(7), 506.
[9] Han, G. Q. *et al.*: *Chin. Chem. Lett.* **1993,** 4(1), 33.
[10] Gao, C. Y. *et al.*: *Bopuxue Zazhi* **1994,** 11(1), 57.
[11] Zhang, S. X. *et al.*: *Huanan Yixueyuan Xuebao (Zhongyi Zhongyao Zhuanji)* **1958,** 117.
[12] Feng, G. H. *et al.*: *Zhonghua Yixue Zazhi* **1956,** 42(10), 969.
[13] Kimura, M. *et al.*: *Yakugaku Zasshi* **1965,** 85(7), 570.
[14] Nakashima, S. *et al.*: *Takeda Kenkyusho Shobo* **1981,** 40(1/2), 27.
[15] Xue, C. S. *et al.*: *Zhongyao Yaoli Yu Yingyong* **1983,** 540.
[16] Sun, C.: *Zhonghua Pifuke Zazhi* **1958,** 3(6), 210.
[17] Hu, F.: *Tianjing Yixue Kexue Lunwen Xuanbian* **1959,** (1), 321.

[J.X. Guo]

440.   *Myristica fragrans* **Houtt.**   (Myristicaceae)

Rou-dou-kou (C), Yuk-dou-kou (H), Nikuzuku (J), Yuk-du-gu-na-mu (K)

Kernel (CP, KP)
Local Drug Name: Rou-dou-kou (C), Yuk-dou-kou (H), Nikuzuku (J), Yuk-du-gu (K).
Processing: 1) Eliminate foreign matter, wash clean, and dry (C, K).
2) To each clean Semen Myristicae, wrap in a mixture of wheat flour and a quantity of water, or carry out the method of making watered pills, moistern the surface of Semen Myristicae with water, wrap in 3-4 layers of wheat flour. Stir-fry the wrapped drug with heated talc powder or sand until the wheat flour cover showing charred yellow, sift, strip off the cover and cool (C, K).
Method of Administration: Oral (decoction: C, H, K).
Folk Medicinal Uses:
1) Epigastric and abdominal distension and pain (C, H, J, K).
2) Anorexia (C, H, J, K).
3) Vomiting (C, H, J, K).

4) Deficiency-cold of the spleen and stomach with persistent diarrhea (C, H, J).
5) Acute gastroenteritis (J).

Scientific Research:
Chemistry
1) Essential oils: pinene, sabinene, camphene, eugenol, myristicin, isoeugenol, methyl eugenol, methoxyl eugenol, methoxyl isoeugenol, safrol, elemicin, isotrimethoxyl allyl benzene [1], α-thujene, carene [2], dipentene, geraniol [3], β-pinene, γ-terpinene, terpinen-4-ol, trimyristin [4].
2) Teiterpenoids: oleanolic acid [3].
3) Diarylpropanoids: compund I, III [2-(4-allyl-2,6-dimethoxyphenyl-1,4-hydroxy-3-methoxyphenylpropanol-1-ol], IV, V [1-3,4,5-trimethoxyphenyl-and 1-(3-methoxy-4-hydroxyphenyl)-2-(4-allyl-2,6-dimethoxy-phenoxy)-propan-1-ol], VIII, IX (dehydrodiisoeugenol), X, licarin-B, 1-(3,4-dimethoxyphenyl)-2-(4-allyl-2,6-dimethoxyphenoxy)-propan-1-ol [5-10].
4) Diaryl nonanoids: 9-(2,5-dihydroxyphenyl) nonanoyl-2,6-dihydroxybenzene [11], 9-(3,4-dihydroxyphenyl) nonanoyl-2,6-dihydroxybenzene [12].
5) Fatty oils: myristin, olein [13].
6) Sugars: starch [13].
Pharmacology
1) Effect on hepatic microsomal mixed-function oxidase [10].
2) Antitumor activity [12].
3) Effect on hepatic detoxification system [14].
4) Effect on drug-metabolizing enzyme [8,10,15,16].
5) Hallucinogenic effect [17].
6) Cerebral excitatory effect [18].
7) Antioxidant activity [11,19].
8) Antibacterial activity [19].
9) High protease activity [20].
10) Hardened effect on tissues of digestive system [21].
11) Effect on hepatic microsomal monooxygenase [22].

Literature:

[1] Trease, G. E. *et al.*: *"Pharmacognosy"* **1978,** 434.
[2] Sanford, K. J. *et al.*: *Phytochemistry* **1971,** 10(6), 1245.
[3] Varshney, I. P. *et al.*: *Indian J. Chem.* **1968,** 6(8), 474.
[4] Guo, X. S. *et al.*: *Yaowu Fenxi Zazhi* **1985,** 5(5), 258.
[5] *"Index Chemicus"* **1973,** 50, 205879, 206091.
[6] Forrest, J. E. *et al.*: *J. Chem. Soc. Perkin Trans. I* **1974,** 205.
[7] Kuo, Y. H. *et al.*: *J. Chin. Chem. Soc. (Taipei)* **1983,** 30(1), 63.
[8] Shin, K. H. *et al. Arch. Pharmacol. Res.* **1988,** 11(3), 240.
[9] Kim, Y. B. *et al.*: *Arch. Pharmacol. Res.* **1991,** 14(1), 1.
[10] Shin, K. H. *et al.*: *Hanguk Saenghwa Hakhoechi* **1990,** 23(1), 122.
[11] He. G. F.: *Shipin Kexue* **1986,** 84, 43.
[12] Nakajima, I.: *Jpn. Kokai Tokkyo Koho* JP 01 42.440.
[13] *"Zhongyao Zhi"* **1984,** Vol.3, 339.
[14] Singh, A. *et al.*: *Food Chem. Toxicol.* **1993,** 31(7), 517.
[15] Chhabra, S. K. *et al.*: *J. Ethnopharmacol.* **1994,** 42(3), 169.
[16] Sherry, C. J. *et al.*: *Experientia* **1978,** 34(4), 492.
[17] Alexander, T. *et al.*: *U.S., Public Health Serv. Publ.* **1967,** 1645, 202.
[18] Edward, B. T. *et al.*: *J. Neuropsychiatry* **1961,** 2, 205.
[19] Nakatani, N. *et al*: *Gekkan Fudo Kemikaru* **1988,** 4(2), 70.
[20] Khan, M. R. *et al.*: *J. Nat, Sci. Math.* **1983,** 23(2), 223.
[21] Shi, Z. Q.: *Eur. Pat. Appl.* Ep454, 127.
[22] Han, Y. B. *et al.*: *Arch. Pharmacol Res.* **1984,** 7(1), 53.

[J.X. Guo]

441.   *Lindera aggregata* **(Sims) Kosterm**   (Lauraceae)

Wu-yao (C), Woo-yuek (H), Uyaku (J)

Root (CP)
Local Drug Name: Wu-yao (C), Woo-yuek (H), Uyaku (J).
Processing: Eliminate foreign matter; for the drug not sliced remove rootlets, grade according to
size, soften thoroughly, cut into thin slices and dry (C).
Method of Administration: Oral (decoction: C, H).
Folk Medicinal Uses:
1) Distending pain in the chest and abdomen accompanied by dyspnea (C, H, J).
2) Enuresis and frequency of urination due to hypofunction of the urinary bladder
(C, H).
3) Hernia (C, H).
4) Dysmenorrhea (C, H).
5) Abdominal pain (J).
6) Headache (J).

Scientific Researches:
Chemistry
1) Sesquiterpenes: lindestrene, lindenenol, hydroxyisogermafurenolide, isofuranogermacrene [1],
epidihydroisolinderalactone [2], linderoxide, isolinderalactone [3], lindestrenolide,
hydroxylindestrenolide, isolinderoxide, lindenene, lindenenone, isogermafurenolide [4],
linderane, neolinderalactone [4,5], lindersaure [6], 1-borneol [7], linderazulene [8],
furanosesquiterpenes [9].
2) Monoterpenes: α-pinene, β-pinene [10].
Pharmacology
1) Bacteriostatic effect [12].
2) Effect on cerebral cortex and blood pressure [12].
3) Diaphoretic effect [12].
4) Angiectatic effect and palliation of muscular spastic pain [12].
5) Effect on body weight [13].
6) Preventive and therapeutic effects on hepatic injury [14].

Literatures:
[1] Takeda, K. *et al.*: *Tetrahedron* **1964**, 20(11), 2655.
[2] Takeda, K. *et al.*: *Chem. Commun.* **1968**, 7, 318.
[3] Ishii, H. *et al.*: *Tetrahedron* **1968**, 24(2), 625.
[4] Takeda, K. *et al.*: *J. Chem. Soc. Section C. Organic* **1969**, 19, 2786.
[5] Takeda, K. *et al.*: *Chem. Commun.* **1968**, 10, 637.
[6] Suzuke, H.: *Yakugaku Zasshi* **1930**, 50(8), 714.
[7] Kondo, H. *et al.*: *Yakagaku Zasshi* **1939**, 59(7), 504.
[8] Takeda, T. *et al.*: *Chem. Parm. Bull. (Japan)* **1953**, 1, 164.
[9] Tori, K. *et al.*: *Tetrahedron Lett.* **1975**, (51), 4583.
[10] *"Zhongyao Zhi"* **1982**, Vol.2, 298.
[11] Qin, J.F. *et al.*: *Zhongcaoyao* **1983**, 14(11), 492.
[12] *"Quanguo Zhongcaoyao Huibian"* **1975**, Vol.1, 210.
[13] Imamato, K.: *Naika no Ryoiki* **1960**, 8(8), 479.
[14] Yamahara, J. *et al.*: *Shoyakugaku Zasshi* **1983**, 37(1), 84.

[J.X. Guo]

Lindera umbellata **Thunb.** (Lauraceae)

Da-ye-diao-zhang (C), Kuromoji (J)

Related Plant: *L. umbellata* Thunb. var. *membranacea*

Root bark
Local Drug Name: Diao-zhang-gen (root: C), Kuromoji (root bark: J).
Processing: Dry under the sun (C, J).
Method of Administration: Oral (decoction: C, J), topical (decoction: C).
Folk Medicinal Uses:

1) Acute gastroenteritis (C, J).
2) Scabies (C).
3) Traumatic injury (C).
4) Rheumatic arthritis (C).
5) Eczema (C).
6) Beriberi (J).

Scientific Researches:
Chemistry

1) Flavonoids: 2',4',6'-Trihydroxydihydrochalcone [11], 2',6'-dihydroxy-4'-methoxy-3'-(3''-methyl-6''-methylethyl-2''-cyclohexenyl) chalcone [1,11] and 2,4,6-trihydroxy chalcone[2], kaempferol, quercetin, afzerin, avicularin, quercitrin, hyperin, isoquercitrin and rutin [12], linderatin, linderatone, methyllinderatone [14, 18], isolinderatone, neolinderachalcone and neolinderatin [17].
2) Phenolic compounds: hexahydrodibenzofurane from the barks [3], 5,6-dehydrokawain [4], and pinocembrin [16].
3) Essential oil: 1,8-cineole, limonene, linalool, α-pinene [5], β-pinene, β-caryophyllene, carvone, γ-terpineol, geraniol, geranyl acetate, myrcene, 2-bornanol and 3-carene [10, 15].
4) Alkaloids: Bulbocapine, launobine [6], laurolitsine, boldine and laurotetanine [13].
5) Steroids: β-Sitosterol, stigmasterol and campesterol [8].
6) Others: Palmitone (=16-hetriacontane) [7], paraffins [9].

Pharmacology

1) Melanin formation inhibitor in melanoma B16 cells (2',6'-dihydroxy-4'-methoxy-3'-(3''-methyl-6''-methylethyl-2''-cyclohexenyl) chalcone, hexahydrodibenzofurane) [1, 3, 20].
2) UV-Absorbing agent as cosmetic (2,4,6-trihydroxy chalcone, 5,6-dehydrokawain) [2, 4].
3) Activity against house dust mites (essential oil) [19].

Literatures:
[1] Fujii, A. *et al.*: *Jpn Kokai Tokkyo Koho*, JP 08112521 A2, **1996**, Japan.
[2] Fujii, A. *et al.*: *Jpn Kokai Tokkyo Koho*, JP 08112522 A2, **1996**, Japan.
[3] Sashita, Y. *et al.*: *Jpn Kokai Tokkyo Koho*, JP 08134058 A2, **1996**, Japan.
[4] Fujii, A. *et al.*: *Jpn Kokai Tokkyo Koho*, JP 08133941 A2, **1996**, Japan.
[5] Hayashi, N. *et al.*: *Z. Naturforsch. Teil C*, **1973**, 28, 227.
[6] Tomita, M. *et al.*: *Yakugaku Zasshi* **1969**, 89(5), 737.
[7] Hayashi, N. *et al.*: *J. Indian Chem. Soc.* **1971**, 48(3), 288.
[8] Komae, H. *et al.*: *Phytochem.* **1971**, 10(11), 2834.
[9] Hayashi, N. *et al.*: *Z. Naturforsch. B* **1972**, 27(11), 1438.
[10] Hayashi, N. *et al.*: *Z. Naturforsch. C* **1973**, 28(3-4), 227.
[11] Tanaka, H. *et al.*: *Phytochem.* **1984**, 23(5), 1198.
[12] Takizawa, N.: *Shoyakugaku Zasshi* **1984**, 38(2), 194.
[13] Kozuka, M. *et al.*: *J. Nat. Prod.* **1985**, 48(1), 160.
[14] Tanaka, H. *et al.*: *Chem. Pharm. Bull.* **1985**, 33(6), 2602.
[15] Nii, Hiromichi: *Koryo* **1986**, 152, 53.
[16] Shimomura, H. *et al.*: *Phytochem.* **1988**, 27(12), 3937.
[17] Ichino, K. *et al.*: *Chem. Lett.* **1989**(2), 363; *Tennen Yuki Kagobutsu Toronkai Koen Yoshishu* **1988**, 30, 9.

[18] Ichino, K. *et al.*: *Heterocycles* **1990**, 31(3), 549.
[19] Furuno, T. *et al.*: *Mokuzai Gakkaishi* **1994,** 40(1) 78.
[20] Mimaki, Y. *et al.*: *Chem. Pharm. Bull.* **1995**, 43(5) 893.

[T. Kimura]

443.   *Litsea cubeba* **(Lour.) Pers.**   (Lauraceae)

Shan-ji-jiao (C), Aomoji (J)

Fruit (CP)
Local Drug Name: Bi-cheng-qie (C), But-dung-cair (H), Hicchoka (J).
Processing: Eliminate foreign matter, and dry in the sun (C, J). Dry in shade (H).
Method of Administration: Oral (decoction: C, H, J).
Folk Medicinal Uses:
                    1) Epigastric pain accompanied by feeling of cold (C, H, J).
                    2) Nausea and vomiting due to cold in the stomach (C, J).
                    3) Abdominal colic of cold type (C).
                    4) Turbid urine caused by cold-damp (C).
                    5) Indigestion (H).

Root
Local Drug Name: Dou-see-keung-gun (H).
Processing: Dry in shade (H).
Method of Administration: Oral (decoction: H).
Folk Medicinal Uses:
                    1) Rhoumatic bone pain (C, H).
                    2) Low back pain (C, H).
                    3) Traumatic injury (C, H).
                    4) Cold (C, H).
                    5) Headache (C, H).
                    6) Gastric pain (C, H).

Leaf
Local Drug Name: Dou-see-keung-yip (H).
Processing: Use in fresh (H).
Method of Administration: Topical (used as poultice: H).
Folk Medicinal Uses:
                    1) Boils (C, H).
                    2) Pyodermas (C, H).
                    3) Mastitis (C, H).
                    4) Snake bites (C, H).

Scientific Researches:
Chemistry
   1) Essential oils: citral, methyl heptenone, linalool, limonene, citronellal, camphene, α-pinene, α-terpineol, geraniol, geranyl acetate, camphor, safrole, α-humulene, β-pinene, *p*-cymene, β-methylhepteneketone, methylheptyketone [1-3].
   2) Fatty acids: lauric acid, cis-4-decenoic acid, cis-4-dodecenoic acid, cis-4-tetradecenoic acid [4].
   3) Lignans: *l*-cubebin, *l*-hinokinin, *l*-clusin, *l*-dihydrocubebin, (2R,3R)-2-(3", 4", 5-trimethoxybenzyl)-3-(3',4'-methylenedioxybenzyl)-1,4-butanediol (*l*-dihydroclusin), (3R,4R)-3,4-bis (3,4,5-trimethoxybenzyl) tetrahydro-2-furanol (*l*-cubebinin) [5], *l*-cubebinone, *l*-isoyatein, *l*-thujaplicatin, *l*-yatein, *l*-cubebininolide, (2R,3R)-2-(3",4"-methylene dioxybenzyl)-3-(3',4'-dimethoxy benzyl butyrolactone) [6].

Pharmacology
1) Relieving asthma and removing the phlegm [7].
2) Antiallergic effect [7].
3) Antischistosomal effect [8].
4) Effect against cardiac arrhythmia [9].
5) Antifungal effect (citral) [10-12].
6) Inhibiting Trichomonas vaginalis [13].

Literatures:
[1] *"Zhongguo Jingji Zhiiwuzhi"* **1961,** 753, 1338.
[2] Research Group for Essential Oils: *Zhiwu Xuebao* **1975,** (17), 35.
[3] Zhan, Y. X. *et al.: Sepu* **1985,** 2(4), 190.
[4] Wang, J. P. *et al.: Zhiwu Xuebao* **1983,** 25(3), 245.
[5] Prabhu B. R. *et al.: Phytochemistry* **1985,** 24, 329.
[6] Badheka L. P. *et al.: Phytochemistry* **1986,** 25, 487.
[7] Qing, B. C. *et al.: Yaoxue Xuebao* **1980,** 15(10), 584.
[8] *"Quanguo Zhongcaoyao Huibian"* **1975,** Vol.1, 104.
[9] Zhang, F. W.: *Zhongcaoyao* **1985,** 16(6), 254.
[10] Zhou, Y. *et al.: Zhongxiyi Jiehe Zazhi* **1984,** 4(9), 558.
[11] Tu, X. Y. *et al.: Zhongyao Tongbao* **1985,** 10(5), 231.
[12] Li, K.Q.: *Zhongguo Yiyuan Yaoxue Zazhi* **1986,** 6, 483.
[13] Tu, X.Y. *et al.: Zhongyao Tongbao* **1986,** 11, 694.

[J.X. Guo]

444.   *Nigella glandulifera* Freyn   (Ranunculaceae)

Liu-guo-hei-zhong-cao (C)

Seed (CP)
Local Drug Name: Hai-zhong-cao-zi (C)
Processing: Eliminate foreign matter, and dry in the sun (C).
Method of Administration: Oral (decoction: C).
Folk Medicinal Uses:
       1) Tinnitus for forgetfulness (C).
       2) Amenorrhea (C)
       3) Inadequate secretion of milk (C).
       4) Urinary infection, urolithiasis (C).
Contraindications: Contraindicated in pregnancy and in patients with febrile diseases (C).

Scientific Researches:
Chemistry
1) Flavonoids: Nigeglanoside, nigeglanose[1]
2) Triterpenes: 3-O- [β-D-xylopyranosyl (1→3)-α-L-rhamnopyranosyl (1→2)-α-L-arabino-pyranosyl]-28-O-[α-L-rhamnopyranosyl(1→4)-β-D-glucopyranosyl(1→6)-β-D-gluco-pyranosyl] hederagenin[1]
3) Sugars: Sucrose[1]
4) Sterols: β-Sitosterol[1]
5) Alkaloids: N,N-Dimethyl-1,2-dimethoxy-10.11-dihydroxyaporphine quaternary ammonium chloride[1]

Literatures:
[1] Hao, H. et al.: *Yaoxue Xuebao* **1996,** 31(9), 659.

[J.X. Guo]

445.   *Pulsatilla cernua* Sprengel   (Ranunculaceae)

Okinagusa (J), Ga-neun-ip-hal-mi-ggot (K)

Related plants: *Pulsatilla chinensis* Spreng., Hiroha-okinagusa (J); *P. koreana* Nakai, Hal-mi-ggot (K).

Root
　　Local Drug Name: Hakuto-o (J), Baek- du-ong (K).
　　Processing: Dry under the sun (J, K).
　　Method of Administration: Decoction (J, K).
　　Folk Medicinal Uses:
　　　　　　　　1) Febrile diseases (J, K).
　　　　　　　　2) Traumatic injury (J, K).
　　　　　　　　3) Diarrhea, melena (J, K).
　　　　　　　　4) Nasal hemorrhage (J, K).
　　　　　　　　5) Abdominal pain (J, K).
　　　　　　　　6) Toothache (J).

Scientific Researches:
　　Chemistry
　　　　1) Saponins: Sapindoside [1].
　　Pharmacology
　　　　1) Skin lightening (saponin) [2].
Literatures:
　　[1] Shimizu, M. *et al.*: *Chem. Pharm. Bull.* **1978**, 26(6), 1666.
　　[2] Maeda, N. *et al.*: *Japan Kokai Tokkyo Koho,* JP 08133955 A2, **1996** Japan.

[T. Kimura]

446.   *Pulsatilla chinensis* (Bge.) Regel   (Ranunculaceae)

Bai-tou-weng (C), Hiroha-okinagusa (J)

Related plants: *P. cernua* (Thunb. ex Murry) Spreng.: Okinagusa (J); *P. koreana* Nakai ex Mari: Hal-mi-ggot (K).

Root (CP)
　　Local Drug Name: Bai-tou-weng (C), Bark-ton-yung (H), Hakuto-o (J), Baek-du-ong (K).
　　Processing: Eliminate foreign matter, wash clean, soften thoroughly, cut into thick slices and dry (C).
　　Method of Administration: Oral (decoction: C, H, J).
　　Folk Medicinal Uses:
　　　　　　　　1) Amoebic dysentery (C, H, J, K).
　　　　　　　　2) Pudendal itching with excessive leukorrhea (C, H).
　　　　　　　　3) Toothache (J, K).
　　　　　　　　4) Abdominal pain (J, K).
　　　　　　　　5) Traumatic injury (J).
　　　　　　　　6) Sputum (K).
　　　　　　　　7) Fever (K).
　　　　　　　　8) Acute gastritis (K).
　　　　　　　　9) Cough (K).
　　　　　　　　10) Spasm (K).
　　　　　　　　11) Fracture of bone (K).

Scientific Researches:
Chemistry
  1) Triterpenoid saponins [1,2].
  2) Lactones: anemonin [3].
Pharmacology
  1) Antiamebic effect [4].
  2) Antibacterial effect [5-7].

Literatures:
[1] Zhu, R. H. *et al.*: *Huaxue Xuebao* **1955**, 21(3), 328.
[2] Chen, W. K. *et al.*: *Huaxue Xuebao* **1983**, 41(8), 739.
[3] *"Zhongcaoyao Youxiaochengfen De Yanjiu"* **1972**, Vol.1, 388.
[4] Jiang, M. X. *et al. Wuhan Yixueyuan Xuebao* **1958**, (1), 1.
[5] Wang, Y. *et al.*: *Zhiwu Xuebao* **1954**, 2, 121.
[6] Wang, W. S. *et al.*: *Yaoxue Xuebao* **1959**, 7, 522.
[7] Cao, R. L. *et al.*: *Zhonghua Pifuke Zazhi* **1957**, (4), 286.

[J.X. Guo]

447.   *Ranunculus ternatus* **Thunb.**   (Ranunculaceae)

Xiao-mao-gen (C), Gae-gu-ri-gat (K)

Root tuber (CP)
  Local Drug Name: Mao-zhao-cao (C), Mour-jour-cho (H), Myo-jo-cho (K).
  Processing: Eliminate foreign matter, and dry in the sun (C, K).
  Method of Administration: Oral (decoction: C, H, K).
  Folk Medicinal Uses:
        1) Tuberculosis of lymph nodes without alceration (C, H, K).

Scientific Researches:
Chemistry
  1) Amino acids [1].
  2) Organic acids [1].
  3) Sugars [1]: Diacylated D-glucose [2].
Pharmacology
  1) Bacteriostatic effect on drug-resistant *Mycobacterium tuberculosis* [3].

Literatures:
[1] *"Quanguo Zhongcaoyao Huibian"* **1975**, Vol.1, 791.
[2] Iriki, Y. *et al.*: *Nippon Nogei Kagaku Kaishi* **1975**, 49(1), 7.
[3] Pan, Z. H.: *Zhongyiyao Xinxi* **1986**, (5), 26.

[J.X. Guo]

448.   *Berberis thunbergii* **DC.**   (Berberidaceae)

Zi-bo (C), Megi(J)

Related plant: *B. amurensis* Rupr.: Mae-bal-top-na-mu (K), *B. koreana* Palibin: Mae-ja-na-mu (K).

Stem
  Local Drug Name: Xiao-bo (C), Shobeki (J).
  Processing: Dry under the sun (C, J).
  Method of Administration: Decoction (C, J), topical (paste: C).
  Folk Medicinal Uses:
                          1) Gastrointestinal disorder (C, J).
                          2) Eye diseases (C, J).
                          3) Gastroenteritis (C).
                          4) Dysentery (C).
                          5) Paratyphoid (C).
                          6) Jaundice (C).
                          7) Ascites due to cirrhosis (C).
                          8) Stomatitis (C).
                          9) Urinary tract infection (C).
                          10) Acute nephritis (C).
                          11) Tonsillitis (C).

Scientific Researches:
  Chemistry
    1) Alkaloids: Berberine [1], oxyberberine, berbamine, oxyacanthine [2], isotetrandrine [4].
    2) Anthocyanins [3].

Literatures:
  [1] Kawashima, Y.: *Yakugaku Zasshi*, **1969**, 89(10), 1386.
  [2] Brazdovicova, B. *et al.*: *Chem. Zvesti*, **1980**, 34(2), 259.
  [3] Mamaev, S. A. *et al.*: *Rast. Resur.*, **1971**, 7(2), 280.
  [4] Tomita, M. *et al.*: *Yakugaku Zasshi*, **1960**, 80, 845.

[T. Kimura]

449.   *Mahonia bealei* **(Fort.) Carr.**   (Berberidaceae)

Kuo-ye-shi-da-gong-lao (C), Hiiragi-nanten (J)

Related plant: *M. fortunei* (Lindl.) Fedde: Xi-ye-she-da-gong-lao (C), Jung-guk-nam-cheon (K); *M. japonica*
                DC: Bbul-nam-cheon (K).

Stem (CP)
  Local Drug Name: Gong-lao-mu (C), Gung-loh-muk (H).
  Processing: Cut into pieces, and dry (C).
  Method of Administration: Oral (decoction: C, H, K); Topical (decoction: C, H).
  Folk Medicinal Uses:
                          1) Acute dysentery (C, H, K).
                          2) Icteric hepatitis (C, H).
                          3) Conjunctivitis (C, H).
                          4) Ulcers (C).
                          5) Boils (C).
                          6) Carbuncles (C).
                          7) Toothache due to fire in the stomach (C).

Scientific Researches:
  Chemistry
  1) Alkaloids: Berberine [1].

43

Pharmacology
  1) Antibacterial effect [2].

Literatures:
[1] Nanjing College of Pharmacy: *"Zhongcaoyao Xue"* **1976,** Vol.2, 279.
[2] *"Zhongyao Dacidian"* **1977,** Vol.1, 11.

[J.X. Guo]

450.   *Stauntonia hexaphylla* **Thunb.**   (Lardizabalaceae)

Liu-teng (C), Mube (J), Meol-ggul (K)

Stem and root
  Local Drug Name: Liu-teng (C), Yamokka (J), Ya-mok-gwa (K).
  Processing: Dry under the sun (C, J, K).
  Method of Administration: Oral (decoction: C, J, K).
  Folk Medicinal Uses:
                1) Pain (C, J, K).
                2) Edema (J, K).

Scientific Researches:
  Chemistry
    1) Saponins: Mubenin A, B, C [1] and mubenoside A [2].   Staunoside A, B, D and E [3].
    2) Cardiac glycoside: Stauntonin.
    3) Lignans: Staunoside C [4].
    4) Anthocyanins [5].

Literatures:
[1] Takemoto, T. *et al.: Ann.* **1965,** 685, 237.
[2] Ikuta, A. *et al.: Phytochem.* **1991,** 30(7), 2425.
[3] Wang, H. B. *et al.: Phytochem.* **1993,** 33(6), 1469; **1993,** 34(5), 1389.
[4] Wang, H. B. *et al.: Phytochem.* **1993,** 34(6), 1621.
[5] Ishikura, N. *et al.: Phytochem.* **1976,** 15(3), 442.

[T. Kimura]

451.   *Stephania tetrandra* **S. Moore**   (Menispermaceae)

Fen-fang-ji (C), Fun-fong-gay (H), Shima-hasunohi-kazura (J), Bun-bang-gi (K)

Root (CP)
  Local Drug Name: Fang-ji (C), Fun-fong-gay (H), Funboi (J), Bun-bang-gi (K).
  Processing: Use in fresh or slice and dry under the sun (C, H, J, K).
  Method of Administration: Oral (decoction: C, H, J, K).
  Folk Medicinal Uses:
                1) Edema (C, H, J, K).
                2) Rheumatic arthritis (C, H, J, K).
                3) Gastric ulcer, duodenal ulcer (C, H, K).
                4) Neuralgia (H, J, K).
                5) Hypertension (H, C, J).
                6) Acute gastroenteritis, dysentery (C, H, K).
                7) Snake bite, boils, furuncles (Topical: C, H).

8) Oliguria (C, H)
9) Genitourinary tract infection (H, K).
10) Parotitis, tonsillitis (C, H).
11) Beriberi (C).
12) Leucorrhea (H).

Scientific Research:
Chemistry
1) Alkaloids: tetrandrin (hanfangchin A or fanchinin), fangchinoline (hanfangchin B or demethyltetrandrine) [1, 30], flavonoid glycoside, phenols, volatile oil, organic acid [30].
Pharmacology
1) Calcium antagonistic effect [2-4, 16-18].
2) Anti-inflammatory and antiallergic effect [4–9].
3) Sedative effect [5].
4) Anti-hypertension effect [2, 10-12, 33].
5) Antiarrhythmic effect [2, 13-15].
6) Relaxation effect on smooth muscles [2, 16-19, 32].
7) Antibacterial effect [20].
8) Protective effects on myocardium [2, 16-19].
9) Inhibiting platelet aggregation [25-26].
10) Inhibiting immune hemolysis [27].
11) Anti-fibrosis effect [28-29].
12) Protective effect on cerebral ischemia [31].

Literature:
[1] Yang, L.H. *et al.: Yaowu Fenxi Zazhi*   **1989,** 9, 216.
[2] Fang, D.C. *et al.: Zhonghua Yixue Zazhi*, **1983**, 63, 772.
[3] Fang, D.C. *et al.: Zhongguo Yaoli Xuebao*, **1982**, 3, 233.
[4] Hong, J.L. *et al.: Zhongguo Yaoli Xuebao*, **1989**, 10, 533.
[5] Berezhinskaya, V.V. *et al.: Izuch. i Ispol'z. Lekarstv. Rastit. Resursov SSSR (Leningrad: Med.) Sb.* , **1964**, 320.
[6] Li, W. *et al.: Zhongguo Yaoli Xuebao*, **1987**,   8, 450.
[7] Lu, F.H. *et al.: Yaoxue Xuebao*, **1957**, 5, 113.
[8] He, F.C. *et al.: Zhongguo Yaoli Xuebao*, **1989**, 10, 249.
[9] Zhang, M. *et al.: Zhongguo Yaoli Xuebao*, **1993**, 14, 529.
[10] Hu, G.X. *et al.: Zhongguo Yaoli Xuebao,* **1987**, 8, 325.
[11] Lu, X.S. *et al.: Chinese Journal of Experimental Surgery*, **1987**, 4(3), 124.
[12] Miao, C.Y. *et al.: Zhongguo Yaoli Xuebao*, **1991**, 12, 352.
[13] Li, G.Z. *et al.: Zhongguo Yiyao Xuebao*, **1990**, 5, 348.
[14] Lou, J.S. *et al.: Zhongguo Yaoli Xuebao*, **1988**, 9, 412.
[15] Yao, W.X. *et al.: Zhongguo Yaoli Xuebao*, **1986**, 7, 128.
[16] Yao, W.X. *et al.: Zhongguo Yaoli Xuebao*, **1983**, 4, 130.
[17] Qian, Y.M. *et al.: Zhongguo Yaoli Xuebao*, **1992**, 13, 243.
[18] Yao, W. *et al.: Zhongguo Yaolixue Tongbao*, **1991**, 7, 357.
[19] Masahiro, O. *et al.: Ann. Rept. ITSUU Lab. (Tokyo)*, **1957**, 8, 25.
[20] Hsu, C.L. *et al.: Zhonghua Yixue Zazhi*, **1947**, 33(3,4), 71.
[21] Deng, K.Y. *et al.: Yaoxue Xuebao*, **1993**, 28, 886.
[22] Xia, G.J. *et al.: Tongji Yike Daxue Xuebao*, **1994**, 23, 446.
[23] Miao, N. *et al.: Chinese Journal of Anesthesiology*, **1991**, 11, 275.
[24] Miao, N. *et al.: Chinese Journal of Anesthesiology*, **1989**, 9, 228.
[25] Qian, Y.M. *et al.: Zhongguo Yaoli Xuebao*, **1989**, 10, 61.
[26] Lin, A.P. *et al.: Journal of Chinese Medicine* (Taiwan), **1993**, 4, 73.
[27] Tanaka, N. *et al.: Japan. J. Exptl. Med.,* **1952**, 22, 87.
[28] Jin H. *et al.: Chinese Journal of Tuberculosis and Respiratory Disease*, **1991**, 14, 359.
[29] Li, D.G. *et al.: Chinese Journal of Digestion*, **1994**, 14, 339.

[30] Jiangsu Xinyi Xueyuan: *Zhongyao Dacidian*, **1978**, 1984.
[31] Qi, S.T. *et al.*: *Zhongguo Yaolixue Yu Dulixue Zazhi*, **1993**, 7, 49.
[32] Li, Y.Q. *et al.*: *Zhongguo Yaolixue Xubao*, **1987**, 8, 529.
[33] Wang, H.L. *et al.*: *Zhongguo Yaolixue Yu Dulixue Zazhi*, **1994**, 8, 246.

[P.P.H. But]

452. *Tinospora sinensis* **(Lour.) Merr.**   (Menispermaceae)

Zhong-hua-qing-niu-dan (C), Foon-gun-teng (H)

Vine
Local Drug Name: Kuan-jin-teng (C), Foon-gun-teng (H).
Processing: Wash, slice, and dry under the sun (C, H).
Method of Administration: Oral (decoction: C, H).
Folk Medicinal Uses:
      1) Rheumatic arthritis (C, H).
      2) Sciatica (C, H).
      3) Traumatic injury (C, H).
      4) Lumbago (C).
Contraindications: Pregnancy and puerperium.

Scientific Research:
Chemistry
  1) Glucosides: tinosinen [1], tinosineside A and B [2].
  2) Amino acids, sugars [5].
Pharmacology
  1) Antidiabetic activity [3-4].

Literature:
[1] Yonemitsu, M. *et al.*: *Planta Med.* **1993,** 59, 552.
[2] Yonemitsu, M. *et al.*: *Liebigs Ann.* **1995,** (2), 437.
[3] Gupta, S.S. *et al.*: *Indian J. Med. Res.* **1967,** 55, 733.
[4] Broker, R. *et al.*: *Indian J. Pharm.* **1953,** 15, 309.
[5] Guangzhoushi Yaopin Jianyansuo: *Nongcun Zhongcaoyao Zhiji Jishu* **1971,** 247.

[P.P.H. But]

453. *Piper kadsura* **(Choisy) Ohwi**   (Piperaceae)

Feng-teng (C), Futokazura (J), Hu-chu-deung (K)

Stem (CP)
Local Drug Name: Hai-feng-teng (C), Hoi-fung-tunk (H), Nanto (J), Hae-pung-deung (K).
Processing: Eliminate foreign matter, soak, soften thoroughly, cut into thick slices, and dry in the sun (C, K).
Method of Administration: Oral (decoction: C, H, K).
Folk Medicinal Uses:
      1) Rheumatic or rheumatoid arthritis with joint pain (C, H, J, K).
      2) Muscular contracture (C, H, J, K).
      3) Ankylosis (C, H).
      4) Traumatic pain (J).

Scientific Researches:
Chemistry
  1) Steroids: stigmasterol [1].
  2) Xylans: futoxide, futoenone, futoquinol, futoamide [1], isofutoquinol A, B, isodihydro-
     futoquinol A, B [2], piperenone [3].
  3) Lignans: kadsurenone, kadsurin A, B [4], kadsurenin K, L [5].
  4) Essential oils: α-thujene, α-pinene, camphene, β-pinene, myrcene, α-phellandrene, α-terpinene,
     β-phelandrene, γ-terpinene, α-terpinolene, linalol, terpinen-4-ol, α-terpineol, bornyl acetate, 2-
     undecanone, δ-elemene, copaene, β-elemene, trans-caryophyllene, humulene, α-elemene,
     guaiene, γ-elemene, δ-cadinene, elemol, β-bisabolene, β-eudesnol [6].
Pharmacology
  1) Antitumor effect [1].
  2) Specific inhibitory effect [7].

Literatures:
  [1] Shuji, T.: *Phytochemistry* **1969**, 8(1), 321.
  [2] Matsui, K. *et al.*: *Tetra. Lett.* **1976**, (48), 4371.
  [3] Matsui, K. *et al.*: *Agric. Biol. Chem.* **1976**, 40(6), 1113.
  [4] Chang, M. N.: *Phytochemistry* **1985**, 24(9), 2079.
  [5] Ma, Y. *et al.*: *Yaoxue Xuebao* **1993**, 28(3), 207.
  [6] Fan, S. T. *et al.*: *Zhongyaocai* **1987**, (4), 40.
  [7] Shen, T. Y. *et al.*: *Proc. Natl. Acad. Sci.* **1985**, 82, 672.

[J.X. Guo]

454.   *Piper longum* L.   (Piperaceae)

Bi-bo (C), But-boot (H), Hihatsu (J), Pil-bal (K)

Fruit-spike (CP)
Local Drug Name: Bi-bo (C), But-boot (H), Hibatsu (J), Pil-bal (K).
Processing: Eliminate foreign matter. Break to pieces befere use (C, K).
Method of Administration: Oral (decoction: C, H, K); Topical (powder: C, H, K).
Folk Medicinal Uses:
            1) Epigastric pain, vomiting and diarrhea caused by cold (C, H, J, K).
            2) Migraine (C, H, J, K).
            3) External use for toothache (C, H, J, K).
            4) Acute gastroenteritis (J).

Scientific Researches:
Chemistry
  1) Orangic acids: palmitic acid, tetrahydropiperic acid [1].
  2) Essential oils: *n*-tridecane, *n*-tridecene, *n*-pentadecane, *n*-pentadecene, β-bisabolene, α-
     caryophyllene, *n*-heptadecane, *n*-heptadecene, *n*-nonadecane, *n*-nonadecene [2].
  3) Alkaloids: piperidine [1], piperine, N-isobutyl-decatrans-2-trans-4-dienamide [3], piplartin,
     piperlonguminine [4].
  4) Others: 1-undecylenyl-3,4-methyl-enedioxy benzene [1], sesamin [5].
Pharmacology
  1) Antibacterial effect [6].
  2) Effect on central nervous system [7].
  3) Antifertilitic activity [8].
  4) Antagonist acute myocardial ischemia [9].

5) Relaxation effect on smooth muscle [10].

Literatures:
[1] Gokhale, V. G. *et al.*: *J. Univ. Bombay* **1948,** 16A, 47.
[2] Sun, Y. F. *et al.*: *Zhongyi Zazhi* **1981,** 22(12), 65.
[3] Dhar, K. L. *et al.*: *Indian J. Chem.* **1967,** 5(11), 588.
[4] Chatterjee, A. *et al.*: *Tetrahedron* **1967,** 23, 1769.
[5] Atal, C. K. *et al.*: *Indian J. Chem.* **1966,** 4, 252.
[6] Bhargava, A. K. *et al.*: *Ind. J. Pharm.* **1968,** 30(6), 150.
[7] Singh, N. *et al.*: *J. Res. Indian Med.* **1973,** 8(1), 1.
[8] Prakash, A. O.: *Int. J. Crude Drug Res.* **1986,** 24(1), 19.
[9] Bi, Y. F.: *Neimenggu Yaoxue* **1986,** 5(2), 17.
[10]Zhuang, Z. K.: *Guowai Yixue Zhongyi Zhongyao Fence* **1987,** 9(1), 57.

[J.X. Guo]

455.   *Piper nigrum* L.   (Piperaceae)

Hu-jiao (C), Woo-jiu (H), Kosho (J)Hu-chu-na-mu (K)

Fruit (CP, KP)
Local Drug Name: Hu-jiao (C), Woo-jiu (H), Kosho (J), Hu-chu (K).
Processing: Eliminate foreign matter, break to fine powder before use (C, J, K).
Method of Administration: Oral (decoction: C, H, K); Topical (powder: C, H, K).
Folk Medicinal Uses:
> 1) Vomiting, abdominal pain, diarrhea and anorexia due to cold in the stomach (C, H, J, K).
> 2) Epilepsy with much phlegm (C, H).
> 3) Acute gastroenteritis (J).
> 4) Common cold (K).
> 5) Cough (K).

Root and stem
Local Drug Name: Woo-jiu-gun (H).
Method of Administration: Oral (decoction: H).
Folk Medicinal Uses:
> 1) Vomiting, abdominal pain (H).

Scientific Researches:
Chemistry
> 1) Alkaloids: piperine [1], piperyline, piperoleine A, B, C [2], piperanine [3].
> 2) Essential oils: piperonal, dihydrocarveol, caryophyllene oxide, cryptone [1,5], *cis-p-2-*menthenl-ol, *cis-p-2*,8-menthadien-1-ol, *trans*-pinocarrol [6].
> 3) Others: pipercide [4].

Pharmacology
> 1) Anticonvulsive effect [7-11].
> 2) Antioxidation [12].
> 3) Pesticidal effect [13].
> 4) Heparic drug metabolizing enzyme induction [14]. (The derivant of piperine, antiepilepsirine.)
> 5) Anti-inflammatory effect [11].
> 6) Antithermic effect [11,15].

Literatures:
[1] "*Zhongguo Jingji Zhiwuzhi*" **1961,** 1644,1291.

[2] Grewe, R. *et al.*: *Chem. Ber.* **1970,** 103(12), 3752.
[3] Traxler, J. T.: *J. Agr. Food Chem.* **1971,** 19(6), 1135.
[4] Miyakado, M. *et al.*: *Agric. Biol. Chem.* **1979,** 43(7), 1609.
[5] Torsten, H. *et al.*: *J. Agr. Food Chem.* **1957,** 5, 53.
[6] Richard, H. M. *et al.*: *J. Food Sci.* **1971,** 36(4), 584.
[7] Dept. of Pharmacology: *Beijing Yixueyuan Xuebao* **1974,** (4), 217.
[8] People's Hospital: *Beijing Yixueyuan Xuebao* **1974,** (4), 214.
[9] People's Hospital: *Beijing Yixueyuan Xuebao* **1977,** (4), 234.
[10] Pei, Y. Q. *et al.*: *Yaoxue Xuebao* **1980,** 15(4), 198.
[11] Lee, E. B. *et al.*: *Arch. Pharmacol. Res.* **1984,** 7(2), 127.
[12] Nakatni, N. *et al.*: *Environ. Health Perspect* **1986,** 67, 135.
[13] Srivastava, M. C. *et al.*: *Ind. J. Pharm.* **1968,** 30(3), 65.
[14] Lou, Y. Q. *et al.*: *Zhongguo Yaoli Xuebao* **1984,** 5(2), 76.
[15] Sollmann, T.: *A Manual of Pharmacology* **1957,** 8, 162.

[J.X. Guo]

456.   *Actinidia polygama* **Miquel**   (Actinidiaceae)

Ge-zao (C), Matatabi (J), Gae-da-rae (K)

Fruit gall
Local Drug Name: Mutianliao-zi (C), Mokutenryo (J), Mok-cheon-ryo-ja (K)
Processing: Collect fruits metamorphosed by infection of *Pseudasphondylia matatabi* Yukawa.
Method of Administration: Decoction (J), liquor (J)
Folk Medicinal Uses:
                1) Feeling of cold (J, K).
                2) Uses for cat (J, K).
                3) Pain, colic (J).

Fruit
Local Drug Name: Ge-zao (C), Matatabi (J), Gae-da-rae (K)
Processing: Dry under the sun (C), fresh fruits (J).
Method of Administration: Oral (decoction) (C, J), liquor (J).
Folk Medicinal Uses:
                1) Weakness (J, K).
                2) Lumbago (C).
                3) Hernia pain (C).

Branch and Leaf
Local Drug Name: Mutianliao (C).
Processing: Dry under the sun (C, J).
Method of Administration: Oral (decoction)(C, J).
Folk Medicinal Uses:
                1) Leprosy (C).
                2) Weakness (J).

Scientific Researches:
Chemistry
     1) Iridoids: Iridomyrmesin, isoiridomyrmesin, actinidine [1], dihydronepetalactone, isodihydro-nepetalactone, neonepetalactone [2]. α-, β-, γ- and δ-iridodiol [3], actinidiolide, actinidol, dihydroactinidiolide [4], matatabiether, isoneomatatabiol, isodihydroiridodiol [5], dehydroiridodial as the pungent principle [6], iridodial gentiobioside and dehydroiridodial gentiobioside [7], actinidialactone, isoactinidialactone, isoepiiridomyrmecin,

49

isoneonepetalactone and neonepetalactone[8].
2) Triterpenoids [9].
3) Polysaccharides. [10].
4) Vitamins: *l*-ascorbic acid, 98mg/100g fresh fruits [11].
Pharmacology
1) Ulcer protection [12].
2) Choresterol lowering, antidiabetic and anti herpes activity (lipopolysaccharides) [13].

Literatures:
[1] Sakan, T. *et al.*: *Bull. Chem. Soc. Jap.*, **1959**, 32, 315; **1959**, 32, 1154; 1155; *Nippon Kagaku Zasshi*, **1960**, 81, 1320; 1324; 1327; 1444; 1445; *Bull. Chem. Soc. Japan*, **1960,** 33, 712; Isoe, S.: *Kagaku* , **1965**, 20, 145.
[2] Sakan, T. *et al.*: *Tetrahedron Letters*, **1965**, 4097; *Bull. Chem. Soc. Japan*, **1959**, 32, 1155.
[3] Sakan, T. *et al.*: *Bull. Chem. Soc. Japan*, **1964**, 37, 1888.
[4] Sakan, T. *et al.*: *Tetrahedron Letters*, **1967**, 1623.
[5] Isoe, J. *et al.*: *Tetrahedron Letters*, **1968**, 5319; Hyeon, S. B. et al.: *ibid.* **1968**, 5325.
[6] Yoshihara, K. *et al.*: *Chem. Lett.* **1978**, 4, 433.
[7] Murai, F. *et al.*: Planta Med., 1979, 37(3), 234; *Koryo*, **1994**, 182, 73.
[8] Sakai, T. *et al.*: *Bull. Chem. Soc. Japan*, **1980**, 53(12), 3683; *Tetrahedron*, **1980,** 36(20-21), 3115.
[9] Sashida, Y. *et al.*: *Phytochem.* **1992**, 31(8), 2801; **1994**, 35(2), 377.
[10] Redgwell, R. J.: *Phytochem.* **1983**, 22(4), 951.
[11] Anetai, M. *et al.*: *Hokkaido Eisei Kenkyushoho*, **1996**, 46, 34.
[12] Inagawa, H. *et al.*: *Chem. Pharm. Bull.*, **1992,** 40(4), 994.
[13] Soma, G. *et al.*: *European Pat.*: EP 462021 A2 911218; EP 91401622 910617; JP 90155425 900615; *Ibid.*: *European Pat.*: EP 462022 A2 911218; EP 91401623 910617; JP 90155428 900615; *Ibid.*: *European Pat.*: EP 462020 A2 911218; EP 91401621 910617; JP 90155426 900615.

[T. Kimura]

457.   *Cratoxylon ligustrinum* **(Spach) Bl.**   (Guttiferae)

Huang-niu-mu (C), Wong-ngau-muk (H)

Young Leaf, Root or Bark
Local Drug Name: Huang-niu-cha (C), Wong-ngau-char (H).
Processing: Wash, slice and dry under the sun (C, H).
Method of Administration: Oral (decoction: C, H).
Folk Medicinal Uses:
1) Colds (C, H).
2) Fever (C, H).
3) Enteritis (C, H).
4) Jaundice (C, H).
5) Heliosis (C).
6) Hoarseness (H).
7) Prevention of heat stroke and dysentery (H).
8) Diarrhea (H).
9) Cough (H).

Scientific Research:
Chemistry
1) Terpenes: α-ocimene, γ-terpinene, linalool, terpine-4-ol, (–)-α-terpineol, δ-elemene, copaene, zingiberene, β-caryophyllene, β-farnesene, α-caryophyllene, γ-cadinene, β-cubebene, γ-elemene, δ-cadinene, ledol, δ-cadinol [1].

Literature:

[1] Zhu L.F. *et al.*: *Aromatic Plants and Essential Constituents.* South China Institute of Botany, Chinese Academy of Sciences, Guangzhou, **1993**, 261.

[P.P.H. But]

458.　　　　　*Garcinia hanburyi* **Hooker f.**　　(Guttiferae)

Deung-hwang-na-mu(K)

Resin
Local Drug Name: To-ou(J), Deung-hwang(K)
Processing: Dry under the sun(K)
Method of Administration: Oral(decoction, K)
Folk Medicinal Uses:

　　　　　　　　1) Constipation(J)
　　　　　　　　2) Bleeding(K)
　　　　　　　　3) Edema(K)

Scientific Research:
Chemistry
　1) Xanthones: Gambogic acid[1-3], neogambogic acid[1, 3], isogambogic acid, isomorellinol[2], gambogin, morellin dimethyl acetal, isomoreollin B, moreollic acid, gambogenic acid, gambogenin, isogambogenin, desoxygambogenin, gambogenin dimethyl acetal, gambogellic acid, hanburin, isomorellin, morellic acid, desoxymorellin[5]
Phamacology
　1) Antitumor activity[4]

Literature:

[1] Lu, G. B. and Fang, J.: *Zhongcaoyao* **1988**, 19(7), 198.
[2] Lin L. J. *et al.*: *Magn. Res. Chem.* **1993**, 31(4), 340.
[3] Lu, G. B. *et al.*: *Yao Hsueh Hsueh Pao* **1984**, 19(8), 636.
[4] Belkin M. and Fitzgerald, D. B.: *J. Nat. Cancer Inst.* **1952**, 13, 139.
[5] Asano, J. *et al.*: *Phytochemistry* **1996**, 41(3), 815.

[C. K. Sung]

459.　　　　　*Hypericum erectum* **Thunb.**　　(Guttiferae)

Xian-lian-qiao (C), Otogiriso (J), Go-chu-na-mul (K)

Whole herb
Local Drug Name: Xiao-dui-ye-cao (C), Sho-rengyo (J), So-yeon-gyo (K).
Processing: Dry under the sun (C, J, K).
Method of Administration: Oral (decoction: C, J, K), topical (juice, bath: J, K).
Folk Medicinal Uses:

　　　　　　　　1) Bleeding (C, J, K).
　　　　　　　　2) Hematemesis (C, J, K).
　　　　　　　　3) Menstrual disorder (C, J, K).
　　　　　　　　4) Traumatic injury (C, J, K).
　　　　　　　　5) Epistaxis (J, K).
　　　　　　　　6) Rheumatism (J, K).

7) Neuralgia (J, K).
8) Snake bite (C).
9) Metrorrhagia (J).
10) Gout (J).
11) Bruise (J).
Contraindication: Dermatitis.

Scientific Researches:
Chemistry
1) Hypericin [7].
2) Flavonoids: Quercetin [2].
3) Phloroglucinols: Otogirine and otogirone [5].
4) Terpenoids: Erectumin A and B [6].
Pharmacology
1) Hair growth stimulant (fatty acid, naphthalene sulfonic acid and benzophenone sulfonic acid) [1].
2) Hemostatic and antihemorrhagic acitivity (wedelolactone, demethylwedelolactone) [3].
3) Bacterial sialidase inhibition (fatty acids) [4].
4) Antibiotic and antiallergenic activity (otogirin, otogirone) [5].
5) Vasodilator (erectumin A, B) [6].

Literatures:
[1] Okamoto, Y.: *Jpn. Kokai Tokkyo Koho*, JP 08040835, A2 (**1996**) Japan. ; *Ibid*. JP 08040836.
[2] Palamarchuk, O. P.: *Farm. Zh. (Kiev)* **1975**, 30(2), 77.
[3] Kosuge, T. *et al.*: *Chem. Pharm. Bull.* **1985,** 33(1), 202; Hokuriku Pharm. Co. Ltd.: *Japan Kokai Tokkyo Koho*, JP 60120879, 850628; Appl. JP 83228353, 831205.
[4] Furuya, T. *et al.*: *Shoyakugaku Zasshi*, **1989**, 43(3), 204.
[5] Tada, M. *et al.*: *Phytochem.* **1991**, 30(8), 2559.
[6] Jokura, Y. *et al.*: *Japan Kokai Tokkyo Koho*, JP 92211676 A2 JP 04211676, 920803; Appl. JP 9136890, 910206.
[7] Brockmann, H. *et al.*: *Ann.* **1942**, 553, 1; Chem. Ber. 1957, 90, 2302.

[T. Kimura]

460.   *Macleaya cordata* **R. Br.**   (Papaveraceae)
                [= *Bocconia cordata* R. Br.]

Bo-luo-hui (C), Takenigusa (J), Juk-ja-cho (K)

Whole herb
Local Drug Name: Bo-luo-hui (C), Hakurakukai (J), Bak-rak-hoi (K).
Processing: Fresh or dried under the sun (C, J, K).
Method of Administration: Topical (decoction or powder: C, J). Crushed fresh herb (topical; K).
Folk Medicinal Uses:
1) Carbuncle (C, J, K).
2) Traumatic injury (C, J).
3) Rheumatism (C).
4) Ulcer of lower limb (C).
5) Trichomonas vaginalis (C).
6) Eczema (C).
7) Scald (C).
Contraindication: Poisonous in excess use.

Scientific Researches:

Chemistry
1) Alkaloids: Protopine, α-alloprotopine, chelerythrine, sanguinarine, oxysanguinarine, coptisine,berberine, corysamine, macarpine, chelitutine, chelirubine, bocconine [1]. dehydrocheilan-thifoline [2].

Pharmacology
1) Nematicidal and anti fungal activities (chelerythrine and sanguinarine) [3].

Literatures:
[1] Tani, C. *et al.*: *Yakugaku Zasshi* **1962**, 82, 755; Slavik, J. et al.: *Coll. Czech. Chem. Comm.* **1965**, 30, 887.
[2] Takao, N. *et al.*: *Yakugaku Zasshi*, **1973**, 93, 242.
[3] Onda, M. *et al.*: *Nippon Nogei Kagakukaishi*, **1965**, 39, 168.

[T. Kimura]

461.   *Papaver rhoeas* **L.**   (Papaveraceae)

Li-chun-hua (C), Hinageshi (J), Gae-yang-gwi-bi (K)

Flower
Local Drug Name: Li-chun-hua (C), Reishunka (J), Yeo-chun-hwa (K).
Processing: Dry under the sun (C, J, K).
Method of Administration: Oral (decoction: C, J, K).
Folk Medicinal Uses:
1) Cough (C, J, K).
2) Pain (C, J, K).
3) Dysentery, diarrhea (C, K).
4) Sore throat(J)..

Scientific Researches:
Chemistry
1) Alkaloids: Rhoeadine [1], rhoeagenine, isorhoeagenine, isorhoeagenine glucoside, (-)-sinactine, isorhoeadine [2], protopine, glaudine, chelerythrine, sanguinarine, papaverrubine-A, -B, -D, -E[3], (-)-N-methylstylopine, coptisine and adlumidiceine [4], rhoearubine [5], adlumidiceine[6], corydine, fagaline, berberine, palmatine, and 1,2,3,4-tetrahydro-6-methoxy-2-methyl-β-carboline [7], asimilobine, stylopine, isocorydine [8].
2) Triterpenoids and steroids: α- and β-amyrin, β-sitosterol, campesterol and stigmasterol [9].
3) Wax: docosane-1,3-diol, hexacosane-1,7-diol, octacosane-1,9-diol, nonacosane-1,10-diol and triacontane-1,11-diol [10], cyclolaudenol and (+)-10-nonacosanol [11].
4) Flavonoids: Seven heterosides of kaempferol, quercetin and luteolin [12].

Pharmacology
1) Cytotoxicity (alkaloids) [13].
2) Toxic principle (alkaloids) [14].

Literatures:
[1] Santavy, F. *et al.*: *Coll. Czech. Chem. Comm.* **1960**, 25, 1901; Awe, W. et al.: *Naturwissenschaften* **1960**, 47, 107.
[2] Winkler, W. *et al.*: *Arch. d. Pharm.* **1961**, 294, 301.
[3] Nemeckova, A. *et al.*: *Coll. Czech. Chem. Comm.* **1962**, 27, 1210; *Naturwissenschaften* **1967**, 54, 45; Pfeifer, S. *et al.*: *Pharmazie* **1965,** 20, 240; 394; **1964**, 19, 280; *Arch. d. Pharm.* **1965**, 298,385; Santavy, F. *et al.*: *Coll. Czech. Chem. Comm.* **1965**, 30, 3479; **1967,** 32, 4452.
[4] Preininger, V. *et al.*: *Phytochem.* **1973**, 12, 2513; Cvejic, A. *et al.*: *Zb. Prir. Nauke, Matica Srp.*, **1972**, 185; Gasic, O. *et al.*: *Glas. Hem. Drus., Beograd* **1974**, 39(7-8), 499.
[5] Awe, W. *et al.*: *Arzneim. Forsch.* **1959**, 9, 773.

[6] Preininger, V. *et al.*: *Phytochem.* **1973**, 12, 2513.

[7] Slavik, J.: *Coll. Czech. Chem. Comm.* **1978**, 43(1), 316.

[8] El-Masry, S. *et al.*: *Planta Med.* **1981**, 41(1), 61.

[9] Afifi, M. S. *et al.*: *Bull. Pharm. Sci., Assiut Univ.*, **1995**, 18(2), 95.

[10] Jetter, R. *et al.*: *Phytochem.*, **1996**, 74(1), 419.

[11] Drozdz, *et al.*: *Dissertationes Pharm.* **1965**, 17, 527.

[12] Nung, V. *et al.*: *Plant. Med. Phytothr.* **1971**, 5, 177.

[13] Guerkan, E. *et al.*: *Fitoterapia*, **1995,** 66(6), 544.

[14] Biswas, P. *et al.*: *Indian J. Dairy Sci.* **1995**, 48(4), 277.

[T. Kimura]

462.　　　　*Brassica campestris* **L. var.** *nippo-oleifera* **DC.**　　(Cruciferae)

Yuntai(C), Wun-tong-gee (H), Aburana (J), Yu-chae (K)

Seed
Local Drug Name: Yuntaizi (C), Wun-toy-zee (H), Untaishi (J), Un-dae-ja (K).

Processing: Dry under the sun (C, H, J, K).

Method of Administration: Decoction (C, H, J, K).

Folk Medicinal Uses:

1) Night emission (H, J).

2) Traumatic injury (H).

3) Lochia (H).

4) Burn (J)

5) Melena (K).

6) Abdominal pain (K).

Stem and Leaf
Local Drug Name: Untai (J), Un-dae (K).

Processing: Dry under the sun (J, K).

Method of Administration: Decoction (J, K).

Folk Medicinal Uses:

1) Suppurative inflammation (J).

2) Masthopathy (J).

3) Hematemesis (K).

Scientific Researches:
Chemistry

1) Flavonoids: rutin, quercitrin [1].

2) Steroids and triterpenoids: β-sitisterol, campesterol, brassicasterol, cycloaltenol [2].

3) Seed Oil [3].

Literatures:
[1] Classen, D. *et al.*: *Can. J. Bot.* **1981**, 59(8), 1382.

[2] Tamura, T. *et al.*: *Nippon Kagaku Kaishi*, **1958**, 79.

[3] Davik, J. *et al.*: *J. Sci. Food Agric.* **1993**, 63(4), 385; Tanhuanpaa, P. K. *et al.*: *Theor. Appl. Genet.* **1995**, 91, 477; **1996**, 92, 952.

[T. Kimura]

463.　　　　*Brassica juncea* **Czern. et Coss.**　　(Cruciferae)

Jie(C), Gie-choi(H), Karashina(J), Gat(K)

Seed(CP)

Local Drug Name: Jie-zi(C), Gie-gee(H), Gaishi(J), Gae-ja(K)

Processing: 1) Eliminate foreign matter, break to pieces before use(C, K), 2) Stir-fry the seed until it becomes deep yellow and pungent scented. Break to pieces before use(C)

Method of Administration: Oral(decoction, C, K), topical(decoction, C), External(plaster,J)

Folk Medicinal Uses:

1) Cough, asthma and distending pain of the chest caused by cold-phlegm(C)
2) Arthralgia accompanied by numbness due to obstruction of collaterals by phlegm(C)
3) Deep abscess(C)
4) Dyspepsia(J)
5) Boil(J)
6) Arthritis(J)
7) Lumbago(K)
8) Neuralgia(K)
9) Stegnotic(K)
10) Ascariasis(K)
11) Cerebral hemorrhage(K)
12) Menostasis(K)
13) Lumbar-spinal pain(K)
14) Rheumatism(K)
15) Emmenagogue(K)

Scientific Research:

Chemistry

1) Flavonoids: astragalin[1]
2) Steroids: brassicasterol, 22-dehydrocampesterol[2]
3) Indole alkaloids: brassilexin[3]
4) Carotenoids: crocetin[4]
5) Glucosinolates: sinigrin[5]

Phamacology

1) Antitumor-promoting activity[6]
2) Lipid peroxide formation inhibition activity[6]
3) Catalase stimulation activity[7]
4) Desmutagenic activity[7]
5) Hair stimulant activity[8]
6) Platelet activating factor binding inhibition[9]
7) Antibacterial activity[10]
8) Antifungal activity[10]

Literature:

[1] Aguinagalde, I.: *Bot. Mag. Tokyo* **1988**, 101, 55.
[2] Matsumoto, T. *et al.*: *Phytochemistry* **1983**, 22(3), 789.
[3] Devys, M. *et al.*: *Tetrahedron Lett.* **1988**, 29(49), 6447.
[4] Wall, M. E. *et al.*: *J. Nat. Prod.* **1988**, 51(1), 129.
[5] Palmer, M. V. *et al.*: *J. Agr. Food Chem.* **1987**, 35(2), 262.
[6] Maeda, H. *et al.*: *Jap. J. Cancer Res.* **1992**, 83(9), 923.
[7] Yamaguchi, T. *et al.*: *Agr. Biol. Chem.* **1980**, 44(4), 959.
[8] Kubo, M. *et al.*: *Yakugaku Zasshi* **1988**, 108(10), 971.
[9] Han, B. H. *et al.*: *Yakhak Hoe Chi* **1994**, 38(4), 462.
[10] Prasad, Y. R. *et al.*: *Fitoterapia* **1993**, 64(4), 373.

[C. K. Sung]

464.   *Isatis indigodica* **Fort.**   (Cruciferae)

Song-lan (C), Taisei (J)

Related plant: *I. tinctoria* L: Dae-cheong (K).

Root (CP)
  Local Drug Name: Ban-lan-gen (C), Banrankon (J), Pan-ram-geun (K).
  Processing: Eliminate foreign matter, wash clean, soften thoroughly, cut into thick slices, and dry
        (C, K).
  Method of Administration: Oral (decoction: C, K).
  Folk Medicinal Uses:
          1) Pharyngitis, laryngitis, scarlet fever (C, J, K).
          2) Erysipelas (C, J).
          3) Carbuncle (C, J).
          4) Mumps (C, K).
          5) Eruptive epidemic diseases with dark red or purplish tongue (C).
          6) Nasal hemorrhage (J).
          7) Hematemesis (J).
          8) Common cold (K).

Scientific Researches:
  Chemistry
    1) Sugars: sucrose [1].
    2) Alkaloids: adenosine [1].
    3) Organic acids: palmitic acid [1]
    4) Steroids: β-sitosterol [1,2], γ-sitosterol [2].
    5) Amino acids: L-arginine, L-glutamic acid, L-tyrosine, L-proline, L-valine, γ-aminobutyric acid
       [2].
    6) Sulfocompounds and nitrogen compounds: 1-thiocyanato-2-hydroxy-3-butene, epigoitrin,
       adenosine [1], indigotin, indirubin [2], tryptanthrin [3].
  Pharmacology
    1) Antibacterial effect [3,4].
    2) Virucidal effect [5].

Literatures:
  [1] Huang, C. S. *et al.*: *Yao Hsueh Tung Pao* **1981,** 16(3), 54; *Planta med.* **1981,** 42(3), 308.
  [2] Zhang, S. H.: *Zhongcaoyao* **1983,** 14(6), 246.
  [3] Li, Q. H. *et al.*: *Zhongcaoyao* **1983,** 14(10), 440.
  [4] Gui, C. H. *et al.*: *Yaoxue Tongbao I1959,* 7, 236.
  [5] Li, W. W. *et al.*: *Huanan Yike Daxue Xuebao* **1994,** 19(4), 309.

                                                                       [J.X. Guo]

465.   *Lepidium apetalum* **Willd.**   (Cruciferae)

Du-hang-cai (C), Da-dak-naeng-i (K)

Related Plant: *Descurainia sophia* (L.) Webb ex Prantl: Bo-liang-hao (C), Jae-ssuk (K).

Seed (CP)
  Local Drug Name: Ting-li-zi (C), Ting-lik-gee (H), Teirekishi (J), Jeong-ryuk-ja (K).
  Processing: 1) Eliminate foreign matter (C, K).

2) Stir-fry the clean Semen Lepidii or Semen Descurainiae (C).
Method of Administration: Oral (decoction: C, H, K).
Folk Medicinal Uses:
        1) Cough with profuse expectoration and fullness sensation in the chest, accompanied by hydrothorax, ascites and oliguria (C, H, J).
        2) Dyspnea or orthopnea (C, H, K).
        3) Edema in plumonary heart disease (C, K).
        4) Constipation (J).

Scientific Researches:
Chemistry
  1) Fatty oils [1].
  2) Proteins [1].
  3) Sugars [1].
  4) Alkaloids [2].
  5) Essential oils [2].
  6) Glycosides; sinigrin [1], flavonoid glycosides, isothiocyanic glycoside [2], evomooside (digitoxigenin 3-O-α-L-rhamnoside) [3].
Pharmacology
  1) Cardiac effect [4,5].
  2) Diuretic effect [6].

Literatures:

[1] *"Zhongcaoyao Youxiaochengfen De Yanjiu"* **1972,** Vol.1, 375.
[2] *"Zhongyao Zhi"* **1984,** Vol.3, 625.
[3] Hyun, J. W. *et al.: Planta Med.* **1995,** 61(3), 294.
[4] Bi, Q. Y. *et al.: Wuhan Yixueyuan Xuebao* **1963,** (2), 9.
[5] Liu, S. F.: *Yaoxue Xuebao* **1964,** 11,454.
[6] Nanjing College of Pharmacy: *"Zhongcaoyao Xue"* **1978,** Vol.2, 369.

[J.X. Guo]

466.   *Raphanus sativus* **L.**   (Cruciferae)

Luo-bo(C), Daikon(J), Mu-u(K)

Root
  Local Drug Name:Luo-bo(C), Nae-bok(K)
  Processing: Dry under the sun(K)
  Method of Administration: Oral(decoction, K)
  Folk Medicinal Uses:
        1) Pneumonia(K)
        2) Beriberi(K)
        3) Sputum(K)
        4) Bronchitis(K)
        5) Nicotine toxication(K)
        6) Apepsia(K)
        7) Headache(K)
        8) Appendicitis(K)
        9) CO gas poisoning(K)
        10) Antitussive(K)
        11) Asthma(K)

Seed(CP)

Local Drug Name:Lai-fu-zi(C), Raifukushi(J), Nae-bok-ja(K)
Processing: 1) Dry under the sun(K)
2) Eliminate foreign matter, wash clean and dry. Break to pieces before use (C).
3) Stir-fry the seeds to slightly expanded. Break to pieces before use (C).
Method of Administration: Oral(decoction, K)(C).
Folk Medicinal Uses:
1) Apepsia(J, K)
2) Acute gastritis(J, K)
3) Retention of undigested food with epigastric and abdominal distention and pain, and constipation (C).
4) Diarrhea due to stagnation of undigested food (C).
5) Cough and dyspnea with copious expectoration (C).
6) Epilepsy(K)
7) Headache(K)
8) Jaundice(K)

Scientific Research:
Chemistry
1) Lipids: Phospholipids[1], stearic acid[42]
2) Anthocyanin[2]
3) Carotenoids: β-carotene[2, 28], violaxanthin[28]4
4) Amines: dimethyl amine, N-pentyl amine, aniline, benzylamine, ethylamine, methylamine, N-methyl phenethylamine, phenethylamine, pyrrolidine, pyrroline[23], N-methyl β-phenethylamine[34]
5) Vitamins: ascorbic acid[24]
6) Sulfur compounds: glucocapparin, sinigrin[25], raphanusol B[39], glucoraphenin[40]
7) Indole alkaloids: β-carboline[26], 5-hydroxy indole-3-acetic acid, 5-methoxy indole-3-acetic acid, melatonin, 6-hydroxy melatonin[27]
8) Flavonoids: kaempferol[29, 30], 4',7-dimethoxy kaempferol, 4'-methoxy kaempferol[29], cyanidin-3-sophorobiose-5-O-β-D-glucoside[31], pelargonidin glycoside[32], caffeyl pelargonidin-3-sophoroside-5-glucoside, ferulyl perlargonidin-3-sophoroside-5-glucoside[33], raphanusin A, B[38]
9) Proteins: raphanus antifungal protein NS-LTP[35], raphanus ferredoxin A-1, A-2, B, L-FDB[36]
10) Carbohydrates: raphanus sativus L-arabino-D-galactan, raphanus sativus L-arabino-d-galactan proteoglycan[37]
11) Steroids: β-Sitosterol[41], campesterol, cholesterol, cholesterl 24-methylene[44], teasterone, 28-homoteasterone[45]
12) Phenyl propanoids: L-malic acid 2-O-cafeoyl ester, L-malic acid 2-O-feruloyl ester, L-malic acid 2-O-p-coumaroyl ester, L-malic acid 2-O-sinapoyl ester[43]
Phamacology
1) Antihemolytic activity[3]
2) Antibacterial activity[4, 13, 15]
3) Anticlastogenic activity[5]
4) Antimutagenic activity[6, 10, 16, 19]
5) Antiinflammation activity[7, 8, 21]
6) Antiimplantation activity[9]
7) Antiallergic activity[11]
8) Diuretic activity[12]
9) Platelet aggregation inhibition[14]
10) Thromboxane B-2 synthesis inhibition[14]
11) Antitumor-promoting and anticarcinogenic activity[17, 18]
12) Antioxidant activity[18]
13) Antiviral activity[20]
14) Antihepatotoxic activity[22]
15) Antifungal activity[35]

Literature:

[1] Rakhimov, M. M. and Babaev, M. U.: *Otkrytiya, Izobret., Prom. Obraztsy, Tovarnye Znaki* **1984**, (12), 7. SU1082374 A1 840330
[2] Lichtenthaler, Hartmut K. and Thiess, Dorothea E.: *Physiol. Plant.* **1974**, 30(3), 260.
[3] Kausalya, S. *et al.*: *Clinician* **1984**, 48(12), 460.
[4] Chen, C. P. *et al.*: *Shoyakugaku Zasshi* **1987**, 41(3), 215.
[5] Lim-Sylianco, C. Y. *et al.*: *Philippine J. Sci.* **1986**, 115(1), 23.
[6] Morita, K. *et al.*: *Agr. Biol. Chem.* **1978**, 42(6), 1235.
[7] Yasukawa, K. *et al.*: *Phytother. Res.* **1993**, 7(2), 185.
[8] Dabral, P. K. and Sharma, R. K.: *Probe* **1983**, 22(2), 120.
[9] Matsui, A. D. S. *et al.*: *Med. Pharmacol. Exp.* **1967**, 16, 414.
[10] Kada, T. *et al.*: *Int. Z. Klin. Pharmakol. Ther. Toxikol.* **1971**, 5(1), 65.
[11] Mitchell, J. C. and Jordan, W. P.: *Brit. J. Dermatol.* **1974**, 91, 183.
[12] Caceres, A. *et al.*: *J. Ethnopharmacol.* **1987**, 19(3), 233.
[13] George, M. and Pandalai, K. M.: *Indian J. Med. Res.* **1949**, 37, 169.
[14] Kasjanovova, D. and Macejka, J.: *Pharmazie* **1992**, 47(11), 876.
[15] Abodou, I. A. *et al.*: *Qual. Plant Mater. Veg.* **1972**, 22(1), 29.
[16] Shinohara, K. *et al.*: *Agr. Biol. Chem.* **1988**, 52(6), 1369.
[17] Hertog, M. G. L. *et al.*: *J. Agr. Food Chem.* **1992**, 40(12), 2379.
[18] Maeda, H. *et al.*: *Jap. J. Cancer Res(GANN)* **1992**, 83(9), 923.
[19] Rojanapo, W. and tepsuwan, A.: *Environ. Health Perspect. Suppl.* **1993**, 101(3), 247.
[20] Khurana, S.M.P. and Bhargava, K. S.: *J. Gen. Appl. Microbiol.* **1984**, 16, 225.
[21] Han B. H. *et al.*: *Korean J. Pharmacog.* **1972**, 4(3), 205.
[22] Hong, N. D. *et al.*: *Korean J. Pharmacog.* **1982**, 13, 33.
[23] Neurath, G. B. *et al.*: *Food Cosmet. Toxicol.* **1977**, 15, 275.
[24] Yao, G. *et al.*: *Yingyang Xuebao* **1983**, 5(4), 373.
[25] Schnitzler, W. H.: *Gartenbauwissenschaft* **1974**, 39, 21.
[26] Ozawa, Y. *et al.*: *Agr. Biol. Chem.* **1990**, 54(5), 1241.
[27] Hattori, A. *et al.*: *Biochem. Mol. Biol. Int.* **1995**, 35(3), 627.
[28] Becker, K. and Lichtenthaler, H. K.: *Z. Pflanzenphysiol.* **1975**, 75, 303.
[29] Daniel, M.: *Curr. Sci.* **1989**, 58(23), 1332.
[30] Bilyk, A. and Sapers, G. M.: *J. Agr. Food Chem.* **1985**, 33(2), 226.
[31] Tian, J. L. *et al.*: *Hua Hsueh Chin Ji* **1992**, 33(3), 114.
[32] Liebstein, A. M.: *Amer. Med.* **1927**, 33, 33.
[33] Lu, X. L.: *Shipin Yu Jajiao Gongye* **1985**, 6, 19.
[34] Marquardt, P. *et al.*: *Arzneim-Forsch.* **1976**, 26, 201.
[35] Terras, F.R.G. *et al.*: *Plant Physiol.* **1992**, 100(2), 1055.
[36] Obata, S. *et al.*: *Arch. Biochem. Biophys.* **1995**, 316(3), 797.
[37] Tsumuraya, Y. *et al.*: *Carbohydr. Res.* **1987**, 161(1), 113.
[38] Fuleki, T.: *J. Food Sci.* **1969**, 34(4), 365.
[39] Hasegawa, K. and Hase, T.: *Plant Cell Physiol.* **1981**, 22, 303.
[40] Brinker, A. M. and Spencer, G. F.: *J. Chem. Ecol.* **1993**, 2279.
[41] Wang, C. T. *et al.*: *Shan-His Hsin I Yao* **1979**, 8(11), 50.
[42] Han, B. H. *et al.*: *Ann. Rep. Nat'l Prod. Res. Inst. Seoul Nat'l Univ.* **1981**, 20, 49.
[43] Nielsen, J. K. *et al.*: *Phytochemistry* **1984**, 23(8), 1741.
[44] Duperon, P.: *C. R. Acad. Sci. Ser. D.* **1967**, 265(5), 409.
[45] Schmidt, J. *et al.*: *Phytochemistry* **1993**, 34(2), 391.

[C. K. Sung]

467.   *Liquidambar formosana* **Hance**   (Hamamelidaceae)

Feng-xiang-shu (C), Fung-shu (H), Fuu (J)

Resin (CP)

Local Drug Name: Feng-xiang-zhi (C), Bai-jiao-xiang (H), Fukoushi (J).
Processing: Dry in the shade (C, H).
Method of Administration: Oral (pills or powder: C, H); Topical (C).
Folk Medicinal Uses:

1) Swelling and pain of carbuncle and boil (C, H, J).
2) Traumatic injuries (C, H).
3) Spitting of blood (C, H).
4) Epistaxis (C, H).
5) Traumatic hemorrhage (C, H).

Contraindication: Pregnancy (H).

Fruit (CP)

Local Drug Name: Lu-lu-tong (C), Low-low-tung (H), Rorotsu (J).
Processing: Eliminate foreign matter and dry (C, H).
Method of Administration: Oral (decoction: C, H).
Folk Medicinal Uses:

1) Lumbago (C, H).
2) Urticaria (C, H).
3) Lack of lactation (C, H).
4) Dysuria (C, H).
5) Rheumatic arthralgia (C, H).
6) Arthralgia with numbness and muscular contracture (C, J).
7) Amenorrhea (C, J).
8) Irregular menstruation (H).
9) Edema (C).

Scientific Researches:
Chemistry

1) Organic acids: cinnamic acid [1].
2) Alcohols: cinnamic alcohol [1].
3) Monoterpenes: *l*-borneol [1], bornyl transcinnamate [2], *l*-bornyl cinnamate [9].
4) Sesquiterpenes: caryophyllene oxide [9].
5) Triterpenes: liquidambronal, ambronal [2], liquidambronoric acid [3], liquidambronic acid, hombranic acid, formosolic acid, ambradiolic acid [4,5], liquidambaric acid, 24-ethyl-Δ^5-cholesten-3β-ol [8], 28-noroleanonic acid, betulonic acid (liquidambaronic acid) [9].
6) Essential oils: β-terpinene, β-pinene, limonene, γ-terpinene, myrtenal, α-terpinol, transcarveol, thymol, carvacrol, copaene, β-elemene, trans-β-farnesene, α-muurolene, α-elemene, cadinene, elemol [7].
7) Aromatic compounds: styracin epoxide, isostyracin epoxide, styracin (cinnamyl cinnamate) [9].

Pharmacology

1) Antithrombotic effect [6].
2) Antihepatotoxic effect [9].
3) Antiarthritic effect [10].

Literatures:

[1] Dobashi, R. *et al.*: *Kogyokagaku Kaishi* **1919**, 22, 288.
[2] Liu, C. *et al.*: *Youji Huaxue* **1991**, 11(5), 508.
[3] Pham Truong Thi Tho: *Tap San. Hoa-Hoc* **1975**, 13(4), 34.
[4] Yankov, L.K. *et al.*: *Dokl. Bolg. Akad. Nauk.* **1980**, 33(1), 75.
[5] Yankov, L.K. *et al.*: *Dokl. Bolg. Akad. Nauk.* **1980**, 33(3), 357.
[6] Zhu, L. *et al.*: *Zhongcaoyao* **1991**, 22(3), 404.
[7] Wang, Z.W. *et al.*: *Shanghai Diyi Yixueyuan Xuebao* **1984**, 11(2),147.

[8] Sun, Y.R. *et al.*: *Zhongcaoyao* **1988,** 19(8), 342.
[9] Konno, C. *et al.*: *Planta Med.* **1988,** 54(5), 417.
[10] *"Zhejiang Yaoyong Zhiwuzhi"* **1980,** Vol.1, 469.

[J.X. Guo]

468.   *Liquidamber orientalis* **Mill.**   (Hamamelidaceae)

Su-he-xiang-shu(C), So-hyap-hyang-na-mu(K)

Resin(CP)
Local Drug Name:Su-he-xiang(C), Ryudo-sogoko(J), So-hyap-hyang(K)
Processing: Dry under the sun(K)
Method of Administration: Oral(decoction, K)(pills or powder:C)
Folk Medicinal Uses:

1) Pain with cold sensation in the cheat on abdomen(C).
2) Stroke, sudden loss of consciousness(C).
3) Epilepsy and convulsions(C).
4) Bronchitis(J)
5) Scabies(J: external, K)
6) Epileptic convulsion(K)
7) Abdominal pain(K)
8) Pernio(K)

Scientific Research:
Chemistry
1) Terpenes: Borneol acetate, mentha-2,4(8)-diene, β-phellandrene, α–, β–pinene, terpinen-4-ol, α–, γ-terpinene, α–terpineol, δ-cadinene, trans-caryophyllene, copaene, δ-elemene, allo-aromadendrene[1], abietic acid, dehydroabietic acid[2]
2) Phenylpropanoids: Cinnamic acid, cinnamyl acetate, cinnamyl ricinoleate[2], allo-cinnamic acid[3]
Phamacology
1) Antimutagenic activity[2]
2) Platelet aggregation inhibition[3]
3) Antianginal activity[4]

Literature:
[1] Chen, Y. *et al.*: *Linchan Hua Hsueh Yu Gong Yi* **1991,** 11(2), 157.
[2] Mitscher, L. A. *et al.*: *Mutat. Res.* **1992,** 267(2), 229.
[3] Zhang, W. and Zhuang, L.: *Chung Ts'ao Yao* **1985,** 16(3), 112.
[4] Chen, K.: *Amer. J. Chin. Med.* **1981,** 9, 193.

[C. K. Sung]

469.   *Sedum lineare* **var.** *contractum* **Miq.**   (Crassulaceae)
[= *S. sarmentosum* Bunge]

Dol-na-mul(K)

Whole plant
Local Drug Name: Seok-ji-gap(K)
Processing: dry under the sun(K)

Method of Administration: Oral(decoction, K)
Folk Medicinal Uses:
> 1) Weakness(K)
> 2) Poisoning(K)
> 3) Mastitis(K)
> 4) Child erysipelas(K)
> 5) Malaria(K)

Scientific Research:
Chemistry
1) Cyanogenic glucosides: Sarmentosin[1]
2) Alkaloids[2]
Phamacology
1) Lowering of SGPT(sarmentosin)[1]
2) Suppressive effect on cell-mediated immune response(sarmentosin)[1]
3) Inhibition of the gp 120-CD4 interaction[3]

Literature:
[1] Zhu, D. Y. *et al.*: *Drug Development Research* **1996**, 39(2), 147.
[2] Kim, J. H. *et al.*: *Phytochemistry* **1996**, 41(5), 1319.
[3] Woo, E. R. *et al.*: *Phytomedicine* **1997**, 4(1), 53.

[C. K. Sung]

470. *Hydrangea macrophylla* Seringe var. *thunbergii* Makino
(Saxifragaceae)

Amacha (J), Gam-da(K)

Related plant: *Hydrangea macrophylla* Seringe, Ajisai (J), Su-guk (K).

Leaf (JP)
Local Drug Name: Amacha (J), Gam-da(K)
Processing: Fermentation, crumple up and dry under the sun (J).
Method of Administration: Decoction (J).
Folk Medicinal Uses:
> 1) Diabetes (J, K).
> 2) Sweetener without carbohydrate (J, K).

Scientific Researches:
Chemistry
1) Dihydroisocoumarins: Phyllodulcin [1,2], phyllodulcin-8-*O*-β-D-glucoside [1], thunberginol A, B, C, D, E, G, thunberginol G 3'-*O*-glucoside, (-)- and (+)-hydrangenol 4'-*O*-glucoside [3], skimmin, hydrangeol and umbelliferone [4], phyllodulcin monomethylether [5], macrophylloside A, B and C [6], hydramcroside A and B [7].
2) Phthalides: Hydramacrophyllol A, and B [3, 8]. Thunberginol F [3].
3) Flavonoids: Quercetin [9]. Kaempferol 3-*O*-β-D-glucopyranosyl(1→2)-β-D-glucoside, quercetin 3-*O*-β-D-glucopyranosyl(1→2)-β-D-glucoside, kaempferol 3-*O*-α-L-rhamnopyranosyl(1→6)-β-D-glucoside, kaempferol 3-*O*-β-D-glucopyranosyl(1→2)[α-L-rhamnopyranosyl(1→6)]-β-D-glucoside [3].
Pharmacology
1) Antiulcer, antiallergic, cholagogic and inhibition of intestinal contraction (methanol extract) [10].
2) Antiallergic effect (thunberginol A, B, C, D, E, F, (-)-hydrangeol 4'-*O*-glucoside) [3,11].

3) Inhibition of histamine release from rat mast cells (hydramacrophyllol A, B, hydramacroside A and B)[3,8,7].
4) Antimicrobial activity against oral bacteria (thunberginol C, D, E and G) [3].
5) Cytotoxic activity of polymorphonuclear leukocytes (thunbergianol A) [12].

Literatures:
[1] Asahina, Y. *et al.*: *Yakugaku Zasshi*, **1929**, 49, 117; **1930**, 50, 573; Suzuki, H. *et al.*: *Agric. Biol. Chem.*, **1977**, 41, 1815.
[2] Arakawa, H.*et al.*: *Chem. & Ind.* **1959**, 671.
[3] Yoshikawa, M. *et al.*: *Chem. Pharm. Bull.*, **1992**, 40(12), 3352; **1996**, 44, 1440.
[4] Suzuki, H. *et al.*: *Agric. Biol. Chem.* **1977**, 41(1), 205; 41(4), 719.
[5] Suzuki, H. *et al.*: *Agric. Biol. Chem.* **1979**, 43(3), 653; 43(8), 1785.
[6] Hashimoto, T. *et al.*: *Phytochem.* **1987**, 26(12), 3323.
[7] Yoshikawa, M. *et al.*: *Chem. Pharm. Bull.* **1994**, 42(8), 1691.
[8] Yoshikawa, M. *et al.*: *Chem. Pharm. Bull.*, **1994,** 42, 2225
[9] Kimura, Y. *et al.*: *Nichidaiyakuho* **1960**, 3-4, 51.
[10] Yamahara, J. *et al.*: *Yakugaku Zasshi*, **1994**, 114, 401.
[11] Yoshikawa, M. *et al.*: *Chem. Pharm. Bull.*, **1992**, 40, 3121; Shimoda, H. *et al.*: *Wakan Iyakugaku Zasshi*, **1995**, 12(4), 450.
[12] Kinoshita, K. *et al.*: *Planta Med.* **1992**, 58(2), 137.

[T. Kimura]

471.   *Crataegus cuneata* **Sieb. et Zucc.**   (Rosaceae)

Ye-shan-zha(C), Saan-jar(H), Sanzashi(J), Cham-san-sa-na-mu(K)

Fruit
Local Drug Name: Shan-zha(C), Saan-jar(H), Sanzashi(J), San-sa-ja(K)
Processing: Cut into slices, and dry in the sun(C, H, J, K)
Method of Administration: Oral(decoction, C, H, J, K)
Folk Medicinal Uses:
　　　　　　　　1) Indigestion(C, H)
　　　　　　　　2) Stomachic(H, K)
　　　　　　　　3) Apepsia(J, K)
　　　　　　　　4) Taeniasis(C)
　　　　　　　　5) Frostbite(C)
　　　　　　　　6) Dysentery(C)
　　　　　　　　7) Hypertension(C)
　　　　　　　　8) Fish poisoning(J)
　　　　　　　　9) Stomachache after child birth(K)
　　　　　　　　10) Ascariasis(K)
　　　　　　　　11) Common cold(K)

Scientific Research
Chemistry
1) Flavonoids: (-)-Epi-catechin, quercetin[1], hyperoside, rutin[2]
2) Phenylpropanoid: Chlorogenic acid[1]
3) Miscellaneous: Citric acid, succinic acid, tartaric acid[2], citric acid monomethyl ester, citric acid dimethyl ester, citric acid trimethyl ester[1]
Pharmacology
1) Plant root growth stimulant effect[3]
2) Alcohol dehydrogenase stimulation effect[4]

3) Aldehyde dehydrogenase stimulant effect[4]
4) Narcotic antagonist activity [5]
5) AIDS therapeutic effect [6]
6) Antihepatotoxic activity [7]
7) Antihypercholesterolemic activity [7]
8) Skin pigmentation effect [8]
9) Sunscreen effect [8]

Literature:
[1] Xie, Y.R. *et al.: Chih Wu Hsueh Pao* **1981**, 23, 383
[2] Gao, G.Y. *et al.: Yao Hsueh Hsueh Pao* **1995**, 30 (2), 138
[3] Shimomura, H. *et al.: Shoyakugaku Zasshi* **1981**, 35 (3), 173
[4] Sakai, K. *et al.: Chem. Pharm. Bull.* **1989**, 37 (1), 155
[5] Wu, B.W. *et al.: Patent-Brit.* **1967**, 1 (096, 708), 3pp
[6] Yu, J. *et al.:* Int. J. *Orient. Med.* **1989**, 14 (4), 189
[7] Hong, N. D. *et al.: Korean J. Pharmacog.* **1982**, 13, 33
[8] Watanabe, C. *et al.: Patent-Japan Kokai Tokkyo Koho*-03 **1991**, 193 (712), 7pp

[C. K. Sung]

472.   *Potentilla chinensis* **Ser.**   (Rosaceae)

Wei-ling-cai(C), Kawarasaiko(J), Ddak-ji-ggot(K)

Herb(CP)
Local Drug Name: Wei-ling-cai(C)
Processing: Eliminate foreign matter , wash clean , soften thoroughly , cut into sections , and dry
            under the sun(C).
Method of Administration: Oral(decoction, C), Topical(decoction or paste:C).
Folk Medicinal Uses:
            1) Dysentery with bloody stools, chronic dysentery (C).
            2) Hemorrhoidal bleeding (C).
            3) Carbuncles and sores (C).

Root
Local Drug Name: Ko-saiko(J), Wi-reung-chae(K)
Processing: Dry under the sun(K)
Method of Administration: Oral(decoction, J, K)
Folk Medicinal Uses:
            1) Women's weakness(J, K)
            2) Common cold(J, K)
            3) Drug after child birth(K)
            4) Pyrexia(K)
            5) Hemostatic(K)

Scientific Research
Chemistry
  1) Coumarins: 3,3',4-tri-O-methyl ellagic acid[1]
Pharmacology
  1) Antiallergenic activity [2]
  2) Antieczema effect [3, 4, 5]

Literature:

[1] Kim, H. S.: *Yakhak Hoechi* **1989**, 33(6), 377
[2] Latchman, Y. *et al.*: *Brit. J. Dermatol.* 1995, 132(4), 592
[3] Sheehan, M. P. *et al.*: *Lancet* **1992**, 340(8810), 13
[4] Sheehan, M. P. *et al.*: *Clin. Exp. Dermatol.* **1995**, 20(2), 136
[5] Sheehan, M. P. *et al.*: *Brit J. Dermatol.* **1992**, 126(2), 179

[C. K. Sung]

473.   *Potentilla discolor*   (Rosaceae)

Fan-bai-cao(C), Tsuchiguri(J), Som-yang-ji-ggot(K)

Herb
Local Drug Name:Fan-bai-cao(C), Honpakuso(J), Beon-baek-cho(K),
Processing: Dry under the sun(K)(C).
Method of Administration: Oral(decoction,C,K);Topical(paste or powder:C).
Folk Medicinal Uses:
                1) Female disease(C, J, K)
                2) Dysentery(C).
                3) Spitting blood(C).
                4) Bloody stool(C).
                5) Trauma(C).
                6) Carbuncle(C).
                7) Common cold(J)

Scientific Research
Chemistry
  1) Flavonoids: kaempferol, quercetin, naringenin[1]
  2) Org. acids: fumalic acid, protocatechuic acid, m-phthalic acid, gallic acid[1]
Pharmacology
  1) Antibacterial effect(org. acids)[1]
  2) Antiviral activity [2]

Literature
[1] Liu, Y. and Su, S.: *Zhongcaoyao* **1984**, 15(7), 333
[2] Minshi, Z.: *J. Trad. Chinese Med.* **1989**, 9(2), 113

[C. K. Sung]

474.   *Prinsepia uniflora* **Batal.**   (Rosaceae)

Rui-he (C)

Related Plant: *P. uniflora* Batal. var. *serrata* Rehd.: Ci-ye-bian-he-mu (C).

Kernel (CP)
Local Drug Name: Rui-ren (C), Yui-yun (H).
Processing: Eliminate foreign matter, wash clean, dry in the sun. Break to pieces before use (C).
Method of Administration: Oral (decoction: C, H).
Folk Medicinal Uses:
                1) Conjunctivitis and blepharitis masginolis with impaired vision and
                   photophobia (C, H).

Scientific Researches:
 Chemistry
  1) Fatty oils [1].

Literatures:
 [1] *"Zhongguo Jingji Zhiwuzhi"* **1961**, Vol.1, 529.

[J.X. Guo]

475.   *Rosa chinensis* **Jacq.**   (Rosaceae)

Yue-ji (C), Wol-gye-hwa (K)

Flower (CP)
 Local Drug Name: Yue-ji-hua (C), Yuet-gwai-far (H), Wol-gye-hwa (K).
 Processing: Dry in the shade or at a low temperature (C, K), or used in fresh (H).
 Method of Administration: Oral (decoction: C, H, K); Topical (H).
 Folk Medicinal Uses:
              1) Menstrual disorders (C, H, K).
              2) Dysmenorrhea (C, H, K).
              3) Boils and pyodermas (C, H).
              4) Cervical tuberculous lymphadenopathy (C, H).
 Contraindication: Pregnancy.

Root
 Local Drug Name: Yue-ji-hua-gun (C), Yuet-gwai-far-gun (H).
 Method of Administration: Oral (decoction: C, H).
 Folk Medicinal Uses:
              1) Traumatic injury (C, H).
              2) Leucorrhea (C, H).
              3) Nocturnal emission (C, H).

Scientific Researches:
 Chemistry
  1) Essential oils [1].
  2) Tannins: gallic acid [2].
  3) Flavonoids: quercitrin [2].
  4) Phytochrom [2].
 Pharmacology
  1) Antifungal activity [3].

Literatures:
 [1] *"Zhongyao Da Cidian"* **1977,** Vol.1, 477.
 [2] *"Quanguo Zhongcaoyao Huibian"* **1975,** Vol.1, 215.
 [3] Tripathi, S.C. *et al.: Physiol. Micro-Org. Symp.* **1976,** (Pub. **1977**), 225.

[J.X. Guo]

476.   *Rosa laevigata* **Michx.**   (Rosaceae)

Jin-ying-zi (C), Gum-ying-gee (H), Naniwaibana (J), Geum-aeng-ja (K)

Fruit (CP)

Local Drug Name: Jin-ying-zi (C), Gum-ying-gee (H), Geum-aeng-ja (K).
Processing: 1) Eliminate foreign matter, wash and dry (C, K).
          2) Sock clean Fructus Rosae Laevigatae briefly, soften thoroughly, halve longitudinally, remove hair and achenes, and dry (C).
Method of Administration: Oral (decoction: C, H, K).
Folk Medicinal Uses:
        1) Nocturnal emission, spermatorrhea (C, H, K).
        2) Enuresis, frequent urination (C, H, K).
        3) Abnormal uterine bleeding (C, H, K).
        4) Chronic dysentery (C, H, K).
        5) Protracted diarrhea (C, H).
        6) Excessive leukorrhea (C, H).
        7) Night sweating (C, H).
        8) Rectal prolapse (H).
        9) Prolapse uterus (H).

Root
Local Drug Name: Jin-ying-zi-gun (C), Gum-ying-gun (H).
Processing: Dry in the sun (C, H), or use in fresh (H).
Method of Administration: Oral (decoction: C, H).
Folk Medicinal Uses:
        1) Enteritis (C, H).
        2) Dysentery (C, H).
        3) Pyelitis (C, H).
        4) Leucorrhea (C, H)
        5) Chyluria (C, H).
        6) Elephantiasis (C, H).
        7) Rheumatic althralgia (C, H).
        8) Low back pain (C, H).
        9) Traumatic injury (C, H).
        10) Irregular menses (C, H).
        11) Nephritis (H).

Leaf
Local Drug Name: Jin-ying-zi-ye (C), Gum-ying-gee-yip (H).
Processing: Use in fresh (C, H).
Method of Administration: Topical (fresh leaves: C, H).
Folk Medicinal Uses:
        1) Boils and pyodermas(C, H).
        2) Burns and scalds (C, H).
        3) Wound bleeding (C, H).

Flower
Local Drug Name: Gum-ying-far (H).
Processing: Use in fresh or dry in the sun (H).
Method of Administration: Oral (decoction: H).
Folk Medicinal Uses:
        1) Dysentry (H).

Scientific Researches:
Chemistry
  1) Glycosides: saponin [1].
  2) Resins [2].
  3) Vitamins: vitamin C [1,3], P, B_2, K, E, carotin [3].
  4) Sugars [2,3].

5) Organic acids: malic acid, citric acid [2,3].
6) Lipids[3].
7) Trace elements: Fe [3,4], Zn, Cu, Mn, Mg, Ca, Na, K [4].
8) Tannins [2,3]: sanguiin H-4, pedunculagin, agrimoniin, laevigatin A, B, C, D, E, F, G, agrimonic acid A, B [5,6].
9) Triterpenoids: ursolic acid, euscaphic acid, oleanolic acid, 2α-methoxyursolic acid, 11α-hydroxytormentic acid, tormentic acid 6-methoxy-β-glucopyranosyl ester [7], 2α,3β,19α,23-tetrahydroxyurs-12-en-28-oic acid, 2α,3α,19α,23-tetrahydroxyurs-12-en-28-oic acid, diacetyl-2α, 3β-dihydroxy-lupan-28-oic acid [8].
10) Steroids: stigmasta-3α,5α-diol 3-O-β-D-glucopyanoside [7], β-sitosterol, daucosterol [8].
Pharmacology
1) Bacteriostatic effect [1].
2) Effect on experimental atheroscleorsis [9].
3) Effect on the content of hydroxyproline and the activities of selenium glutathione peroxidase [10].

Literatures:
[1] *"Quangguo Zhongcaoyao Huibian"* **1975,** Vol.1, 543.
[2] *"Zhongcaoyao Youxiaochengfen De Yanju"* **1972,** Vol.1, 437.
[3] Wang, J. R.: *Guoshu* **1987,** (1), 26.
[4] Ma, C. L. *et al.*: *Zhongcaoyao* **1985,** 16(6), 244.
[5] Yoshida, T. *et al.*: *Phytochemistry* **1989,** 28(9), 2451.
[6] Yoshida, T. *et al.*: *Chem. Pharm. Bull.* **1989,** 37(4), 920.
[7] Fang, J. M. *et al.*: *Phytochemistry* **1991,** 30(10), 3383.
[8] Gao, Y. *et al.*: *Zhongguo Zhongyao Zazhi* **1993,** 18(7), 426.
[9]*"Zhongyao Da Cidian"* **1975,** Vol.1, 1407.
[10] Tian, Q. L. *et al.*: *Dongwu Xuebao* **1992,** 38(1), 95.

[J.X. Guo]

477.   *Rosa rugosa* **Thunb.**   (Rosaceae)

Mei-gui (C), Mui-gwai (H), Maikai (J), Hae-dang-hwa (K)

Flower bud (CP)
Local Drug Name: Mei-gui-hua (C), Mai-gwai-far (H), Maikaika (J), Mae-gwue-hwa (K).
Processing: Dry at a low temperature (C, K).
Method of Administration: Oral (decoction: C, H, K).
Folk Medicinal Uses:
1) Epigastric pain, anorexia, nausea and vomiting caused by stagnated qi (C, H, K).
2) Menstrual disorders (C, H, K).
3) Traumatic pain (C, H, K).

Scientific Researches:
Chemistry
1) Essential oils [1-3]: citronellol, geraniol, nerol, eugenol, *n*-phenylethyl alcohol [4], benzyl alcohol, linalool, nonyl alcohol, nonyl aldehyde, phenethyl acetate, *l-p*-menthene [5], β-damascone, roseoxide, α-naglinatene [6], phenylethanol, β-citronellol, citronellyl acetate [7].
2) Organic acids: citric acid [8,9].
3) Phytochroms: cyanin, β-carotene [8,9].
4) Flavonoids: quercetin [8-10], apigenin 7-O-glucoside, luteolin 7-O-glucoside, kaempferol 3-O-rhamnosylgalactoside 7-O-rhamnoside, rutin, quercetin 3,7-O-diglucoside [10].
5) Tannins: qallic acid [8,9], rugosin A, B, C [11], D, E, F, G [12].

6) Triterpenoids: 28-*O*-glucosides of euscaphic acid, tormentic acid, arjunic acid [13].
7) Others: fatty oils, waxes [8,9].
Pharmacology
1) Detoxification [8,14].
2) Choleretic effect [8,14].

Literatures:

[1] Dobson, H. E. M. *et al.*: *Phytochemistry* **1987,** 26(12), 3171.
[2] Dobson, H. E. M. *et al.*: *Isr. J. Bot.* **1990,** 39(1), 143.
[3] Flament, I. *et al.*: *Acs. Symp. Ser.* **1993,** 525, 269.
[4] *"Quanguo Zhongcaoyao Huibian"* **1975,** Vol.1, 476.
[5] *"Zhongyao Zhi"* **1994,** Vol.5, 244.
[6] Liu, Z. J.: *Youjiu Huaxue* **1982,** (2), 83.
[7] Li, Z. L. *et al.*: *Sepu* **1988,** 6(1), 18.
[8] *"Zhongyao Da Cidian"* **1977,** Vol.1, 1224.
[9] Lawrence, B. M.: *Perfumer and Flavorist* 5, Dec **1981,** 41.
[10] Kaneta, N.: *Agric. Biol. Chem.* **1979,** 43(3), 657.
[11] Okuda, T. *et al.*: *Chem. Pharm. Bull.* **1982,** 30(11), 4230.
[12] Okuda, T. *et al.*: *Chem. Pharm. Bull.* **1982,** 30(11), 4234.
[13] Young, H. S. *et al.*: *Arch Pharmacol Res.* **1987,** 10(4), 219.
[14] *"Jianming Zhongyi Cidian"* **1988,** 501.

[J.X. Guo]

478.   *Rubus chingii* **Hu**   (Rosaceae)

Hua-dong-fu-pen-zi (C).

Related plants: *R. coreanus* Mig.: Tokkuri-ichigo (J), Bok-bun-ja-ddal-gi (K).

Fruit (CP)
Local Drug Name: Fu-peng-zi (C), Fuk-poon-gee (H), Fukubonshi (J), Bok-bun-ja (K).
Processing: Eliminate foreign matter, treat the fruit with boiling water for a moment or steam briefly, and dry (C, K).
Method of Administration: Oral (decoction: C, H, K).
Folk Medicinal Uses:
                1) Enuresis (C, H).
                2) Frequent urination (C, H).
                3) Impotence (C, H).
                4) Premature ejaculatim (C, H).
                5) Seminal emission and spermatorrhea (C, H).
                6) Weakness (J, K).
                7) Stomachic (K).
                8) Ophthalmia (K).
                9) Gonorrhoea (K).

Scientific Researches:
Chemistry
1) Sugars [1].
2) Tannins: ellagic acid [2].
3) Steroids: β-sitosterol [2].
4) Essential oils [3].
5) Flavones [3].
6) Vitamins [3,4].

7) Triterpenoids: fupenzic acid [3,5].
Pharmacology
  1) Bacteriostatic effect [1].
  2) Estrogen-like effect [1].

Literatures:
[1] *"Zhongyao Zhi"* **1984,** Vol.3, 702.
[2] Xu, Z. W. *et al.: Zhongcaoyao* **1981,** 12(6), 19.
[3] Liu, M. S., *et al.: Shenyang Yaoxueyuan Xuebao* **1994,** 11(1), 68.
[4] Mar, P. G. *et al.: Chin. J. Physiol* **1936,** 10(2), 273.
[5] Hattori, M. *et al.: Phytochemistry* **1988,** 27(12), 3975.

[J.X. Guo]

479.   *Astragalus complanatus* **R. Br.**   (Leguminosae)

Bian-jing-huang-gi(C) , Sar-yuan-gee(H), Seon-hwang-gi(K)

Seed(CP)
Local Drug Name: Sha-yuan-zi(C) , Sar-yuan-gee(H), Sa-weon-ja(K)
Processing: 1) Dry under the sun(C, K), 2) Stir-fry the clean seed with salt-water to dryness(C)
Method of Administration: Oral(decoction, H, K)
Folk Medicinal Uses:
        1) Spermatorrhea(H, K)
        2) Lumbago(H, K)
        3) Back pain, nocturnal emission and premature ejaculation in deficiency
           syndromes of the kidney(C)
        4) Turbid discharge with urination(C)
        5) Excessive leukorrhea(C)
        6) Dribbling of urine after urination(C)
        7) Dizziness and blurred vision(C)
        8) Frequent urination(H)
        9) Leukorhea(H)
       10) Hematuria(H)
       11) Enuresis(K)
       12) Oliguria(K)

Scientific Research:
Chemistry
  1) Sterols: β-Sitosterol[1]
  2) Fatty acids: heptenoic acid, tetradecanoic acid, pentadecanoic acid, hexadecanoic acid, octadecenoic acid, octadecanoic acid, octadecadienoic acid, linolenic acdi, eicosanoic acid, eicosenoic acid, docosanoic acid[1]
  3) Glycosides: Neocomplanoside, myricomplanoside[2]

Literature:
[1] Chen, M. and Liu, F.: *Chung Kuo Chung Yao Tsa Chih* **1990,** 15(4), 225.
[2] Cui, B. L. *et al.: Yao Hsueh Hsueh Pao* **1989,** 24(3), 189.

[C. K. Sung]

480.   *Caesalpina sappan* **L.**   (Leguminosae)

So-muk(H) , Suo(J), So-bang-mok (K)

Wood
Local Drug Name: So-muk(H), Suo-boku(J), So-mok(K)
Processing: Dry under the sun(K)
Method of Administration: Oral(decoction, H, J, K)
Folk Medicinal Uses:
                1) Hemorrhage(H, J, K)
                2) Diarrhea(J)
                3) Contusion(K)

Scientific Research:
Chemistry
  1) Neoflavanoids: Brazilin[1], tetraacetylbrazilin, protsappanin A[2]
Phamacology
  1) Immunomodulating activity(brazilin)[1]
  2) Prevention of intestinal metaplasia and atypical hyperplasia[3]
  3) Antioxidant activity(brazilin)[4]
  4) Inactivation of human sperm motility[5]

Literature:
[1] Choi, S. Y. *et al.*: *Planta Med.* **1997**, 63(5), 405.
[2] Xu, H. *et al.*: *Chung Kuo Chung Yao Tsa Chih* **1994**, 19(8), 485.
[3] Liu, X. R. *et al.*: *Chung Kuo Chung His I Chieh Ho Tsa Chih* **1992**, 12(10), 602.
[4] Moon, C. K. *et al.*: *Drug Chem. Toxicol.* **1992**, 15(1), 81.
[5] Shih, I. M. *et al.*: *J. Formos. Med. Assoc.* **1990**, 89(6), 466.

[C. K. Sung]

481.   *Crotalaria sessiliflora* **L.** (Leguminosae)

Ye-bai-he (C), Yair-bark-hup (H), Tanukimame (J), Hwal-na-mul (K)

Whole Plant
Local Drug Name: Nong-ji-li (C), Nung-gut-lay (H), Ya-bya-kugo (J), Ya-baek-hap (K).
Processing: Use in fresh or cut into segments and dry under the sun (C, H, J, K).
Method of Administration: Oral (decoction: C, H, K); Topical (crushed fresh or dry herb: C, H, K);
                    Injection (C).
Folk Medicinal Uses:
                1) Boils and pyodermas (C, H, J, K).
                2) Skin cancer (C, H, K).
                3) Cervical cancer (C, H).
                4) Esophageal cancer (C, H).
                5) Tinnitus, deafness, dizziness, vertigo (H).
                6) Edema (J).
                7) Dysentery (K).
                8) Fever (K).
   Side effects: poisonous, hepatotoxic.

Scientific Research:
Chemistry
  1) Pyrrolizidine alkaloids: monocrotaline [1–3], integerrimine, trichodesmine [1].
  2) Amino acids: glutamic acid, aspartic acid, alanine [4].
Pharmacology
  1) Antitumor activity [2]

Literature:
[1] Rieder, E. *et al.*: *Planta Med.* **1992,** 58, 283.
[2] Huang, L. *et al.*: *Yaoxue Xuebao* **1980,** 15, 278.
[3] Sha, S. Y. *et al.*: *Yaoxue Tongbao* **1980,** 15, 4.
[4] Jing Y. Q. *et al.*: *Zhongyao Tongbao* **1987,** 12, 425.

[P.P.H. But]

482.   *Lespedeza cuneata* **G. Don**   (Leguminosae)

Jie-ye-tie-sao-zhou (C), Tit-soe-zau (H), Medohagi (J), Bi-su-ri (K)

Root or Whole Plant
Local Drug Name: Tie-zao-zhou (C), Tit-soe-zau (H), Ya-kan-mon (J), Ya-gwan-mum (K).
Processing: wash, chop finely and dry under the sun (C, H, J, K)
Method of Administration: Oral (decoction: C, H, J, K); Topical (crushed fresh herb: C, H)
Folk Medicinal Uses:
          1) Stomatitis (C, H, J, K).
          2) Infantile malabsorption and malnutrition (C, H, K).
          3) Gastroenteritis (C, H, J).
          4) Bacillary dysentery (C, H, K).
          5) Chronic bronchitis (C, H, J).
          6) Icteric hepatitis (C, H).
          7) Nephritic edema (C, H).
          8) Leucorrhea (C, H).
          9) Boils, furuncles (C, H).
          10) Herpes zoster (C, H).
          11) Snake bites (C).

Scientific Research:
Chemistry
    1) β-sitosterol, succinic acid, triacontan-1-ol, quercetin, kaempferol, avicularin, juglanin, trifolin,
       D-fructose, myo-inositol, pinitol, 6,8-di-C-pentosylapigenin [1–2].
    2) C-glycosylflavones: isovitexin, isoorientin, vicenin-2, lucenin-2 [3].
    3) Phenolics and tannins [4–7].
    4) Protein [5].
    5) Succinic acid [8].
    6) Potassium lespedezate, potassium isolespedezate [9–10].
    7) Pentacylic triterpene: 3β,22β,24-trihydroxyolean-12-ene [11]
Pharmacology
    1) Exitation effect on uterus in pregnant animals [12].
    2) Antitussive effect [13].
    3) Antibacterial effect [14].

Literature:
[1] Matsuura, S. *et al.*: *Yakugaku Zasshi* **1978,** 98, 1542.
[2] Numata, A. *et al.*: *Chem. Pharm. Bull.* **1979,** 27, 602.
[3] Numata, A. *et al.*: *Chem. Pharm. Bull.* **1980,** 28, 964.
[4] Lindroth, R. L. *et al.*: *J. Chem. Ecol.* **1986,** 12, 713.
[5] Fales, S. L. *et al.*: *Can. J. Plant Sci.* **1984,** 64, 637.
[6] Mosjidis, C. O. *et al.*: *Ann. Bot. (London)* **1990,** 66, 495.
[7] Terrill, T. H. *et al.*: *Corp Sci.* **1990,** 30, 219.
[8] Zhou, F. X. *et al.*: *Zhongcaoyao* **1980,** 11, 523.

[9] Shigemori, H. *et al.*: *Tetrahedron* **1990,** 46, 383.
[10] Shigemori, H. *et al.*: *Tetrahedron Lett.* **1989,** 30, 3991.
[11] Steffens, J. C. *et al.*: *Phytochemistry* **1986,** 25, 2291.
[12] Huang, H. *et al.*: *Yunnan Yixue Zazhi* **1965,** (2), 45.
[13] Hunan Yiyao Gongye Yanjiusuo: *Zhongcaoyao Tongxun* **1972,** (3), 19.
[14] Anonymous: *Zhongcaoyao Tongxun* **1972,** (1), 13.

[P.P.H. But]

483.   *Sophora subprostrata* **Chun. et T. Chen.**   (Leguminosae)

Shan-dou-gen(C), Sarn-dou-gun(H), Gwang-du-geun(K)

Related plants: *S. tonkinensis* Gapnep.: Yae-nan-huai(C); *Indigofera kirilowii* Max.: Ddan-bi-ssa-
        ri(K)

Root and Rhizome(CP)
Local Drug Name: Shan-dou-gen(C), Sarn-dou-gun(H), Sanzukon(J), San-du-geun(K)
Processing: Dry under the sun(K) Eliminate foreign matter, soak in water, wash clean, soften
        thoroughly, cut into thick slices, and dry in the sun(C)
Method of Administration: Oral(decoction, C, H, J, K)
Folk Medicinal Uses:
              1) Jaundice(H, J, K)
              2) Diarrhea(J, K)
              3) Hemorrhoid(J, K)
              4) Sore throat and painful swelling of the gums due to accumulation of toxic
                 heat(C)
              5) Common cold(H)
              6) Sore throat(H)
              7) Febrile diseases(J)
              8) Tumor(J)
Side effects: Excessive dose would induce serious vomiting or even death

Scientific Research:
Chemistry
    1) Triterpenes: Abrisapogenol C, D, E, H, I, kadzusapogenol A, cantoniensistriol, melilotigenin,
        sophoradiol, soyasapogenol A, B, subprogenin A, B, C, D, wistariasapogenol A[1], abrisaponin
        I, kudzusaponin A-3, dehydro soyasaponin I, subproside I, II, subproside III[2], soyasaponin
        II[2, 3], kaikasaponin I, III, 3-O-(α-rhamnopyranosyl(1-2)-β-D-galactopyranosyl(1-2)-D-
        glucopyranosyl), kudzusapogenol A, soyasaponin A-3, saoyasaponin I[3], subproside IV, V, VI,
        VII[4]
    2) Flavonoids: Bayin, sophoraflavone A, B[5], 2-((2'-hydroxy-1-methyl-ethyl)-7'-(3-methyl-but-3-
        enyl)-2',3'-dihydro-benzofuran)-5-yl)-7-hydroxy-8-(3-methyl-but-2-enyl) chroman-4-one, 2-
        ((3'-hydroxy-2',2'-dimethyl-8'-(3-methyl-but-2-enyl)-chroman-6'-yl)-7-hydroxy-8-(3-methyl-
        but-2-enyl) chroman-4-one, daidzein[6], 4',7-dihydroxy flavone, (-)-maackiain, trifolirhizin-6'-
        monoacetate[7], (-)-pterocarpin[7, 8], trifolirhizin[8], sophoranone[9], sophoradin[9, 10]
    3) Alkaloids: Anagyrine, methyl cytisine[8, 11], matrine[8, 11, 12, 13, 14], oxymatrine[11, 13],
        matrine-N-oxide[8, 12, 14], sophocarpine[15]
    4) Steroids: Daucosterol[7], β-sitosterol[11]
    5) Carbohydrates: Sophora polysaccharide SSA[16]
Phamacology
    1) Cytotoxic activity[17]
    2) Antiulcer activity[9, 22]
    3) Antibacterial activity[18]

4) Adrenergic receptor blocking activity[19]
5) Calcium channel blocking activity[19]
6) Antimitogenic activity[20]
7) Immunostimulant activity[20]
8) Psoriasis treatment[21]
9) Plaque formation suppressant activity[23]
10)Tumor necrosing factor induction[24]
11) Hypothermic activity[25]

Literature:
[1] Takeshita, T. *el al.*: *Chem. Pharm. Bull.* **1991**, 39(7), 1908.
[2] Ding, Y. *et al.*: *Chem. Pharm. Bull.* **1992**, 40(1), 139.
[3] Sakamoto, S. *et al.*: *Phytochemistry* **1992**, 31(4), 1339.
[4] Ding, Y. *et al.*: *Chem. Pharm. Bull.* **1992**, 40(7), 1831.
[5] Shirataki Y. *et al.*: *J. Nat. Prod.* **1986**, 49(4), 645.
[6] Kyogoku, K. *et al.*: *Chem. Pharm. Bull.* **1973**, 21, 1436.
[7] Komatsu, M. *et al.*: *Phytochemisty* **1976**, 15, 1089.
[8] Shibata, S.: *Some recent Developments in the chemistry of Natural Products*(Rangaswamt, S. and N.V. Subbas Rao, Ed), Prentice Hall, New Delhi **1972**, 1972, 1.
[9] Sasajima, M. *et al.*: *Nippon Yakugigaku Zasshi* **1978**, 74, 897.
[10] Saziki, R. *et al.*: *J. Pharmacobio Dyn.* **1983**, 6(3), S59.
[11] Shibata, S.: *Yakugaku Zasshi* **1961**, 81(11), 1635.
[12] Fukushima, S. *et al.*: *Patent-Japan*-72 03,749 **1972**
[13] Cui, J. F. and Zhang, G.: *Zhongyao Tongbao* **1986**, 11(2), 102.
[14] Willaman, J. J. and Li, H. L.: *Lloydia* **1970**, 33S, 1.
[15] Jiang, Z. Y.: *Chung Yao T'ung Pao* **1982**, 7(5), 29.
[16] Zhang, L. *et al.*: *Chung Ts'ao Yao,* **1993**, 24(1), 8.
[17] Kosuge, T. *et al.*: *Yakugaku Zasshi* **1985**, 105(8), 791.
[18] Franzblau, S. G. and Cross, C.: *J. Ethnopharmacol.* **1986**, 15(3), 279.
[19] Han, G. Q. *et al.*: *Int. J. Chinese Med.* **1991**, 16(1), 1.
[20] Mori, H. *et al.*: *Jap. J. Pharmcol.* **1989**, 49(3), 423.
[21] Zhu, R. K. *et al.*: *Chung I Tsa Chih* **1981**, 22(4), 22.
[22] Yamazaki, M. *et al.*: *Shoyakugaku Zasshi* **1981**, 35, 96.
[23] Namba, T. *et al.*: *Shoyakugaku Zasshi* **1984**, 38(3), 253.
[24] Xu, Q. *et al.*: *Int. J. Immunopharmcol.* **1989**, 11(6), 607.
[25] Chuang, C. Y. *et al.*: *Proc. Natl. Sci. Counc. Repub. China Part B* **1983**, 7(3), 536.

[C. K. Sung]

484.   *Vigna umbellata* **Ohwi et Ohashi**   (Leguminosae)
[= *Phaseolus calcaratus* Roxb.]

Chixiaodou (H), Tsuruazuki (J), Deong-gul-pat (K)

Related plants: *Vigna anguralis* (Willd.) Ohwi et Ohashi; Azuki (J), Pat (K).

Seed
Local Drug Name: Chixiaodou (C), Sekishozu (J), Jeok-so-du (K).
Processing: Dry under the sun (C, J, K).
Method of Administration: Decoction (C, J, K).
Folk Medicinal Uses:
1) Edema (C, J, K).
2) Carbuncle (C, J, K).
3) Beriberi (C, J, K).

4) Diarrhea (C).
5) Melena (C).
6) Jaundice with dark urine (C).
7) Acute rheumatic arthritis (C).
8) Bils, appendicitis (C).

Scientific Researches:
Chemistry
1) Flavonoids: Coumestrol, phaseollidin and kievitone [2, 4].
2) Amino acids and proteins: Globulins [1, 5].
3) Carbohydrates [3].
Pharmacology
1) Antifungal activity (isoflavonoids) [2].

Literatures:
[1] Sayanova, V. V.: *Izv. Akad. Nauk. Mold. SSR, Ser. Biol. Khim. Nauk* **1976**, (6), 23.
[2] Sukumaran, K. *et al.*: *Indian J. Microbiol.* **1980**, 20(3), 204.
[3] Yasui, T. *et al.*: *Bot. Mag.* **1985**, 98(1049), 75.
[4] Seneviratne, G. *et al.*: *Biochem. Syst. Ecol.* **1992**, 20(5), 459.
[5] Gomathinayagam, P. *et al.*: *J. Plant Biochem. Biotechnol.* **1994,** 3(2), 149; Fujihara, S. *et al.*: *Plant Cell Physiol.* **1994**, 35(8), 1127.

[T. Kimura]

485.   *Averrhoa carambola* L.   (Oxalidaceae)

Yang-tao (C), Yeung-toe (H), Gorenshi (J)

Fruit
Local Drug Name: Yang-tao (C), Yeung-toe (H), Yoto (J).
Processing: Use in fresh or dried (C, H).
Method of Administration: Oral (decoction: C, H, J).
Folk Medicinal Uses:
1) Cough (C, H, J).
2) Sorethroat (C, H).
3) Malarial splenomegaly (C, H).
4) Food poisonng (J).

Root
Local Drug Name: Yang-tao-gen (C), Yeung-toe-gun (H).
Processing: Use in fresh or dried (C, H).
Method of Administration: Oral (decoction: C, H).
Folk Medicinal Uses:
1) Arthralgia (C, H).
2) Chronic headache (C, H).
3) Epistaxis (C).
4) Spermatorrhea (C).

Leaf
Local Drug Name: Yang-tao-ye (C, H).
Processing: Use in fresh or dried (C).
Method of Administration: Oral (decoction: C, H); Topical (crushed fresh leaves: C, H).
Folk Medicinal Uses:
1) Colds (C, H).

2) Gastroenteritis (C, H).
3) Oliguia (C, H).
4) Traumatic injury (C, H).
5) Boils and Pyodermas (C, H).
6) Postpartum edema (C).

Flower
Local Drug Name: Yang-tao-hua (C), Yeung-toe-far (H).
Processing: Use in fresh or dried (C).
Method of Administration: Oral (decoction: C, H).
Folk Medicinal Uses:
        1) Subcalorism and fever (C).
        2) Malaria (H).

Scientific Research:
Chemistry
1) 4 isomeric megastigma-4,6,8-trienes, megastigma-5,8(E) and (Z)-dien-4-one, megastigma-4,6,8-trien-3-ones, 2,2,6,7-tetramethylbicyclo[4.3.0]nona-1(9),4,7-triene and its isomers, the (E) and (Z)-theaspiranes, retro-α-ionones, megastigma-4,6,8-trien-3-ols [1–2], megastigma-6,7-diene-3,5,9-triol, β-damascenone; ionone derivs: 4-hydroxy-β-ionol, 3-hydroxy-β-ionol, 4-oxo-β-ionol, 3-hydroxy-β-ionone, 3-oxo-α-ionol, 3-oxo-retro-α-ionol, 3-oxo-4,5-dihydro-α-ionol, 3-oxo-7,8-dihydro-α-ionol, 3-hydroxy-β-damascone, 3,5-dihydroxy-megastigma-6,7-diene-9-one, 3-hydroxy-5,6-epoxy-β-ionone, 3-hydroxy-5,6-epoxy-β-ionol, 3,4-dihydro-3-hydroxyactinidol, vomifoliol, 4,5-dihydrovomifoliol, 7,8-dihydrovomifoliol [17].
2) Polygalacturonase [3], polyphenoloxidase [8].
3) Aascorbic acid) [4-7], oxalic acid, malic acid [10-11].
4) Carbohydrates: glucose, fructose [9-11], dietary fiber [9], sucrose [11].
5) Cyanidin-3-O-β-D-glucoside, cyanidin-3,5-O-β-D-diglucoside [12].
6) Pectin [13].
7) (E)-hex-2-enal, methyl benzoate [14].
8) Lutein, cryptoxanthin, lycopene, α-, γ– and β-carotene [15].
9) (1′S, 4E)-2,3-dihydroabscisic alcohol [16].

Literature:
[1] MacLeod, G. *et al.*: *Phytochemistry* **1990**, 29, 165.
[2] MacLeod, G. *et al.*: *Flavour Sci. Technol. Weurman Symp.* **1990**, 6th, 81.
[3] Ghazali, H. M. *et al.*: *Food Chem.* **1987**, 24, 147.
[4] Tee, E. S. *et al.*: *Pertanika* **1988**, 11, 39.
[5] Liu, L. J. *et al.*: *Guangpuxue Yu Guangpu Fenxi* **1989**, 9(4), 78.
[6] Ali, S. H. *et al.*: *N. Z. J. Corp. Hortic Sci.* **1992**, 20(2), 6.
[7] Liu, H. I. *et al.*: *Zhonghua Nongye Yanjiu* **1991**, 40, 280.
[8] Adnan, T. A.B.T. *et al.*: *Pertanika* **1986**, 9, 219.
[9] Nahar, N. *et al.*: *J. Sci. Food Agric.* **1990**, 51, 185.
[10] Campbell, C. A. *et al.*: *J. Am. Soc. Hortic Sci.* **1989**, 114, 455.
[11] Campbell, C. A. *et al.*: *HortScience* **1989**, 24, 472.
[12] Gunasegaran R. *et al.*: *Fitoterapia* **1992**, 63, 89.
[13] Roy, P. *et al.*: *Sci. Cult.* **1989**, 53, 110.
[14] Froehlich, O. *et al.*: *Flavour Fragrance J.* **1989**, 4, 177.
[15] Tee, E. S. *et al.*: *Food Chem.* **1991**, 41, 309.
[16] Lutz, A. *et al.*: *Phytochemstry* **1994**, 36, 811.
[17] Herderich, M. *et al.*: *Flavour Fragrance J.* **1992**, 7, 179.

[P.P.H. But]

486.   ***Linum usitatissimum* L.**   (Linaceae)

Ya-ma (C), Ama (J), A-ma (K)

Seed (KP)
   Local Drug Name: Ya-ma-zi (C), Ama-nin (J), A-ma-in (K).
   Processing: Dry under the sun (C, J, K). Break to pieces or grind after stir-frying (C).
   Method of Administration: Oral (decoction: C, K).
   Folk Medicinal Uses:
                    1) Constipation (C, J, K).
                    2) Catarrhal enteritis (J, K).
                    3) Dryness and itching of the skin (C).
                    4) Withering and loss of hair (C).
   Contraindication: Contraindicated in patients with loose bowels (C).

Scientific Researches:
   Chemistry
      1) Terpenoids abd steroids: Cycloartenol [1,2], tocopherol, carotenoids and steroids [3], β-
         sitosterol, stigmasterol, campesterol, fucosterol and 24-methylenecycloartan-3-ol [2].
      2) Phenolic compounds: Isoorientin, 4-hydroxy-3,5-dimethoxy cinnamic acid, 1-*O*-coumaroyl-
         glucose, 1-*O*-feruloylglucose, 1-*O*-caffeoylglucose, glucoferulic acid (= ferulic acid gluco-
         pyranoside), glucocaffeic acid, vicenin 2, lucenin 2, lucein 2-7-*O*-α-L-rhamnopyranoside and
         orientin 7-*O*-α-L-rhamnopyranoside [4], aryltetralin lignans [5].
      3) Flavonoids: Glycosylflavonoids [6], lucenin 7-rhamnoside, vicenin 7-rhamnoglucoside,
         vicenin 5-glucoside-7-rhamnoside, orientin 7-rhamnoside and isoorientin 7-glucoside [7],
         orientin, isoorientin, vitexin, isovitexin, lucenin-1, lucenin-2, vicenin-1 and -2 [8].
      4) Peptide methylesters [9].
      5) Fatty acids and fatty oil [10, 11].
      6) Polysaccharides: mucin [12].
   Pharmacology
      1) Antimicrobial activity against *Streptomyces pneumonia* (extract) [13].
      2) Peroxidase inhibition (phenolic compounds) [14].
      3) Vitamin B_6 antagonist [15].

Literatures:
   [1] Capella P.: *Nature* **1961**, 190, 167.
   [2] Middleditch, B. S. *et al.*: *Phytochem.* **1972**, 11(3) 1183.
   [3] Malyshevaa, A. G.: *Masloboino-zhirovaya Prom.* **1961**, 27(9), 7.
   [4] Ibrahim, R. K. *et al.*: *Phytochem.* **1970**, 9(8), 1855.
   [5] Konuklugil, B.: *Fitoterapia*, **1996**, 67(4), 379.
   [6] Dubois, J. *et al.*: *Phytochem.* **1971**, 10(11), 2839.
   [7] Okuntsov, M. M. *et al.*: *Biol. Nauki.* **1969**, 69.
   [8] Dubois, J. *et al.*: *Phytochem.* **1971**, 10, 2839.
   [9] Kaufman, H. P. *et al.*: *Chem. Ber.* **1959**, 92, 2805.
   [10] Bhatia, I. S. *et al.*: *Indian J. Biochem.* **1970**, 7(3), 215; Sekhon, K. S. et al.: *Oleagineux* **1973**,
        28(11), 525.
   [11] Guillaumin, R. *et al.*: *Rev. Franc. Corps Gras* **1964**, 11, 91.
   [12] Kalac, J. *et al.*: *Biol. Pr.* **1974,** 20(4), 58.
   [13] Alkofahi, A. *et al.*: *Alexandria J. Pharm. Sci.* **1996**, 10(2), 123.
   [14] Tyson, H. *et al.*: *Z. Pflanzenphysiol.* **1971**, 66(5), 385; Fieldes, M. A. et al.: *Phytochem.* **1973**,
        12(9), 2133.
   [15] Tjostem, J. L.: *Proc. Iowa Acad. Sci.* **1965**(1967), 72, 51.

                                                                    [T. Kimura]

487.   *Breynia fruticosa* **(Linn.) Hook.**   (Euphorbiaceae)

Hei-mian-shu (C), Hark-min-sun (H)

Root
  Local Drug Name: Hei-mian-shu (C), Hark-min-sun (H)
  Processing: Slice, dry under the sun (C, H)
  Method of Administration: Oral (decoction: C, H)
  Folk Medicinal Uses:
          1) Acute gastroenteritis (C, H).
          2) Tonsillitis (C, H).
          3) Bronchitis (C, H).
          4) Urinary tract stones (C, H).
          5) Post-partum uterine contraction pain (C, H).
          6) Rheumatic arthritis (C, H).
  Remarks: Overdose produces vomiting, dizziness, toxic hepatitis, even death.
  Contraindication: Pregnancy.

Leaf
  Local Drug Name: Hei-mian-ye (C), Hark-min-sun-yip (H)
  Processing: Use in fresh (C, H).
  Method of Administration: Topical (decoction for washing or juice for application in lesion: C, H).
  Folk Medicinal Uses:
          1) Burns (C, H).
          2) Eczema (C, H).
          3) Allergic dermatitis (C, H).
          4) Pruritus (C, H).
          5) Vaginitis (C, H).

Scientific Research:
  Pharmacology
  1) Inhibitory effects on the activities of murine retroviral reverse transcriptase and human DNA polymerases [1].
  2) Inhibitory effect on mutagenic activity of benzo{a}pyrene [2].

Literature:
  [1] Ono, K. *et al.*: *Chem. Pharm. Bull.* **1989,** 37, 1810.
  [2] Meng, Z.M. *et al.*: *Shoyakugaku Zasshi* **1990**, 44, 225.

[P.P.H. But]

488.   *Phyllanthus emblica* **L.**   (Euphorbiaceae)

Yu-gan-zi (C), Yau-gum-gee (H), Yukan (J)

Fruit (CP)
  Local Drug Name: Yu-gan-zi (C), Yau-gum-gee (H), Amarolcu (J)
  Processing: Eliminate foreign matter, and dry (C). Use fresh or preserved (H).
  Method of Administration: Oral (pills or powder: C; decoction: H).
  Folk Medicinal Uses:
          1) Cough (C, H, J).
          2) Sore throat (C, H, J).
          3) Vitamin C deficiency (C, H).
          4) Cold (C, H).
          5) Fever (C, H).

6) Toothache (C, H).
7) Liver and gall bladder diseases (C, J).
8) Heat in the blood and blood stasis (C).
9) Dyspepsia, abdominal pain (C).
10) Dryness of the mouth (C).
11) Diabetes (H).

Root
Local Drug Name: Yu-gan-zi-gen(C), Yau-gum-gee-gun(H).
Processing: Use fresh or dry and store (C, H).
Method of Administration: Oral(decoction: C, H).
Folk Medicinal Uses:
1) Hypertension (C, H).
2) Epigastric pain (C, H).
3) Enteritis (C, H).
4) Tuberculous lymphadenopathy (C, H).

Leaf
Local Drug Name: Yu-gan-zi-ye(C), Yau-gum-gee-yip(H).
Processing: Use fresh or dry and store (C, H).
Method of Administration: Oral(decoction: C, H); Topical(decoction for washing: C, H).
Fold Medicinal Uses:
1) Edema (C, H).
2) Eczema (C, H).

Scientific Researches:
Chemistry
1) Vitamins: Vitamin C [1-3], carotene [4].
2) Phenols: Emblicol [5].
3) Organic acids: Phyllemblic acid [5], mucic acid [6].
4) Tannins [7,8]: Chebulinic acid, chebulagic acid, corilagin, terchebin, chebulic acid, gallic acid, ellagic acid [9], putranjivain A, 1,6-di-O-galloyl-β-D-glucose, 1-O-galloyl-β-D-glucose, digallic acid [10].
5) Flavonoids: Kaempterol-3-O-β-D-glucoside, quercetin-3-O-β-D-glucoside [10].
Pharmacology
1) Inhibitory effect on human immunodeficiency virus (HIV) [10].
2) Effect on the glycogen level of myocardium [11].
3) Antispasmodic effect and weak inhibitory effect on the central nervous system [12].
4) Hepatoprotective effect [13].

Literatures:
[1] Mukerji: *The Indian Pharm. Codex* **1953**, 1, 156.
[2] Margaret, J. M.: *Food Research* **1952**, 17, 31.
[3] Julia, F. M.: *Econ. Botany* **1960**, 14, 119.
[4] Satyanarayana, M. N. *et al.*: *Indian J. Med. Res.* **1963**, 51(4), 764.
[5] Pillay, P. P. *et al.*: *Current Sci, (India)* **1958**, 27, 266.
[6] Soman, R. *et al.*: *Current Sci. (India)* **1962**, 31, 13.
[7] *"Zhongguo Jingji Zhiwuzhi"* **1961**, 1177.
[8] Srivastava, R. P. *et al.*: *Sci. Cult.* **1964**, 30(9), 446.
[9] Theresa, Y. M. *et al.*: *Leather Sci.* **1965**, 12(9), 327.
[10] El-Mekkawy, S. *et al.*: *Chem. Pharm. Bull.* **1995**, 43(4), 641.
[11] Tariq, M. *et al.*: *Indian J. Exp. Biol.* **1977**, 15(6), 485.
[12] Rao, M. R. R. *et al.*: Indian J. Exptl. Biol. **1964**, 2(1), 29.
[13] Gulati, R. K. *et al.*: *Indian J. Exp. Biol.* **1995**, 33(4), 261.

[J.X. Guo]

489. *Dictamnus albus* L. subsp. *dasycarpus* Kitagawa (Rutaceae)
[= *D. dasycarpus* Turcz.]

Hakusen(J), Baek-seon(K)

Root bark
 Local Drug Name: Hakusenhi(J), Baek-seon-pi(K)
 Processing: Dry under the sun(K)
 Method of Administration: Oral(decoction, K)
 Folk Medicinal Uses:
>>> 1) Jaundice(J, K)
>>> 2) Menstrual disorder(J)
>>> 3) Contusion(K)
>>> 4) Tineapedis(K)

Scientific Research:
 Chemistry
  1) Sesquiterpenes: Dictamnol[1, 2], dictamnosides A-E[4]
  2) Alkaloids: 6β-hydroxy fraxinellone[3]
  3) Limonoids[3]
 Phamacology
  1) Antifungal activity(limonoids)[3]

Literature:
 [1] Koike, T. *et al.*: *Chem. Pharm. Bull.* **1996**, 44(4), 646.
 [2] Piet, D. P. *et al.*: *Chem. Pharm. Bull.* **1996**, 44(7), 1400.
 [3] Zhao, W. M. *et al.*: *Phytochemistry* **1998**, 47(1), 7.
 [4] Zhao, W. M. *et al.*: *Phytochemistry* **1998**, 47(1), 63.

[C. K. Sung]

490. *Choerospondias axillaris* Burtt et Hill (Anacardiaceae)

Nan-suan-zao (C), Larm-shuan-joe (H),

Bark
 Local Drug Name: Larm-shuan-joe-pay (H).
 Processing: Scrape off the rough surface and dry under the sun (H).
 Method of Administration: Topical (decoction for washing or powder blended in sesame oil: H).
 Folk Medicinal Uses:
>>> 1) Burns (H).
>>> 2) Scalds (H).
>>> 3) Wound bleeding(H).
>>> 4) Psoriasis (H).
>>> 5) Scrotal eczema (H).
>>> 6) Boils (H).
>>> 7) Ulcers (H).

Fruit
 Local Drug Name: Guang-zao (C), Larm-shuan-joe (H).
 Processing: Use in fresh (H) or dried (C).
 Method of Administration: Oral (chew and suck: H).
 Folk Medicinal Uses:

1) Stagnation of qi and blood with pectoral pain, palpitation and shortness of breath (C).
2) Restlessness (C).
3) Indigestion (H).
4) Distention (H).

Seed
Local Drug Name: Larm-shuan-joe-yan (H).
Processing: Use in fresh or dry under the sun (H).
Method of Administration: Oral (decoction: H).
Folk Medicinal Uses:
1) Insomnia (H).

Scientific Research:
Chemistry
1) Flavonoids [1–3]: naringenin, quercetin, kaempferol, kaempferol-5-O-arabinoside, quercetin-3-O-rhamnoside, myricetin, myricetin-3-O-rhamnoside [4, 6, 8].
2) Steroids: daucosterol, β-sitosterol [4, 8].
3) Phenols: protocatechuic acid, gallic acid, ellagic acid, 3,3'-dimethoxyellagic acid, p-dihydroxybenzene[5], (+)-catechin hydrate [6].
4) Flavonoids: kaempferol-7-O-glucoside [4, 8].
5) Sugars [9]: salicylic acid [4, 8], citric acid [5].
6) Glucoside: choerospondin [7, 12].
Pharmacology
1) Immunostimulatory effect [1].
2) Antiarrhythmic effect [2]
3) Enhancement of the tolerance of mice to hypoxia [3, 11].
4) Antagonistic effect on myocardial ischemia [3, 11].
5) LD_{50} of total glavones from fruits: 112 mg/kg i.v. in mice [2–3]
6) Inhibitory effect on ADP-induced platelet aggregation [5].
7) Therapeutic value in second degree burns [10].

Literature:
[1] Wang, Y. Z. *et al.*: *Zhongguo Yaolizue Tongbao* **1991**, 7, 214.
[2] Li, Z. X. *et al.*: *Zhongguo Yaoli Xuebao* **1984**, 5, 251.
[3] Li, Z. X. *et al.*: *Zhongcaoyao* **1984,** 15, 265.
[4] Deng, L. J. *et al.*: *Zhongcaoyao* **1989,** 20, 104.
[5] Wang, N. L. *et al.*: *Zhongcaoyao* **1987,** 18, 482.
[6] Phan,T. S. *et al.*: *Tap Chi Hoa Hoc* **1993,** 31(3), 76.
[7] Lu, Y. Z. *et al.*: *Yaoxue Tongbao* **1982,** 17, 120.
[8] Khabir, M. *et al.*: *Indian J. Chem., Sect. B* **1987,** 26B, 85.
[9] Maskey, K. *et al.*: *J. Nepal Chem. Soc.* **1982,** 2, 23.
[10] Ngyuyen, D. D. *et al.*: *Scandinavian J. Plastic & ReconstructiveSurgery & Hand Surgery* **1996,** 30, 139.
[11] Li, Z. X. *et al.*: *Zhongyao Tongbao* **1985**, 10, 138.
[12] Li, Z. X. *et al.*: *YaoxueXuebao* **1983**, 18, 199.

[P.P.H. But]

491.   *Rhus javanica* **L.**   (Anacardiaceae)

Nurude(J), Buk-na-mu(K),

Related plants: *R. chinensis*

Gall
  Local Drug Name: Gobaishi(J), O-bae-ja(K)
  Processing: Dry under the sun(K)
  Method of Administration: Oral(decoction, J, K)
  Folk Medicinal Uses:

                    1) Acute gastritis(J, K)
                    2) Dry sputum(J, K)
                    3) Diarrhea(J, K)
                    4) Diphtheria(K)
                    5) Hematemesis(K)
                    6) Emetics(K)
                    7) Apoplexy(K)
                    8) Eye disease(K)
                    9) Tape worm(K)
                    10) Hemorrhoid(K)
                    11) Tonsillitis(K)
                    12) Leucorrhea(K)

Scientific Research
  Chemistry
    1) Tannins: Peta-m-digalloyl-β-D-glucose, 1,2,3,4,6-penta-O-galloyl-β-D-glucose, gallic acid[1]
    2) Triterpenes: Rhuslactone[2]
  Pharmacology
    1) Inhibition of replication of murine and human cytomegalovirus[3, 4, 5]
    2) Anti-Herpes simplex virus activity[3, 4, 5]
    3) Plant growth inhibition(ethanol extract)[6]

Literature
  [1] Nishizawa, M. *et al.*: *J. Chem. Soc. Perkin Trans.* **1982**, 1(12), 2963.
  [2] Sung, C. K. *et al.*: *J. Chem. Soc. Chem. Comm.* **1980**, 909.
  [3] Shiraki, K. *et al.*: *Nippon Rinsho* **1998**, 56(1), 156.
  [4] Yukawa T. A. *et al.*: *Antiviral Res.* **1996**, 32(2), 63.
  [5] Kurokawa M. *et al.*: *Antiviral Res.* **1995**, 27(1-2), 19.
  [6] Shimomura, H. *et al.*: *Shoyakugaku Zasshi* **1982**, 36(2), 132.

                                                                              [C. K. Sung]

492.   *Rhus verciniflua* **Stokes**   (Anacardiaceae)

               Qi-shu(C), Gon-chut(H), Urushinoki(J), Ot-na-mu(K)

Balsam
  Local Drug Name: Gan-gi(C), Gon-chut(H), Kanshitsu(J), Geon-chil(K)
  Processing: Dry under the sun(C, K)
  Method of Administration: Oral(decoction, K,H   pills or powder:C)
  Folk Medicinal Uses:

                    1) Rheumatism(C, H, K)
                    2) Ascariasis(C)
                    3) Menstrual disorder (C)
                    4) Filariasis(C)
                    5) Menstrual disorder(J)
                    6) Cough(J)
                    7) Ascaris(J)

8) Neuralgia(K)
Contraindications: during pregnancy
Side Effects: urticaria

Scientific Research
Chemistry
  1) Phenols: urushiol[1, 3], urushiol diacetate[3], anacardic acid[4]
  2) Catechols: 3-10'Z,13'E,15'E-heptadecatrienyl catechol[3], 4-8'Z,11'E,13'Z-pentadecatrienyl catechol[5], stellacyanin[6]
  3) Proteins: Rhus verniciflua antigen[7]
Pharmacology
  1) Dermatitis producing effect[8]
  2) Cytotoxic activity[9, 10]

Literature

[1] Yamaguchi, Y. *et al.*: *J. Chromatogr.* **1981**, 214(3), 343.
[2] Hashimoto, O. and Minami, K.: *Mokuzai Gakkaishi* **1980**, 26, 49.
[3] Yamauchi, Y. and Oshima, R.: *J. Chromatogr.* **1980**, 198(1), 49.
[4] Tyman, J. H. P. and Lam. S. K.: *Chem. Nat. Prod. 11th* **1978**, 2, 190.
[5] Du, Y. and Oshima, R.: *J. Chromatogr.* **1984**, 284(2), 463.
[6] Hill, H. A. and Lee, W. K.: *Biochem. Soc. Trans.* **1979**, 7(4), 733.
[7] Wen, Y. Y. *et al.*: *Chih Wu Hsueh Pao* **1984**, 26(5), 523.
[8] Shiohara, T. *et al.*: *J. Amer. Acad. Dermatol.* **1990**, 22(4), 647.
[9] Sato, A.: *Yakugaku Zasshi*, **1989**, 109(6), 407.
[10] Lee, J. H. *et al.*: *Korean J. Pharmacog.* **1986**, 17(4), 286.

[C. K. Sung]

493.   *Cardiospermum halicacabum* **L.**   (Sapindaceae)

Dao-de-ling (C), Doe-day-ling (H), Pung-seon-deong-gul (K)

Whole Plant
Local Drug Name: Dao-de-ling (C), Doe-day-ling (H), Ga-go-gwa (K).
Processing: Use in fresh or dry under the sun (C, H).
Method of Administration: Oral (decoction: C, H); Topical (decoction or crushed fresh herb: C, H).
Folk Medicinal Uses:
        1) Snake bite (C, H, K).
        2) Pyodermas and carbuncles (C, H).
        3) Traumatic injury (C, H).
        4) Scabies (C, H).
        5) Eczema (C, H).
        6) Urinary tract infection (H, K).
        7) Edema (H, K).
        8) Colds and fever (H).
        9) Nephritis (H).
      10) Oliguria (H).
      11) Diabetes mellitus (H).
      12) Pertussis (H).
      13) Jaundice (K).

Scientific Research:
Chemistry
  1) Alkaloids [1].

2) Lipids: Fatty acids ($C_{20:1}$, arachidic, linoleic, stearic) [2], diesters [3], ester ($C_9H_{18}O_5$) [4].

3) β-Sitosterol [2], β-sitosterol-β-D-galactoside [5], (+)-pinitol, apigenin-7-O-glucuronide, chrysoeriol-7-O-glucuronide [6], luteolin-7-O-glucuronide [2, 6].

4) Protein, amino acid [7].

Pharmacology
   1) Antibacterial effect [1].
   2) Cardiac inhibitory effect [1].
   2) Hypotensive effect [1].
   3) Anti-spasmolytic effect [1].
   4) Atypical tonic effect on rat uterus [1].
   5) Biphasic effect on the frog rectus abdominis muscle [1].
   6) Antiinflammatory effect [8].
   7) Insecticidal effect [9–10].

Literature:
[1] Shukla, S. D. *et al.: Indian J. Pharm.* **1973,** 35(1), 40.
[2] Ahmed, I. *et al.: Sci. Int. (Lahore)* **1993**, 5(1), 67.
[3] Mikolajczak,, K. L. *et al.: Lipids* **1970**, 5, 812.
[4] Hopkins, C. Y. *et al.: Phytochemistry* **1968**, 7, 619.
[5] Khan, M. S. Y. *et al.: Indian Drugs* **1990**, 27, 257.
[6] Rao, C. V. *et al.: Acta Cienc. Indica, Chem.* **1987**, 13, 169.
[7] Prakash, D. *et al.: Plant Foods Hum. Nutr. (Dordrecht, Neth.)* **1988**, 38, 235.
[8] Chandra, T. *et al.: Arogya (Manipal, India)* **1984**, 10(1), 57.
[9] Shabana, M. M. *et al.: Bull. Fac. Pharm. (Cairo Univ.)* **1990**, 28(2), 79.
[10] Khan, M. W. Y. *et al.: JAOCS, J. Am. Oil Chem. Soc.)* **1983**, 60, 949.

[P.P.H. But]

494.   *Litchi chinensis* **Sonn.**   (Sapindaceae)

Li-zhi (C), Lai-gee (H), Yeo-ji (K)

Seed (CP)
   Local Drug Name: Li-zhi-he (C), Lai-gee-wut (H), Reishi (J), Yeo-ji-haek (K).
   Processing: 1) Eliminate foreign matter, wash clean and dry. Break to pieces before use (C, K).
                   2) Stir-fry the clean Semen Litchi with salt water to dry (C).
   Method of Administration: Oral (decoction: C, H, K).
   Folk Medicinal Uses:
                   1) Hernial pain of cold type (C, H, K).
                   2) Swelling and pain of the testis (C, H, K).
                   3) Weakness (J).

Scientific Researches:
   Chemistry
   1) Amino acids: α-(Methylenecyclopropyl)-glycine [1,2].
   2) Acids: Levulinic acid, malic acid, citric acid, lactic acid, malonic acid, fumaric acid, succinic acid, phosphoric acid, glutaric acid [3], cyclopropene fatty acids (CPFA), dihydroxterculic acid[4], palmitic acid, oleic acid, linoleic acid [5].
   3) Sugars: Fructose, glucose, sucrose [6].
   Pharmacology
   1) Antimutagenic effect [2].
   2) Hypoglycemic effect [1,7,8].

Literatures:
[1] Gray, D. O. *et al.*: *Biochem. Jour.* **1962,** 82, 385.
[2] Minakata, H. *et al.*: *Experientia* **1985,** 41(12), 1622.
[3] Chan, H. T. *et al.*: *J. Food Sci.* **1974,** 39(4), 792.
[4] Vickery, J. R.: *J. Am. Oil Chem. Soc.* **1980,** 57(2), 87.
[5] Gaydou, E. M. *et al.*: *J. Agric. Food Chem.* **1993,** 41(6), 886.
[6] Chan, H. T. *et al.*: *J. Food Sci.* **1975,** 40(4), 772.
[7] Deng, G. M.: *Guangxi Yixue* **1982,** 4(4), 172.
[8] Shen, W. Y. *et al.*: *Zhejiang Yaoxue* **1986,** (4), 8.

[J.X. Guo]

495.   *Gossypium nanking* Meyen   (Malvaceae)
                     [= *G. indicum* Lam.]

Wata(J), Mok-hwa(K)

Seed
Local Drug Name: Menjitsu(J), Myeon-hwa-ja(K)
Processing: Dry under the sun(K)
Method of Administration: Oral(decoction, J, K)
Folk Medicinal Uses:
                    1) Galactagogue(J, K)
                    2) Erisipelas(K)
                    3) Jaundice(K)
                    4) Cancer(K)
                    5) Glossitis(K)
                    6) Neuralgia(K)
                    7) Dermatopathy(K)
                    8) Mastitis(K)
                    9) Hemostyptic(K)
                    10) Yellow phlegm(K)

Root
Local Drug Name: Menkonpi(J), Myeon-hwa-geun(K)
Processing: Dry under the sun(K)
Method of Administration: Oral(decoction, J, K)
Folk Medicinal Uses:
                    1) Menstrual disorder(J)
                    2) Gonorrhoea(K)
                    3) Appendicitis(K)
                    4) Furuncle(K)
                    5) Hernia(K)
                    6) Cough(K)
                    7) Hysterocele(K)
                    8) Wart(K)

Scientific Researches:
Chemistry
1) Anthocyans: Betaines[1]

Literatures:
[1] Zhang, J. et al.: *Bunseki Kagaku* **1997**, 46(4), 275.

[C. K. Sung]

496.   *Hydnocarpus anthelmintica* **Pierre**   (Flacourtiaceae)

Da-feng-zi (C), Tai-fung-gee (H), Daifushi (J), Dae-pung-ja-na-mu (K)

Kernel
Local Drug Name: Da-feng-zi-ren (C), Tai-fung-gee (H), Daifushi (J), Dae-pung-ja (K).
Processing: 1) Eliminate foreign matter and remaining testa (C).
              2) Pound the clean kernels into pieces, remove the oils, then pulverize into frost-like
                 powder (C).
Method of Administration: Oral (pills or powder made by frost-like powder: C, H, K); Topical
              (paste: C).
Folk Medicinal Uses:
              1) Leprosy (C, J, K).
              2) Scabies (C, K).

Scientific Researches:
Chemistry
    1) Lipids [1]: Chaulmoogric acid, gorlic acid, hydrocarpic acid, dehydrochaulmoogric glyceride,
       oleic glyceride, palmitic glyceride [2], cyclopentenyl fatty acids [3,4], α-ketodicarboxylic acids
       [5], β-cyclopent-2-enyltridec-4-enoic acid , C_{13}-4-hexadecenoic acid, C_{16} and C_{18} cyclopentyl
       fatty acids[6].
    2) Amino acids: Cyclopentenylglycine [4,7].
    3) Glycosides: Taraktophyllin, epivolkenin [8].
Pharmacology
    1) Bacteriostasis [9,10].
    2) Toxicity [10].

Literatures:
    [1] Radwan, S. S. *et al.: Chem. Phys, Lipids* **1974,** 13(1), 103.
    [2] Cole, H. L. *et al.: J. Am. Chem. Soc.* **1939,** 61, 3442.
    [3] Cramer, V. *et al.: Biochem. Biophys. Acta* **1976,** 450(2), 261.
    [4] Cramer, V. *et al.: Eur. J. Biochem.* **1977,** 74(3), 495.
    [5] Tober, I. *et al.: Dev. Plant Biol.* **1980,** 6 (*Biog. Funct. Plant Lipids),* 227.
    [6] Christie, W. W. *et al.: Lipids* **1989,** 24(2), 116.
    [7] Cramer, V. *et al.: Biochemistry* **1980,** 19(13), 3074.
    [8] Jaroszewske, J. W. *et al.: Tetrahedron* **1987,** 43(10), 2349.
    [9] Cao, R. L. *et al.: Zhonghua Pifuke Zazhi* **1957,** 5, 286.
    [10] Chaopia, R. N. *et al.: Chopra's Indigenous Drugs of Inida* **1958,** 417.

[J.X. Guo]

497.   *Gymnostemma pentaphyllum* **Makino**   (Cucurbitaceae)

Jiao-gu-lan(C), Chut-yip-darm(H), Amachazuru(J), Dol-oe(K)

Whole plant
Local Drug Name: Chut-yip-darm(H), Amachazuru(J), Chil-yeop-dam(K)
Processing: Dry under the sun(K, J)
Method of Administration: Oral(decoction, H, J, K)
Folk Medicinal Uses:
              1) Chronic bronchitis(J, K)
              2) Diabetes(J, K)
              3) Debility(H)

4) Furuncle(K)

Rhizome
Local Drug Name: Jiao-gu-lan(C)
Processing: Wash clean, dry in the sun and ground into powder(C)
Method of Administration: Oral(decoction, C)
Folk Medicinal Uses:
>>> 1) Infectious hepatitis(C)
>>> 2) Pyelitis(C)
>>> 3) Gastroenteritis(C)

Scientific Research:
Chemistry
1) Triterpenes: 12-Oxo-2α,3β,20(S)-trihydroxydammar-24-ene[1], (20S)-3β-20, 23-trihydroxy-dammar-24-en-21-oic acid-21,23-lactone, (20R)-3β-20, 23-trihydroxydammar-24-en-21-oic acid-21,23-lactone, (20S)-dammar-23-ene-3β,20, 25,26-tetraol, (20R)-dammar-25-ene-3β,20,21,24–tetraol[2]
2) Inorganics: Zn[3]
Phamacology
1) Radiation protective effect[4]
2) Esophageal cancer prevention effect[5]
3) Tumor cell inhibition effect[6]

Literature:
[1] Hu, L. *et al.*: *J. Nat. Prod.* **1996**, 59(12), 1143.
[2] Piacente, S. *et al.*: *J. Nat. Prod.* **1995**, 58(4), 512.
[3] Xie, L. *et al.*: *Chung Kuo Chung Yao Tsa Chih* **1990**, 15(6), 348.
[4] Chen, W. C. *et al.*: *Am. J. Chin. Med.* **1996**, 24(1), 83.
[5] Wang C. *et al.*: *Hua His I Ko Hsueh Hsueh Pao* **1995**, 26(4), 430.
[6] Han M. Q. *et al.*: *Chung Kuo Chung His I Chieh Ho Tsa Chih* **1995**, 15(3), 147.

[C. K. Sung]

498. *Lagenaria siceraria* **Standl. var.** *hispida* **Hara** (Cucurbitaceae)

Hyotan(J), Jong-gu-ra-gi-bak(K)
Fruit
Local Drug Name: Koro(J), Ho-ro(K)
Processing: Dry under the sun(K)
Method of Administration: Oral(decoction, K)
Folk Medicinal Uses:
>>> 1) Edema(K)
>>> 2) Jaundice(K)
>>> 3) Gonorrhea(K)

Scientific Research:
Chemistry
1) Triterpenes: Bryonolic acid [1]

Literature:
[1] Cho, H. J. *et al.*: *Phytochemistry* **1992**, 31(11), 3893.

[C. K. Sung]

499.   *Momordica grosvenori* **Swingle**   (Cucurbiaceae)

Luo-hang-guo (C), Law-hon-gwor (H)

Fruit (CP)
Local Drug Name: Luo-hang-guo (C), Law-hon-gwor (H), Rakanka (J).
Processing: Dry in the air for several days, and dry at a low temperature (C).
Method of Administration: Oral (decoction: C, H).
Folk Medicinal Uses:
  1) Dry cough, sore throat and hoarsness of voice due to heat to the lung (C, H).
  2) Constipation (C).

Scientific Researches:
Chemistry
  1) Triterpenoids: mogroside IV, V, VI [1-3], triterpene I [4], mogroester [5].
  2) Sugars: fructose [6].
  3) Amino acids: [6].
  4) Flavones [6].

Literatures:
  [1] Takemoto, T. *et al.*: *Yakugaku Zasshi* **1983,** 103(11), 1151.
  [2] Takemoto, T. *et al.*: *Yakugaku Zasshi* **1983,** 103(11), 1155.
  [3] Takemoto, T. *et al.*: *Yakugaku Zasshi* **1983,** 103(11), 1167.
  [4] Hu, G.Q. *et al.*: *Faming Zhuanli Shenqing Gongkai Shuomingshu* CN 87,101,850, 16 Dec **1987,** Appl. 09 Mar **1987;** 5pp.
  [5] Wang, Y.P. *et al.*: *Zhongcaoyao* **1992,** 23(2), 61.
  [6] *"Zhongyao Zhi"* **1984,** Vol.3, 455.

[J.X. Guo]

500.   *Cleistocalyx operculatus* **(Roxb.) Merr. et Perry**   (Myrtaceae)

Shui-rong (C), Shui-yung (H)

Flower Bud
Local Drug Name: Shui-rong-hua (C), Shui-yung-far (H).
Processing: Dry under the sun (C, H).
Method of Administration: Oral (decoction: C, H).
Folk Medicinal Uses:
  1) Colds and fever (C, H).
  2) Summer heat and indigestion (C, H).
  3) Acute gastroenteritis (C, H).
  4) Bacillary dysentery (C, H).

Root
Local Drug Name: Shui-rong-gen (C), Shui-yung-gun (H).
Processing: Dry under the sun (C, H).
Method of Administration: Oral (decoction: C, H).
Folk Medicinal Uses:
  1) Hepatitis (C, H).

Bark
Local Drug Name: Shui-rong-pi (C), Shui-yung-pay (H).
Processing: Use in fresh or dry under the sun (C, H).

Method of Administration: Topical (dicoction for washing or macerated fresh herb: C, H).
Folk Medicinal Uses:
    1) Scalds (C, H).
    2) Pruritus (C, H).
    3) Tinea pedis (C, H).
    4) Pyoderma (C, H).
    5) Leprosy (C).

Leaf
Local Drug Name: Shui-rong-ye (C), Shui-yung-yip (H).
Processing: Use in fresh or dry under the sun (C, H).
Method of Administration: Topical (macerated fresh herb or dicoction: C, H).
Folk Medicinal Uses:
    1) Acute mastitis (C, H).

Scientific Research:
Chemistry
 1) Leaf: β-ocimene, myrcene, β-caryophyllene, (E)-β-ocimene [1].
 2) Bark: arjunolic acid [2].
 3) Flower bud: 2,4'-dihydroxy-6'-methoxy-3',5'-dimethylchalcone, 5,7-dihydroxy-6,8-dimethyl-flavanone, 7-hydroxy-5-methoxy-6,8-dimethylflavanone, ethyl gallate, gallic acid, ursolic acid, β-sitosterol, cinnamic acid[3].
Pharmacology
 1) Antifungal activity (arjunolic acid) [2].

Literature:
 [1] Dung, N.X. *et al.*: *J. Essent. Oil Res.* **1994**, 6, 661.
 [2] Nomura, M. *et al.*: *Shoyakugaku Zasshi* **1993**, 47, 408.
 [3] Zhang, F.X. *et al.*: *Zhiwu Xuebao* **1990**, 32, 469.

                   [P.P.H. But]

501.   *Rhodomyrtus tomentosa* (Ait.) Hassk (Myrtaceae)

Tao-jin-niang (C), Toe-gum-leung (H)

Root
Local Drug Name: Tao-jin-niang (C), Toe-gum-leung (H).
Processing: Slice and dry under the sun (C, H).
Method of Administration: Oral (decoction: C, H).
Folk Medicinal Uses:
    1) Chronic dysentery (C, H).
    2) Hepatitis (C, H).
    3) Low back pain (C, H).
    4) Lumbar muscle strain (C).
    5) Acute and chronic gastroenterities (C).
    6) Stomachache (C).
    7) Dyspepsia (C).
    8) Rheumatic arthritis (C).
    9) Uterine bleeding (C).
   10) Proctoptosis (C).
   11) Burns (C).

Leaf

Local Drug Name: Tao-jin-niang-ye (C), Toe-gum-leung-yip (H).
Processing: Dry under the sun (C, H).
Method of Administration: Oral (decoction: C, H).
Folk Medicinal Uses:

      1) Acute gastroenteritis (C, H).
      2) Dyspepsia (C).
      3) Dysentery (C).
      4) Wound bleeding (C).

Fruit
Local Drug Name: Tao-jin-niang-guo (C), Toe-gum-leung-gwor (H).
Processing: Steam and dry under the sun (C, H).
Method of Administration: Oral (decoction: C, H).
Folk Medicinal Uses:

      1) Anemia of pregnancy (C, H).
      2) Debility after illness (C, H).
      3) Neurasthenia (C, H).
      4) Tinnitus (C).
      5) Spermatorrhea (C).

Scientific Research:
Chemistry
  1) Lupeol, β-amyrin, β-amyrenonol, betulin, friedelin, α-amyrin, taraxerol [1].

Literature:
[1] Hui, W.H. *et al.: Phytochemistry* **1975,** 14, 833.

[P.P.H. But]

502.   *Syzygium aromaticum* **Merr. et Perry**   (Myrtaceae)
                [= *Eugenia caryophyllata* Thunb.]

Ding-xiang (C), Ding-heung (H), Choji (J), Jeong-hyang(K)

Flower bud(CP, JP, KP)
Local Drug Name: Ding-xiang (C), Ding-heung (H), Choji (J), Jeong-hyang(K)
Processing: Dry in the shade (C, J: imported).
Method of Administration: Oral (decoction: C, H, J), topical (oil: C, H, J).
Folk Medicinal Uses:

      1) Toothache (C, H, J, K).
      2) Dyspepsia, anorexia, diarrhea, epigastric and abdominal pain with cold sensation (C, J, K).
      3) Hiccup and vomiting (C, J, K).
      4) Fever (J, K).
      5) Impotence due to deficiency of kidney yang (C).

Scientific Researches:
Chemistry
  1) Essential oil: Eugenol, acetyl eugenol, α- and β-caryophyllene, humulene, α-ylangene, furfural, methyl salicylate, vanillin, chavicol, caryophylla-4(12)-,8(13)-dien-5β-ol and caryophylla-3,8(13)-dien-5α-ol [1], zonarene [2], coniferyl aldehyde [13].
  2) Flavonoid: Kaempferol, rhamnetin [3].
  3) Tannins: Eugenin, 1-desgalloyleugenin, 2-desgalloyleugenin, syzyginin A and B [4].

4) Triterpenoid and steroids: Oleanolic acid and 2α-hydroxyoleanolic acid, stigmasterol glucoside, β-sitosterol glucoside and campesterol glucoside [5].

5) Chromones: Eugenoside I and II [6].

Pharmacology

1) Antimicrobial activity (essential oil) [7].

2) Inhibition of the growth of Herpes simplex virus (flower buds) [8]. Antivirus activity (eugeniin) [4].

3) Growth inhibitory activity against Gram-negative anaerobic periodontal oral pathogens (methanol extract of flower buds) [9].

4) Cholagogic (eugenol) [10]

5) Inhibition of platelet aggregation and production of tromboxane (eugenol, acetyleugenol) [11].

6) Antispamodic and sedative (eugenol, acetyleugenol) [12].

Literatures:

[1] Deyama, T. *et al.*: *Yakugaku Zasshi* **1971**, 91, 1383.

[2] Andersen, N. H. *et al.*: *Phytochem.* **1973**, 12, 827.

[3] Shanghai Zongyiyo Zazhi **1957**(5), 224.

[4] Nonaka, G. *et al.*: *Chem. Pharm. Bull* **1978**, 28, 685; Takechi, M. *et al.*: *Planta Medica* **1981**, 42, 69; Tanaka, T. *et al.*: *Phytochem.* **1996,** 43(6), 1345.

[5] Brieskorn, C. H. *et al.*: *Phytochem.* **1975**, 14, 2308.

[6] Saito, T. *et al.*: *Nippon Shoyaku Gakkai Koen Yoshishu* 30th, **1983**, 77

[7] Deans, S. G. *et al.*: *Flavour Fragrance J.*, **1995**, 10(5), 323.

[8] Kurokawa, M. *et al.*: *Wakan Iyakugaku Zasshi*, **1995**, 12(3), 187.

[9] Cai, L. *et al.*: *J. Nat. Prod.*, **1996**, 59(10), 987.

[10] Yamahara, J. *et al.*: *J. Pharm. Dyn.* **1983**, 6, 281.

[11] Leakman, G. M. *et al. Phytother. Res.* **1990**, 4, 90.

[12] Wagner, H. *et al.*: *Deut. Apoth -Ztg.* **1973**, 113, 1159; *Planta Med.* **1979**, 37, 9.

[13] Wahba, S. K. *et al.*: *J. Pharm. Sci.* **1964**, 53, 829.

[T. Kimura]

503.　　　*Melastoma candidum* **D. Don**　　(Melastomataceae)

Ye-mu-dan (C), Yair-mou-darn (H)

Whole Plant

Local Drug Name: Ye-mu-dan (C), Yair-mou-darn (H).

Processing: Wash, slice, use in fresh or dried (C, H).

Method of Administration: Oral (decoction: C, H); Topical (crushed fresh leaves or ground dry leaves: C, H).

Folk Medicinal Uses:

　　　　1) Dyspepsia (C, H).

　　　　2) Enteritis (C, H).

　　　　3) Bacillary dysentery (C, H).

　　　　4) Hepatitis (C, H).

　　　　5) Nose-bleeding (C, H).

　　　　6) Burns and bleeding wounds (C, H).

　　　　7) Thromboangiitis (C, H).

　　　　8) Traumatic injury (C, H).

　　　　9) Hematochezia (C).

　　　10) Melena (H).

Scientific Research:

Chemistry

1) Castalagin, procyanidin B-2, helichrysoside [1].
Pharmacology
1) Antihypertensive effect [1].

Literature:
[1] Cheng, J.T. *et al.*: *Planta Med.* **1993**, 59, 405.

[P.P.H. But]

504.   *Terminalia chebula* **Retzius**   (Combretaceae)

He-zi (C), Mirobaran, Myrobalan (J), Ga-ri-reuk (K)

Fruit(CP)
Local Drug Name: He-zi (C), Hor-gee (H), Kashi (J), Ga-ja (K).
Processing: 1) Eliminate foreign matter, wash clean and dry. Break to pieces before use (C).
           2) Macerate dried clean fruit briefly, core to soften, remove the kernels and dry (C).
Method of Administration: Decoction (C, H, J, K).
Folk Medicinal Uses:
            1) Diarrhea (C, H, J, K).
            2) Cough (C, H, J).
            3) Loss of voice (H).
            4) Bloody stool (H).
            5) Weakness (K).
            6) Fever (K).

Scientific Researches:
Chemistry
    1) Tannins: Tannins [1], chebulinic acid, neochebulinic acid [2].
    2) Carbohydrates: Galacturonic acid, glucose, mannose and xylose [3].
    3) Anthraquinones: Sennoside A [4].
    4) Guanidines: 9-(2-hydroxyethoxymethyl)guanidine [5].
    5) Steroids: β-Sitosterol [6].
    6) Tritepenoids: Chebuloside I and II [7], arjungenin and arjunglucoside [8].
    7) Fatty acids: Ricinoleic acid [9].
Pharmacology
    1) Prevention of herpes virus infection recurrence (9-(2-hydroxyethoxymethyl)-guanidine) [5].
        Anti-herpes simplex virus [10].
    2) Anti-cytomegalovirus activity (hot water extract) [11].
    3) Inhibition of mutagenicity of Trp-P-1 (aqueous extract) [12].
    4) Skin depigmentation (extract) [13].
    5) Purgative (sennoside A) [4].
    6) Antioxidant and preventive effect on acute liver injury (tannin) [14].
    7) Antitumor (tannins) [15]. Anticancer topoisomerase inhibitor (chebulanin) [16].
    8) Treating AIDS (human immunodeficiency virus) (extract) [17].
    9) Antimicrobial against methicillin-resistant Staphylococus aureus (extract) [18].
    10) Immunosuppressive effects on CTL-mediated cytotoxicity (gallic acid and chebulagic acid)
        [19].

Literatures:
[1] Srivastava, J. C. *et al.*: *Indian Agr.* **1967**, 11, 69; Khaleque, A. *et al.*: *Bangladesh J. Biol. Agr. Sci.*
    1972, 1(1), 59; Bhatia, K. *et al.*: *Indian For.* **1977**, 103, 273; Vivas, N. *et al.*: *J. Sci. Food Agric.*
    1996, 72 309.
[2] Schmidt, O. Th. *et al.*: *Ann.* **1957**, 609, 192, 199.

[3] Hathway, D. E. *et al.*: *Bioch. J.* **1958**, 70, 155.
[4] Gaind, K. N. *et al.*: *Indian J. Pharm.* **1965**, 27, 145: **1968**, 30(10), 233.
[5] Hozumi, T. *et al.*: *Jpn. Kokai Tokkyo Koho* JP 96268901 A2   JP 08268901 (19961015).
[6] Beri, R. M.: *Indian Oil Soap J.* **1970**, 35(12), 274.
[7] Kundu, A. P. *et al.*: *Phytochem.* **1993**, 32(4), 999.
[8] Reddy, B. M. *et al.*: *Int. J. Pharmacogn.* **1994,** 32 (4), 352.
[9]. Hosamani, K. M.: *J. Sci. Food Agric.* **1994,** 64, 275.
[10] Kurokawa, M. *et al.*: *Wakan Iyakugaku Zasshi* **1995**, 12(3), 187; Antiviral Res. **1995**, 27, 19.
[11] Yukawa, T. A. *et al.*: *Antiviral Res.* **1996**, 32(2), 63.
[12] Niikawa, M. *et al.*: *Nat. Med.* **1995**, 49(3), 329.
[13] Hanna, R.: *PCT Int. Appl.* WO 9624327 A1 **(1996)**.
[14] Fu, N.-W. *et al.*: *Zhongcaoyao* **1992**, 23(11), 585.
[15] Lee, S.-H. *et al.*: *Arch. Pharmacal Res.* **1995**, 18(2), 118.
[16] Tokura K. *et al.*: *Japan Kokai Tokkyo Koho*, JP 95138165 A2; JP 07138165 **1995**0530.
[17] Hozumi, T. *et al.*: *Japan Kokai Tokkyo Koho*, JP 9787195 A2; JP 0987195 **1997**0331.
[18] Sato, Y. *et al.*: *Biol. Pharm. Bull.* **1997,** 20 (4), 401.
[19] Hamada, S. *et al.*: *Biol. Pharm. Bull.* **1997,** 20(9), 1017.

[T. Kimura]

505.   *Oenothera stricta* **Ledeb. ex Link**   (Onagraceae)

Dal-ma-ji-ggot(K)

Related plants: *O. odorata* Jacg.: Matsuyoigusa(J)

Seed
  Local Drug Name: Dae-so-ja(K)
  Processing: Dry under the sun(K)
  Method of Administration: Oral(decoction, K)
  Folk Medicinal Uses:
                    1) Common cold(J, K)
                    2) Bronchitis(K)
                    3) Dermatitis(K)
                    4) Sore throat(K)

Scientific Research:
  Chemistry
   1) Lipids: γ-Linolenic acid, prostaglandin F2α[1]

Literature:
  [1] Groenewald, E. G. *et al.*: *Planta Med.* **1994**, 60(1), 84.

[C. K. Sung]

506.   *Camptotheca acuminata* **Decne**   (Nyssaceae)

Xi-shu (C), Hay-shue (H), Kiju (J), Heui-su (K)

Fruit, Leaf, Branch, Bark and Root
  Local Drug Name: Xi-shu (C), Hay-shue (H), Kiju (J), Heui-su (K).
  Processing: Use in fresh or dry under the sun (H, C, K).

Method of Administration: Oral (decoction: C, H, K); Topical (C, H); Extraction of campatothecin (J).

Folk Medicinal Uses:

1) Chronic granulocytic leukemia (C, H, J, K).
2) Gastric cancer (C, H, J).
3) Urinary bladder cancer (C,H, J).
4) Colon cancer (C, H, J).
5) Rectal cancer (C).
6) Psoriasis (C, H).

Remarks: Toxic effects include nausea, vomiting, gastrointestinal bleeding, diarrhea, cystitis, leukopenia, hematuria, alopecia. Severe intoxication may be fatal.

Scientific Research:

Chemistry

1) Alkaloids: Camptothecin [1-4, 6, 10, 18, 20], 10-hydroxycamptothecin [3-5], 11-hydroxy-camptothecin [4, 7-8], 10-methoxycamptothecin [3, 5-8], deoxycamptothecin [4], 20-deoxycamptothecin , 20-hexanoyl-10-methoxycamptothecin[11], 19-O-methylangustoline[12], 20(S)-camptothecin[13], 18-hydroxy-camptothecin[14], 22-hydroxyacuminatine [15], camptacumotine, camptacumanine [16], 10-hydroxy-deoxycamptothecin [17], 11-hydroxy-20(S)-camptothecin [19].
2) Vincoside lactam [3-4].
3) Venoterpine [4, 10].
4) Betulic acid [4].
5) (+)- Abscisic acid [7].
6) Syringaresinol [7].
7) β-Sitosterol [7, 10], β-sitosterol 3- β-D-glucoside [18].
8) Ellagic acid derivs: 3,4-O,O-methyleneellagic acid, 3',4'-O-dimethyl-3,4-O,O-methylene-ellagic acid, 3,4-O,O-methylene-3',4'-O-dimethyl-5'-methoxyellagic acid, 3,4-O,O-methylene-3',4'-O-dimethyl-5'-hydroxyellagic acid [8-10].
9) Syringic acid [9].
10) Strychnolactone, salicylic acid, nonandioic acid [14].
11) Et. Caffeate ursolic acid, betulinic acid, inositol [20].
12) Tannins: Camptothins A and B [21].

Pharmacology

1) Antineoplastic activity (Camptothecin) [5, 22-24].
2) Antiviral action [5, 24].

Literature:

[1] Lopez-Meyer, M. *et al.*: *Planta Med.* **1994,** 60, 558.
[2] Monroe E. W. *et al.*: *J. Am. Chem. Soc.* **1966,** 88, 3888.
[3] He, X. G. *et al.*: *Chih Wu Hsueh Pao* **1978,** 20, 76.
[4] Hsu, J. S. *et al.*: *Hua Hsueh Hsueh Pao* **1977,** 35, 193.
[5] Wani, M. C. *et al.*: *J. Org. Chem.* **1969,** 34, 1364.
[6] Buta, J. G. *et al.*: *Ind. Eng. Chem. Prod. Res. Dev.* **1978,** 17, 160.
[7] Lin, L. Z. *et al.*: *Huaxue Xuebao***1982,** 50, 85.
[8] Lin, L. T. *et al.*: *Hua Hsueh Tung Pao* **1978,** 36, 327.
[9] Lin, L. T. *et al.*: *Hua Hsueh Hsueh Pao* **1979,** 37, 207.
[10] Lin, L. T. *et al.*: *Hua Hsueh Hsueh Pao* **1977,** 35,227.
[11] Adamovics, J. A. *et al.*: *Phytochemistry* **1979,** 18, 1085.
[12] Lin, L. Z. *et al.*: *Phytochemistry* **1990,** 29, 2744.
[13] Hinz, H. R.: *US Appl. 22,091* **1993,** (2), 36.
[14] Lin, L. Z. *et al.*: *Yaoxue Xuebao* **1988,** 23, 186.
[15] Lin, L. Z. *et al.*: *Phytochemistry* **1989,** 28, 1295.
[16] Lin, L. Z. *et al.*: *Huaxue Xuebao* **1988,** 46, 1207.
[17] Lin, L. Z. *et al.*: *Huaxue Xuebao* **1989,** 47, 506.

[18] Wu, T. S. *et al.*: *Ch'eng-kung Ta Hsueh Hsueh Pao* **1980,** 15, 65.
[19] Wall, M. E. *et al.*: *J. Med. Chem.* **1986,** 29, 1553.
[20] Wu, T. S. *et al.*: *J. Chin. Chem. Soc. (Taipei)* **1985,** 32, 173.
[21] Hatano, T. *et al.*: *Tennen Yuki Kagobutsu Toronkai Koen Yoshishu* **1988,** 30, 292.
[22] Anonymous: *Zhonghua Yixue Zazhi* **1978,** 58, 598.
[23] Anonymous: *Zhonghua Yixue Zazhi* **1975,** 55, 274.
[24] Tafur, S. *et al.*: *Lloydia* **1976,** 39, 261.
[25] Torck, M. *et al.*: *J. Pharmacie de Belgique* **1996,** 51, 200.
[26] Ardizzoni, A.: *Lung Cancer* **1995,** 12 Suppl, S177.

[P.P.H. But]

507.   *Fatsia japonica* **Decne. et Planch.**   (Araliaceae)

Yatsude (J), Pal-son-i (K)

Leaf
   Local Drug Name: Yatsude (J), Pal-gak-geum-ban(K)
   Processing: Fresh leaf (J, K).
   Method of Administration: Water extract (J, K), bath (J, K).
   Folk Medicinal Uses:
                    1) Cough (J, K).
   Contraindications: toxic.

Scientific Researches:
   Chemistry
      1) Saponins: α- and β-fatsin [1].
      2) Triterpene glycosides: 3-*O*-α-L-arabinopyranosyl-oleanolic acid, 3-*O*-α-L-arabinopyranosyl-
         hederagenin, 3-*O*-[β-D-glucopyranosyl(1→4)-α-L-arabinopyranosyl]-hederagenin [2].
      3) Cyanidins: Cyanidin 3-lathyroside [3].
   Pharmacology
      1) Neoplasm inhibitor (DNA topoisomerase inhibitor) (triterpene glycosides) [2].
      2) Skin-lightening (saponins) [4].

Literatures:
   [1] Tanemura, M. *et al.*: *Yakugaku Zasshi* **1975,** 95(1), 1.
   [2] Kitanaka, S. et al.: *J. Nat. Prod.* **1995,** 58(11), 1647.
   [3] Terahara, N. *et al.*: *Phytochem.* **1992,** 31(4), 1446.
   [4] Maeda, N. *et al.*: *Jpn. Kokai Tokkyo Koho* **1996** JP 08133955 A2.

[T. Kimura]

508.   *Panax notoginseng* **(Burk) F. H. Chen**   (Araliaceae)

San-gi(c), Sanshichi-ninjin(J), Sam-chil-in-sam(K)

Root(CP)
   Local Drug Name:San-gi(C), Denshichi(J), Sam-chil(K)
   Processing: Dry under the sun(K). Wash clean ,dry ,and pulverize to fine powder(c).
   Method of Administration: Oral(decoction, K powder:C);Topical(powder:C)
   Folk Medicinal Uses:
                    1) Hematemesis(J, K)

2) Traumatic hemorrhage(J, K)
3) Hemoptysis , epistaxis , abnormal uterine bleeding , traumatic bleeding (C).
4) Pucking pain in the cheat and abdomen , traumatic smelling and pain (C).
5) Cerebral apoplexy(J)
6) Bleeding(J)
7) Hematochezia(K)
8) Rhinorrhagia(K)
Contraindications:Used with caution in pregnancy.

Scientific Research:
Chemistry
1) Saponins: Ginsenosides Rb_1, Rb_2, Rc, Rd, Re, Rf, Rg1, Rg_2, Ro, malonylginsenosides Rb_1, Rb_2, Rc[1], notoginsenosides R1[27], R8, R9[24], notoginsenosides-A, -B, -C, -D[4], -E, -G, -H, -I, -J[5]
2) Fatty acids: 2-Hexyldecanoic acid, 8,11-octadecadienoic acid, 9,10-dihydroxyoctadecanoic acid[2]
3) Polysaccharides[21]: PF3111, PF3112, PBGA11, PBGA12[23]
4) Acetylenic compounds: notoginsenic acid β-sophoroside[5]
5) Others: Neuroexitotoxic nonprotein amino acid(β-N-oxalo-L-α,β-diaminopropionic acid, α- N-oxalo-L-α,β-diaminopropionic acid[3]
Phamacology
1) Na^+-K^+-ATPase activation[6]
2) Immunostimulating activity[7](polysaccharide)[21, 23]
3) Improvement of hypoxic damage and cerebral ischemia/reperfusion injury(saponin)[8, 9, 11]
4) Increasing effect of ventricular fiblillation threshold[10]
5) Vasodilation of brain blood vessel[12]
6) Increasing of monophasic action potentials[13]
7) Antiplatelet and anticoagulation[14]
8) Calcium channel blockade action[15, 26]
9) Blocking calcium channel in smooth muscle[16]
10) Inhibition of proliferation of aortic smooth muscle cell[17]
11) Inhibition of Ca^{2+} entry through receptor-operated Ca^{2+} channel(saponin)[18]
12) Treatment of cardiovascular disease[19]
13) Hypotensive effect(saponin)[20](ginsenoside Re, Rg1)[25](chebulinic acid)[28]
14) Antiarrhythmic effect(ginsenoside Rb_1)[22]
15) Increasing fibrinolytic potential(notoginsenoside R1)[27]

Literature:
[1] Chung W. C. et al.: *Planta Medica* **1995**, 61(5), 459.
[2] Lang, A. et al.: *Beijing Shifan Daxue Xuebao, Ziran Kexueban* **1996**, 32(2), 257.
[3] Long, Y. C. et al.: *Int. J. Peptide Protein Res.* **1996**, 47(1-2), 42.
[4] Yoshikawa, M. et al.: Chemical and Pharmaceutical Bulletin **1997**, 45(6), 1039.
[5] Yoshikawa, M. et al.: *Chemical and Pharmaceutical Bulletin* **1997**, 45(6), 1056.
[6] Jing, L. Q. and Shi, L.: *Acta Pharmacologia Cinica* **1991**, 12(6), 504.
[7] Li, X. L.: *Memorias Do Instituto Oswaldo Cruz* **1991**, 86(S2), 159.
[8] Jiang, K. Y. and Qian, Z. N.: *Zhongguo Yaolixue Yu Dulixue Zazhi* **1995**, 9(3), 231.
[9] Jiang, K. Y. and Qian, Z. N.: *Acta Pharmacologica Sinica* **1995**, 16(5), 399.
[10] Wu, W. et al.: *Acta Pharmacologica Sinica* **1995**, 16(5), 459.
[11] Leung, A. W. N. et al.: *Neurochemical Research* **1991**, 16(6), 687.
[12] Wu, J. X. and Sun, J. J.: *Acta Pharmacologica Sinica* **1992**, 13(6), 520.
[13] Chen, J. Q. et al.: *Acta Pharmacologica Sinica* **1992**, 13(6), 538.
[14] Liao, F. L. et al.: *Clinical Hemorheology* **1992**, 12(6), 831.
[15] Jiang, Y. et al.: *Acta Pharmacologica Sinica* **1993**, 14(S), S8.
[16] Dan, H. X. et al.: *Acta Pharmacologica Sinica* **1993**, 14(S), S22.
[17] Lin, S. G. et al.: *Acta Pharmacologica Sinica* **1993**, 14(4), 314.

[18] Guan, Y. Y. et al.: Acta Pharmcologica Sinica **1994**, 15(5), 392.
[19] Zhang, W. J. et al.: Arteriosclerosis and thrombosis **1994**, 14(7), 1040.
[20] Liu, J. et al.: J. Ethnopharmacology **1994**, 42(3), 183.
[21] Gao, H. et al.: Abstract of papers of the American Chemical Socity **1994**, 207(Mar.), 113.
[22] Guan, Y. Y. et al.: Drug Development Research **1996**, 39(2), 179.
[23] Gao, H. et al.: Pharmaceutical Research **1996**, 13(8), 1196.
[24] Zhao, P. et al.: Phytochemistry **1996**, 41(5), 1419.
[25] Prasain, J. K. et al.: Phytomedicine, **1996**, 2(4), 297.
[26] Ma, L. Y. et al.: Acta Pharmacologica Sinica **1997**, 18(3), 213.
[27] Zhang, W. J. et al.: Cellular and Molecular Biology **1997**, 43(4), 581.
[28] Guan, Y. Y. et al.: Clinical & Experimental Pharmacology & Physiology **1996**, 23(8), 747.

[C. K. Sung]

509.　　　　　　　*Tetrapanax papyriferum* **K. Koch**　　(Araliaceae)

Tong-tuo-mu (C), Tung-cho (H), Kamiyatsude (J), Tong-tai-mok (K)

Pith (CP)
Local Drug Name: Tong-cao (C), Tung-cho (H), Tsuso (J), Tong-cho (K).
Processing: Slice like a paper. Eliminate foreign matter, cut into thick slices (C).
Method of Administration: Decoction (C, H, J, K).
Folk Medicinal Uses:
　　　　1) Edema and oliguria (J, C, K).
　　　　2) Dysuria with difficult painful urination (C).
　　　　3) Lack of milk secretion (C).
　　　　4) Amenorrhea (H).
　　　　5) Insect bite (J).
　　　　6) Headache (J).
　　　　7) Poisoning (K).

Scientific Researches:
　Chemistry
　　1) Saponins and triterpenoids: Papyrioside L-IIa [1], L-IIb, L-IIc and L-IId [3,4], papyrioside LA, LB, LC and LD [8], papyriogenin A [1], C, D, E [3,4], F [5], G [2], H and I [4], propapyriogenin A1 and A2 [3], chikusetsusaponin Ib and IV [6], β-D-glucopyranosyl oleanate-(3)- [α-L-arabino-furanosyl-(1→4)]- [β-D-galactopyranosyl-(1→2)]- methyl- (β-D-glucopyranosid) uronate, α-L-rhamnopyranosyl-(1→4)-β-D-glucopyranosyl-(1→6)-β-D-glucopyranosyl oleanate-(3)-α-L-arabinofuranosyl-(1→4)]-methyl-(β-D-glucopyranosid) uronate, β-D-glucopyranosyl oleanate-(3)-β-D- galactopyranosyl-(1→2)-methyl-(β-D-glucopyranosid)uronate, methyl oleanate-(3)-[α-L-arabinofuranosyl-(1→4)]-[β-D-galactopyranosyl-(1→2)]-methyl-(β-D-glucopyranosid)uronate, β-sitosterol β-D-glucopyranoside, Oleanolic acid -(3)-β-D-galactopyranosyl-(1→2)-β-D-fuco-pyranoside [11].
　　2) Flavonoids: Quercitrin [4].
　　3) Essential oil [7].
　　4) Trace elements and amino acids [12].
　Pharmacology
　　1) Antiinflammatory activity (oleanane triterpenoid glycosides) [9].
　　2) Antihepatotoxic activity (papyriogenins, papyriosides and triterpenoids) [10].

Literatures :
[1] Takai, M. et al.: J. Chem. Soc., Perkin Trans. 1 **1977**, (16), 1801.
[2] Ogihara, Y. et al.: J. Chem. Soc., Chem. Commun. **1978**(8), 364.

[3] Amagaya, S. *et al.*: *J. Chem. Soc., Perkin Trans 1* **1979**, (8), 2044.
[4] Amagaya, S. *et al.*: *Shoyakugaku Zasshi* **1979**, 33(3), 166.
[5] Asada, M. *et al.*: *J. Chem. Soc., Perkin Trans. 1* **1980**,(1), 325.
[6] Takabe, S. *et al.*: *Shoyakugaku Zasshi* **1980**, 34(1), 69: *J. Chem. Res., Synop.* **1981**, (1), 16.
[7] Fujita, S.: *Agric. Biol. Chem.* **1980**, 44(8), 1953.
[8] Kojima, K. *et al.*: *Chem. Pharm. Bull.* **1996**, 44(11), 2107.
[9] Sugishita E. *et al.*: *J. Pharmacobio-Dyn.* **1982**, 5(6), 379.
[10] Hikino, H. *et al.*: *J. Ethnopharmacol.* **1984,** 12(2) 231.
[11] Takabe, S. *et al.*: *Chem. Pharm. Bull.* **1985**, 33(11), 4701.
[12] Wang, L.: *Zhongcaoyao* **1986,** 17(8), 369.

[T. Kimura]

510.   *Anethum graveolens* **L.**   (Umbelliferae)

Shi-luo(C), Himeaikyo(J), Si-ra(K)

Fruit
Local Drug Name: Jirashi(J), Si-ra-ja(K)
Processing: Dry under the sun(J, K)
Method of Administration: Oral(decoction, J, K)
Folk Medicinal Uses:

1) Dyspepsia(J)
2) Meteorism(J)
3) Flatulence(K)
4) Emmenagogue(K)
5) Vomiting(K)
6) Hiccoughs(K)
7) Kidney stone(K)
8) Diarrhea(K)

Scientific Research:
Chemistry
1) Coumarins: aesculetin, bergapten[1], 4-methyl-aesculetin[2]
2) Monoterpenes: anethofuran, carvone, limonene[3], β-pinene[12]
3) Sesquiterpenes: β-caryophyllene, β-eudesmol[4], α-cubebene[5]
4) Flavonoids: apigenin, apigenin-7-O-α-D-glucuronide[6], hyperoside[7], kaempferol glyco-flavone, kaempferol-3-O-β-D-glucuronide[8], 4'-methoxy kaempferol[9]
5) Phenylpropanoids: caffeic acid[1], *p*-coumaric acid[10], dillapiole[11]
6) Xanthones: dillanol, dillanoside[13]
7) Lignans: dillfuran[4]
8) Sterols: ergosterl[2]
9) Lipids: petroselinic acid[14]
10) Alkaloids: piperane[15]
11) Oils[23]
Phamacology
1) Cancer chemopreventive activity(anethofuran, carvone, limonene)[3]
2) Antimutagenic activity[16]
3) Antifungal activity[17]
4) Hypotensive activity(essential oil)[18, 20]
5) Spasmolytic activity(essential oil)[18]
6) Antimitotic activity[19]
7) Hypoglycemic activity[20]
8) Antihyperlipemic activity[21]

9) Diuretic activity[22]

Literature:
[1] Dranik, L. I. and Prokopenko, A. P.: *Khim. Prir. Soedin* **1969**, 5(5), 437.
[2] Glowniak, K. and Doraczynska, A.: *Ann Univ. Mariae Curie-Sklodowska Sect D* **1984**, 37, 251.
[3] Zheng, G. Q. *et al.*: *Planta Med.* **1992**, 58(4), 338.
[4] Ahmad, A. *et al.*: *Phytochemistry* **1990**, 29(6), 2035.
[5] Pino, J. A. *et al.*: *J. Essent. Oil Res.* **1995**, 7(2), 219.
[6] Skorikova, Y. G. and Gavrilishina, L. I.: *Konservn Ovoshchlesush PROM-ST* **1979**, 31.
[7] Teuber, H. and Herrmann, K.: *Z. Lebensm-Unters Forsch.* **1978**, 167(2), 101.
[8] Harbone, J. B. and Williams, C. A.: *Phytochemistry* **1972**, 11, 1741.
[9] Daniel, M.: *Curr. Sci.* **1989**, 58(23), 1332.
[10] Schultz, J. M. and Herrmann, K.: *Z. Lebensm-Unters Forsch.* **1980**, 171, 193.
[11] Badoc, A. and Lamarti, A.: *J. Essent. Oil Res.* **1991**, 3(4), 269.
[12] Charles, D. J. *et al.*: *J. Essent. Oil Res.* **1995**, 7(1), 11.
[13] Kozawa, M. *et al.*: *Chem. Pharm. Bull.* **1976**, 24, 220.
[14] Kleiman, R. and Spencer, G. F.: *J. Amer. Oil Chem. Soc.* **1982**, 59, 29.
[15] Jain, A. K. *et al.*: *Indian J. Chem. Ser. B* **1986**, 25(9), 979.
[16] Natake, M. *et al.*: *Agr. Biol. Chem.* **1989**, 53(5), 1423.
[17] Leifertova, I. and Lisa, M.: *Folia Pharm(Prague)* **1979**, 2, 29.
[18] Shipochliev, T.: *Vet. Med. Nauki* **1968**, 5(6), 63.
[19] Gavaudan, P. and Gavaudan, N.: *C R Acad. Sci.* **1940**, 210, 576.
[20] Dhar, M. L. *et al.*: *Indian J. Exp. Biol.* **1968**, 6, 232.
[21] Dil, A. H.: *Proc. Third Asian Symposium on Medicinal Plants and Species,* Colombo Sri Lanka, Feb. 1977 **1977**, 17.
[22] Mahran, G. H. *et al.*: *Phytother. Res.* **1991**, 5(4), 169.
[23] Narzieva, M. D. *et al.*: *Khim. Prir. Soedin.* **1974**, 10(2), 243.

[C. K. Sung]

511.   *Angelica tenuissima* **Nakai**   (Umbelliferae)

Go-bon(K)

Root
Local Drug Name: Go-bon(K)
Processing: Dry under the sun(K)
Method of Administration: Oral(decoction, K)
Folk Medicinal Uses:
        1) Headache(K)
        2) Lumbago(K)
        3) Red colored nose(K)
        4) Swelling leg(K)

Scientific Research:
Chemistry
  1) Coumarins: Isoimperatorin, prangolarin[1]
  2) Steroids: β-Sitosterol[1]
Phamacology[3]
  1) Antiinflammatory activity[2]

Literature:
[1] Ryu, K. S. *et al.*: *Korean J. Pharmacog.* **1971**, 2, 87.
[2] Han, B. H. *et al.*: *Korean J. Pharmacog.* **1972**, 4(3), 205.

[3] Shin, K. H. *et al.*: *Korean J. Pharmacog.* **1980**, 11, 109.

[C. K. Sung]

512.　　　*Ligusticum jeholense* **Nakai et Kitag.**　(Umbelliferae)

Liao-gao-ben (C)

Related Plant:　*L. sinense* Oliv.: Gao-ben (C), Kohon (J); *L. tenuissimum* (Nakai) kitag.: Go-bon (K).

Rhizome and Root (CP)
Local Drug Name: Gao-ben (C, K), Goh-boon (H).
Processing: Eliminate foreign matter, wash, soften thoroughly, cut into thick slices, and dry in the
　　　　　sun (C).
Method of Administration: Oral (decoction: C, H, K).
Folk Medicinal Uses:
　　　　　　　　1) Pain at the top of the head in colds (C, H, J, K).
　　　　　　　　2) Rheumatic arthralgia (C, H, K).

Scientific Researches:
Chemistry
　1) Essential oils [1].
　2) Organic acids: ferulic acid [1].
　3) Phenols and theri derivatives: myristicin [1].
　4) Lactones: ligustilide [2].
Pharmacology
　1) Antifungal effect [4].

Literatures:
[1]　Dai, B.: *Yaowu Fenxi Zazhi* **1993,** 13(4), 237.
[2]　Lu, R.M. *et al.*: *Yao Hsueh Hsueh Pao* **1980,** (6), 371.
[3]　Sun, X.: *Zhonghua Pifuke Zazhi* **1958,** 6, 210.

[J.X. Guo]

513.　　　*Notopterygium forbesii* **Boiss.**　(Umbelliferae)

Kuan-ye-qiang-huo (C)

Related Plant: *N. incisum* Ting ex H.J. Chang: Qiang-huo (C); *Ostericum koreanum* Kit.: Gang-hwal
　　　　　(K).

Rhizome and Root (CP)
Local Drug Name: Qiang-huo (C), Keung-wood (H), Kyokatsu (J), Gang-hwal (K).
Processing: Eliminate foreign matter, wash clean, soften thoroughly, cut into thick slices, and dry in
　　　　　the sun (C, K).
Method of Administration: Oral (decoction: C, H, K).
Folk Medicinal Uses:
　　　　　　　　1) Headache in common cold (C, H, J, K).
　　　　　　　　2) Rheumatic arthralgia (C, H, K).
　　　　　　　　3) Aching of the back and shoulders (C, H).

Scientific Researches:

Chemistry
  1) Organic acids: ferulic acid [1], *trans*-ferulic acid [2].
  2) Steroids: β-sitosteryl-*O*-β-D-glucopyranoside [2].
  3) Coumarins: bergamottin, cnidilin, nodakenetin [2], notopterol, notoptol, anhydronotoptol, isoimperatorin, bergapten, bergaptol, nodakerin, osthenol, demethylfuropinnarin [3]. bergaptol-*O*-β-D-glucopyranoside, 6'-*O*-*trans*-feruloylnodakenin [4], columbianetin [5].
  4) Essential oils: farcarindiol [3].
  5) Others: 4'-hydroxy-3,5-dimethoxystilbene [2], phenethyl ferulate, *p*-hydroxyphenethyl anisate [3].

Literatures:
[1] Lu, R.M. *et al.*: *Chung Ts'ao Yao* **1980,** 11(9), 395.
[2] Yang, X.M. *et al.*: *Zhongguo yaoxue Zazhi* **1994,** 29(3), 141.
[3] Kozawa, M. *et al.*: *Chem. Pharm. Bull.* **1983,** 31(8), 2712.
[4] Gu, Z.M. *et al.*: *Chem. Pharm. Bull.* **1990,** 38(9), 2498.
[5] Xin, L.J. *et al.*: *Zhiwu Xuebao* **1988,** 30(5), 562.

[J.X. Guo]

514.   *Torilis japonica* **Decandolle**   (Umbelliferae)

Qie-yi(C), Yabujirami(J), Sa-sang-ja(K)

Fruit
Local Drug Name: Qie-yi(C), Jashoshi(J), Sa-sang-ja(K),
Processing: dry under the sun(C, K)
Method of Administration: Oral(decoction, C, K), Topical (decoction:C)
Folk Medicinal Uses:
                1) Trichomonas vaginalis(C)
                2) Carbuncle(C)
                3) Ascariasis(C)
                4) Chronic diarrhea(C)
                5) Women's diseases(J)
                6) Impotence(K)
                7) Infertility(K)

Scientific Research:
Chemistry
  1) Flavonoids: chrisoeriol-7-O-β-D-glucoside, cynaroside, luteolin-7-rutinoside[1]
  2) Sesquiterpene: (-)-germacra-4(15)-trans-5-10-(14)-trien-1-beta-ol, (-)-germacrene D, humulene [2], oppositane A,B, C, D, E [3], torilolide, oxytorilolide[4]
Phamacology
  1) Antitumor activity [5, 7]
  2) Antispasmodic activity [6]
  3) Antibacterial activity, Spontaneous activity stimulation [8]
  4) Antihepatotoxic activity [9]

Literature:
[1] Harbone, J. B., Wiliams, C.A.: *Phytochemistry* **1972,** 11, 1741
[2] Itogawa, H. *et al.*: *Chem. Pharm.Bull.***1983,** 31, 1743.
[3] Itogawa, H. *et al.*: *Chem. Lett.* **1983,** 8, 1253.
[4] Itogawa, H. *et al.*: *Chem. Pharm. Bull.* **1986,** 34, 4682.
[5] Itogawa, H. *et al.*: *Shoyakugaku Zasshi* **1982,** 36, 145.
[6] Itogawa, H. *et al.*: *Shoyakugaku Zasshi* **1983,** 37, 223.

[7] Itogawa, H. : *Shoyakugaku Zasshi* **1988**, 108, 824.
[8] Woo, W.S. *et al.: Arch. Pharm. Res.* **1979**, 2, 127.
[9] Kim, Y. S., Park, K. H. : *Korean J. Pharmacog.* **1994**, 25, 388.

[C. K. Sung]

515. *Pyrola calliantha* H. Ans (Pyrolaceae)

Lu-ti-cao (C), Luk-harm-cho (H)

Related Plant: *P. decorata* H. Andres: Pu-tong-lu-ti-cao (C); *P. japonica* Klenz.: Ichiyakuso (J).

Herb (CP)
Local Drug Name: Lu-xian-cao (C), Luk-harm-cho (H).
Processing: Eliminate foreign matter, and cut into sections (C).
Method of Administration: Oral (decoction: C, H, J).
Folk Medicinal Uses:
        1) Arthralgia with weakness of the loins and knees (C, H).
        2) Excessive menstrual flow (C, H).
        3) Chronic phthisical cough (C, H).
        4) Traumatic hemorrhage (J).

Scientific Researches:
Chemistry
  1) Glycosides: arbutin [1], homoarbutin, isohomoarbutin [2], hyperin, 2"-*O*-galloylhyperin, 6'-*O*-galloylhomoarbutin, renifolin [3], hydroxylrenifolin [4].
  2) Tannins: gallotannin [1], catechin [4].
  3) Triterpenoids: ursolic acid [5].
  4) Sugars: sucrose [5].
  5) Enzymes: emulsin [5].
  6) Essential oils [5].
  7) Quinone compunds: chimaphillin [6], methyl hydroquinone [7].
Pharmacology
  1) Tannin activity and anti-oxidation activity [3].
  2) Antibacterial effect [5,7,8].
  3) Cordial effect [9,10].
  4) Inhibit gestation [11].
  5) Effect on tissue volume of blood flow and the content of plasma cyclonucleotide [12].

Literatures:
[1] Zhang, D. *et al.: Zhongyao Tongbao* **1987,** 12(5), 301, 310.
[2] Thieme, H.: *Pharmazie* **1970,** 25(2), 129.
[3] Chen, X. M. *et al.: Tianran Chanwu Yanjiu Yu Kaifa* **1991,** 3(3), 1.
[4] Wang, J. X. *et al.: Zhiwu Xuebao* **1994,** 36(11), 895.
[5] *"Zhejiang Yaoyong Zhiwu Zhi"* **1980,** (3), 956.
[6] Robert, F. *et al.: Arch. Pharm.* **1930,** 268, 185.
[7] *"Zhongcaoyao Tongxun"* **1976,** 7(7), 12.
[8] Suzhou Medical College: *Hubei Keji Ziliao Yiyao Fence* **1971,** (2), 21.
[9] Zhejiang Medical University: *Yixue Keyan Ziliao* **1972,** (6), 39.
[10] Fang, C. *et al.: Kexue* **1946,** 28(6), 266.
[11] *"Zhongguo Shengli Kexuehui Xueshuhui Yilunwen Zhaiyao Huibian"* (Pharmacology) **1964,** 69.
[12] Zheng, Z. Y. *et al.: Zhongyao Tongbao* **1986,** 11, 179.

[J.X. Guo]

516.   *Arctostaphylos uva-ursi* **Sprengel**   (Ericaceae)

Kumakokemomo (J), U-ba-u-ru-shi (K).

Leaf (JP)
Local Drug Name: Uwa-urushi (J), U-ba-u-ru-shi (K).
Processing: Dry under the sun (J, K).
Method of Administration: Decoction, fluid extract (J, K).
Folk Medicinal Uses:
  1) Nephritis, pyelitis (J, K).
  2) Cystitis, pylocystitis, urethritis (J, K).
  3) Bladder stone (J).

Scientific Researches:
Chemistry
  1) Phenolic compounds: Arbutin, methylarbutin, hydroquinone [1], arbutin diacetate, galloyl arbutin, [2], piceoside [8], 4-hydroxyacetophenone-β-D-glucopyranoside [12], 2-hydroxybenzoic acid, 4-hydroxybenzoic acid, 3,4,5-trihydroxybenzoic acid, 3,4-dihydroxybenzoic acid, 3,4-dihydroxyphenyl acetic acid, 4-hydroxy-3-methoxybenzoic acid, 3-(3,4-dihydroxyphenyl)-2-propenoic acid, gentisic acid, 3-(2-hydroxyphenyl)propanoic acid, sinapic acid, isoferulic acid, ferulic acid and 3-(4-hydroxyphenyl)-2-propenoic acid [13].
  2) Tannins: A gallotannin (penta- to hexa-*O*-galloyl-β-D-glucose), ellagitannin, ellagic acid, gallic acid [2].
  3) Triterpenoids and steroids: Ursolic acid [1], β-sitosterol, betulinic acid, oleanolic acid, uvaol, lupeol, α- and β-amyrin [9].
  4) Flavonoids: Quercetin [1,2], corilagin and myricetin [2,15].
  5) Wax alkanes [10].
  6) Saccharides: Oligosaccharides [11].
Pharmacology
  1) Antibacterial activity (hydoquinone, 4-hydroxyacetophenone-β-D-glucopyranoside) [3,12], antivirus(herpes and influenza) (aq. extract) [4].
  2) Increasing of effect of predonisolone and indomethacine on dermatitis (aq. extract and arbutin) [5].
  3) Inhibitor of histamine release from mast cells (extract) [6].
  4) Whitening agent activity, melanin biosynthesis inhibition (50% ethanol extract) [7].
  5) Antifungal activity (phenolic acids) [14].

Literatures:
  [1] Kimura, K. *et al.*: *Yakugaku Zasshi* **1970**, 90, 394.: Sticher, O. *et al,*: *Planta Med.* **1979**, 35, 253; Akada, Y. *et al.*: *Yakugaku Zasshi* **1979**, 99, 98; Christ, B. *et al.*: *Arzneimittel-Forsch.* **1921**, 11, 129.
  [2] Britton, G. *et al.*: *J. Chem, Soc.* **1965**, 7312; Holopainen, M. *et al.*: *Acta Pharm. Fenn.* **1988**, 97(4), 197.
  [3] Frohne, D.: *Planta Med.* **1970**, 18, 1.
  [4] May, G. *et al.*: *Arzneim. Forsch.* **1978**, 28, 1.
  [5] Kubo, M. *et al.*: *Yakugaku Zasshi* **1990**, 110, 59; *Ibid*, 68; *Ibid*, 253; *Ibid*. 673.
  [6] Ogura, K.: *Jpn. Kokai Tokkyo Koho* **1996** JP 08053360 A2
  [7] Matsuda, H. *et al.*: *Yakugaku Zasshi* **1992**, 112, 276; *Biol. Pharm. Bull.* **1996**, 19(1), 153.
  [8] Karikas, G. A. *et al.*: *Planta Med.* **1987**, 53(3), 307.
  [9] Jahodar, L. *et al.*: *Pharmazie* **1988**, 43(6), 442.
  [10] Salasoo, I.: *Biochem. Syst. Ecol.* **1986**, 15(!), 105.
  [11] Leifertova, I. *et al.*: *Farm. Obz.* **1989**, 58(11), 507.
  [12] Jahodar, L. *et al.*: *Pharmazie* **1990**, 45(6), 446.
  [13] Dombrowicz, E. *et al.*: *Pharmazie* **1991**, 46,(9), 680.

[14] Cipollini, M. *et al.*: *Biochem. Syst. Ecol.* **1992**, 20(6), 501.
[15] Belousov, M. V. *et al.*: *Rastit. Resur.* **1994**, 30(4), 44.

[T. Kimura]

517.   *Rhododendron japonicum* **Suringer**   (Ericaceae)

Renge-tsutsuji (J)

Related plant: *Rhododendron molle* (Bl.) G. Don, Nao-yang-hua (C).

Flower and root
   Local Drug Name: Yotekichoku (J).
   Processing: Use in fresh (J)
   Method of Administration: Liquor (J)
   Folk Medicinal Uses:
              1) Rheumatism (C, J).
              2) Pain (C, J).
              3) Gout (J).
   Contraindications: Toxic in overdose. Nausea, vomiting, breath disorder, convulsion and paralysis.

Scientific Researches:
   Chemistry
      1) Diterpenoids: Grayanotoxin I (=andromedotoxin), sparassol [4], rhodojaponin I, II [1,2], III,
         IV, V, VI and VII [2].
      2) Others: β-Sitosterol, β-sitosterol glucoside, quercetin, ursolic acid, oleanolic acid, friedelin,
         α-amyrin, β-amyrin, maslinic acid, coumarin [1,3].

Literatures:
[1] Yasue, M. et al.: *Yakugaku Zasshi*, **1973**, 93, 1668.
[2] Hikino, H. et al.: *Chem. Pharm. Bull.* **1969**, 17, 1078; **1970**, 18, 1071; **1972**, 20, 1090; Iriye, H.
   et al.: *Tetrahedron Lett.* **1972**, 1381.
[3] Takemoto, T. et al.: *Yakugaku Zasshi* **1958**, 78, 304.
[4] Takemoto, T. et al.: *Yakugaku Zasshi* **1958**, 78, 110.

[T. Kimura]

518.   *Rhododendron metternichii* **Sieb. et Zucc. var.** *hondoensis* **Nakai**
(Ericaceae)

Hon-shakunage (J)

Related plant: *Rhododendron simsii* Planch., Du-jian-hua (C).

Leaf
   Local Drug Name: Shakunage-yo (J).
   Processing: Dry under the sun (J).
   Method of Administration: Decoction (J).
   Folk Medicinal Uses:
              1) Gout (J).
              2) Rheumatism (J).
               3) Traumatic injury (C).

4) Menstrual disorder (C).
Contraindications: Toxic in overdose. Nausea, vomiting, convulsion and paralysis.

Scientific Researches:
Chemistry
1) Diterpenoids: Grayanotoxin I (=andromedotoxin) and III [1].
2) Triterpenoids: Lupeol, ursolic acid and betulinic acid [1].
Pharmacology
1) Toxicity (grayanotoxin) [2].

Literatures:
[1] Ohue, H. *et al.*: *Yakugaku Zasshi* **1974**, 94(6), 756.
[2] Hikino, H. *et al.*: *Chem. Pharm. Bull.* **1979**, 27(4), 874.
[3] Takemoto, T. *et al.*: *Yakugaku Zasshi* **1958**, 78, 110; 304.

[T. Kimura]

519.   *Ardisia crenata* **Sims**   (Myrsinaceae)

Yun-chi-zi-jin-niu (C), Chu-sar-gun (H), Baek-ryang-geum (K)

Related plants: *Ardisia bicolor* Walk.: Zi-bei-zi-jin-niu (C).

Root and Leaf
Local Drug Name: Zhu-sha-gen (C), Chu-sar-gun (H), Ju-sa-geun (K).
Processing: Slice and dry under the sun (C, H, K).
Method of Administration: Oral (decoction: C, H, K); Topical (Mashed root or fresh leaf: C, H).
Folk Medicinal Uses:
1) Rheumatic arthritis (C, H, K).
2) Sorethroat (C, H, K).
3) Tonsillitis (C, H, K).
4) Bronchitis (C, H, K).
5) Traumatic injury (C, H, K).
6) Lymphadenitis (C, H).
7) Snake bite (C, H).
8) Upper respiratory tract infections (C, H).
9) Lumbago (C).
10) Diptheria (C).
11) Erysipelas (C).
12) Fracture (C).
13) Swelling pain of wounds (C).
14) Scarlet fever (H).

Scientific Research:
Chemistry
1) Cyclic depsipeptide: FR900395 [13].
2) Sapogenin: cyclamiretin A [4].
3) Bergenin, friedelin, β-sitosterol, rapanone [5], 11-O-syringylbergenin, carotene, demethyl-bergenin, sucrose [6].
4) Ardicrenin [7], ardisiacrispins A and B, ardisicrenosides A-F [8-10].
Pharmacology
1) Inhibitory effect on plaletet aggregation [1, 3].
2) Hypotensive effect [1, 3].
3) Inhibitory activity on cAMP phosphodiesterase [9, 10].

4) Antifertility effect [4, 11]
5) Inhibitory effect on murine retroviral reverse transcriptase and human DNA polymerases [12].
6) Insecticidal effect [13].

Literature:

[1] Fujioka, M.*et al.*: *J. Org. Chem.* **1988,** 53, 2820.
[2] Miyamae, A. *et al.*: Pept. Chem. **1986,** 24, 135.
[3] Fujioka, M. *et al.*: *Tennan Yuki Kagobutsu Koen Yoshishu* **1986,** 28, 160.
[4] Guan, X.T. *et al.*: *Zhongcaoyao* **1987,** 18, 338.
[5] Ni, M.Y. *et al.*: *Zhongyao Tongbao* **1988,** 13, 737.
[6] Han, L. *et al.*: *Zhongguo Zhongyao Zazhi* **1989,** 14, 737.
[7] Wang, M.T. *et al.*: *Planta Med.* **1992,** 58, 205.
[8] Jia, Z.H. *et al.*: *Phytochemistry* **1994,** 37, 1389.
[9] Jia, Z.H. *et al.*: *Chem. Pham. Bull.* **1994,** 42, 2309.
[10] Jia, Z.H. *et al.*: *Tetrahedron* **1994,** 50, 11853.
[11] Wang, H.Z. *et al.*: *Zhongcaoyao* **1988,** 19, 499.
[12] Ono, Katsuhiko *et al.*: *Chem. Pharm. Bull.* **1989,** 37, 1810.
[13] Earth Chemical Co. Ltd.: *Jpn. Kokai Tokkyo Koho JP 59,205,391,* **1984.**

[P.P.H. But]

520.   *Ardisia japonica* **Blume**   (Myrsinaceae)

Zi-jin-niu (C), Gee-gum-ngau (H), Yabukoji (J), Ja-geum-u (K)

Root
Local Drug Name: Zi-jin-niu (C), Gee-gum-ngau (H), Shikingyu (J), Ja-geum-u (K).
Processing: Dry under the sun (C, J, K).
Method of Administration: Oral (decoction: C, H, J, K), topical (decoction: C, H).
Folk Medicinal Uses:
       1) Traumatic injury (C, H).
       2) Bronchitis (C, K).
       3) Sore throat (J, K).
       4) Lobar pneumonia (C).
       5) Infantile pneumonia (C).
       6) Pulmonary tuberculosis (C).
       7) Hepatitis (C).
       8) Dysentery (C).
       9) Acute nephritis (C).
     10) Urinary infection (C).
     11) Dysmenorrhea (C).
     12) Paint dermatitis (C).
     13) Rheumatism (C).
     14) Cutaneous pruritus (C).
     15) Stomach ache (J).

Scientific Researches:
Chemistry
    1) Saponins: Cyclamiretin A 3β-*O*-α-L-rhamnopyranosyl-(1→4)-β-D-glucopyranosyl-(1→2)-[β-D-glucopyranosyl-(1→4)]α-L-arabinopyranoside [1,9], 3β-*O*-α-{L-rhamnopyranosyl-(1→4)-β-D-glucopyranosyl-(1→2)-[β-D-glucopyranosyl-(1→4)]α-L-arabinopyranoside}-16α-hydroxy-13,28-epoxyolean-29-oic   acid   and   3β-*O*-{α-L-rhamnopyranosyl-(1→4)-β-D-glucopyranosyl-(1→2)-[β-D-glucopyranosyl-(1→4)]   α-L-arabinopyranoside}16α-hydroxy-

13,28-epoxy-30,30-dimethoxyoleane [9].
2) Phenolic compounds: Bergenin, norbergenin [1,2], ardisin (=ardicinol I) [3], ardisinol II [4], quercetin, embelin and ilexol [5], ardisianone A, B and maesanin [8].
3) Essential oil [7].
Pharmacology
1) Anti human immunodeficiency virus (HIV) (bergenin, norbergenin) [1].
2) Antitubercular (ardicin and ardicinol II) [4].
3) Antiasthmatic and anti-inflmmtion (1,4-benzoquinones) [6].
4) Inhibition of 5-lipoxygenase (ardisianone A, B and maesanin) [8].

Literatures:

[1] Piacenthe, S. *et al.*: *J. Nat. Prod.* **1996**, 59(6), 565.
[2] Chinese Academy of Medical Sciences: *Chih Wu Hsueh Pao* **1977**, 19(3), 172.
[3] Liang, B.-L. *et al.*: *K'o Hsueh T'ung Pao* **1979**, 24(19), 910.
[4] Hu, Y. *et al.*: *K'o Hsueh T'ung Pao* **1979**, 24(19), 907; *Hua Hsueh Hsueh Pao* **1981**, 39(2), 153.
[5] Huang, P.-H. *et al.*: *Yao Hsueh T'ung Pao* **1980**, 15(10),39; Huang B.-H. et al.: *Yao Hsueh Hsueh Pao* **1981**, 16(1), 27.
[6] Otsuka Pharm. Co. Ltd.: *Japan Kokai Tokkyo Koho* JP 8575442 A2, JP 6075442, 850427.
[7] Yin, L. *et al.*: *Zhongcaoyao* **1989**, 20(10), 437.
[8] Fukuyama, H. *et al.*: *Chem. Pharm. Bull.* **1993**, 41(3), 561.
[9] De Tommasi, N. *et al.*: *J. Nat. Prod.* **1993**, 56(10), 1669.

[T. Kimura]

521.　　　　　*Maesa perlarius* **(Lour.) Merr.**　　(Myrsinaceae)

Ji-yu-dan (C), Juck-yu-darm (H)

Whole Plant
Local Drug Name: Ji-yu-dan (C), Juck-yu-darm (H).
Processing: Use when fresh (H).
Method of Administration: Topical (Macerated fresh herb: C, H).
Folk Medicinal Uses:
　　　　　1) Traumatic wounds and cuts (C, H).
　　　　　2) Pyodermas (H).
　　　　　3) Sore (C).
　　　　　4) Fracture and detumescence (C).

Scientific Research:
Chemistry
1) Alkaloids: $C_{26}H_{54}O_2N_4$, trihydrochloride, tris(p-toluenesulfonate) [1].
2) Catechol [2].

Literature:

[1] Arthur, H.R. *et al.*: *Phytochemistry* **1966, 5**, 379.
[2] Dzhemukhadze, K.M. *et al.*: *Prikl. Biokhim. Mikrobiol.* **1972, 8**, 207.

[P.P.H. But]

522.　　　　　*Lysimachia christinae* **Hance**　　(Primulaceae)

Guo-lu-huang (C)

Herb (CP)

Local Drug Name: Jin-qian-cao (C).

Processing: Eliminate foreign matter, wash briefly, cut into sections, and dry in the sun, or use in fresh (C).

Method of Administration: Oral (decoction: C).

Folk Medicinal Uses:

       1) Acute urinary infections or urolithiasis with difficult painful urination (C).

       2) Jaundice with dark urine (C).

       3) Hepatic or biliary caleules (C).

       4) Carbuncles (C).

       5) Sores (C).

       6) Venomous snake bite (C).

Scientific Researches:

Chemistry

1) Amino acids [1].
2) Alkaloids: choline [2].
3) Steroids [2].
4) Phenols [2].
5) Inorganic salts: nitrite salts, NaCl, KCl [3].
6) Organic acids: hydroxybenzoic acid [4].
7) Naclic acids: uridine [4].
8) Flavonoids: quercetin, quercetin-3-O -glucoside, kaempferol, kaempferol-3-O-galactoside, kaempferol-3-O-lysinachiatrioside, 3,2',4',6'-tetrahydroxy-4,3'-dimethoxychalone [3], rhamnocitrin-3,4'-diglucoside, kaemptferol-3-rutoside, kaempferol-3-rhamnoside-7-rhamnosyl-(1→3)-rhamnoside [4], kaempferol-3-glucoside [4,5], myricetin 3-rhamnosides, kaempferol 3-(2,6-dirhamnopyranosylglucopyranoside), vicenin-2, kaempferol 3-dirhamnosylglucoside [5].

Pharmacology

1) Cholagogic effect [2].
2) Bacteriostasis [6].
3) Effect on immune response [7,8].
4) Effect on ureterolith [9].
5) Inhibit the crystallization of calcium oxalate monohydrate [10].

Literatures:

[1] *"Zhongcaoyao Youxiaochengfen De Yanjiu"* **1972,** Vol.1, 404.
[2] Nanjing College of Pharmacy: *Zhongcaoyao Xue* **1976,** Vol.2, 809.
[3] Shen, L. D. *et al.*: *Zhongyao Tongbao* **1988,** 13(11), 671.
[4] Zhao, S. P. et al.: *Zhongcaoyao* **1988,** 19(6), 245.
[5] Yasukawa, K. *et al.*: *Planta Med.* **1993,** 59(6), 578.
[6] *"Zhongyyao Zhi"* **1988,** Vol.4, 109.
[7] Yao, C. Z. *et al.*: *Zhongyao Yixue Kexueyuan Xuebao* **1981,** 3(2), 123.
[8] Yao, C. Z. *et al.*: *Zhongyao Yixue Kexueyuan Xuebao* **1982,** 4(5), 286.
[9] Mo, L. J. *et al.*: *Xinzhongyi* **1985,** (6), 51.
[10] Li, H. Z. *et al.*: *Shenyang Yaoxueyuan Xuebao* **1988,** 208, 5(3).

[J.X. Guo]

523.   *Primula japonica* **A. Gray**   (Primulaceae)

Kurinso (J)

Related plant: *Primula vittata* Bur. et Franch.: Bao-chun-hua (C).

Leaf
  Local Drug Name: Kurinso (J).
  Processing: Fresh leaf (J).
  Method of Administration: Apply externally (C, J).
  Folk Medicinal Uses:
           1) Breeding (C).
           2) Traumatic injury (J).
           3) Swelling (J).

Scientific Researches:
  Chemistry
    1) Flavonoids: flavone [1].
    2) Saponins and sapogenins: Dihydropriverogenin A, primulagenin A, protoprimulagenin A
       [2, 3].

Literatures:
  [1] Wollenweber, E. *et al.*: *Z. Naturforsch., C, Biosci.* **1988**, 43(3-4), 305.
  [2] Kitagawa, I. *et al.*: *Chem. Pharm. Bull.* **1972**, 20(10), 2226.
  [3] Kitagawa, I. *et al.*: *Chem. & Ind.* **1973**(6), 276.

[T. Kimura]

524.   *Ligustrum japonicum* **Thunb.**   (Oleaceae)

Nezumimochi (J), Gwang-na-mu (K)

Related Plant: *Ligstrum lucidum* Ait. , To-nezumimochi (J), Dang-gwang-na-mu (K).

Fruit
  Local Drug Name: Nyoteishi (J) , Yeo-jeong-sil (K).
  Processing: Dry under the sun (J, K).
  Method of Administration: Decoction (J, K).
  Folk Medicinal Uses:
           1) Eye diseases (J, K).
           2) Weakness (J, K).
           3) Neurasthenia (J).

Leaf
  Local Drug Name: Nyoteiyo (J), Yeo-jeong-yeop (K) .
  Processing: Dry under the sun (J, K).
  Method of Administration: Decoction (J, K). Extract (J).
  Folk Medicinal Uses:
           1) Gastric ulcer (J, K).
           2) Stomatitis (J, K).
           3) Eye diseases (J, K).

Scientific Researches:
  Chemistry
    1) Triterpenoids and steroids: Acetyl oleanolic acid [1,2], β-sitosterol, lupeol [3], ursolic acid,
       acetylursolic acid, oleanolic acid [2], α- and β-amyrin [4]
    2) Lignans: Syringaresinol, [5].
    3) Phenolic compounds: 2(4-Hydroxyphenyl)ethanol, 2(3,4-dihydroxyphenyl)ethanol, salidro-
       side [2], benzoic acid, benzyl alcohol, benzaldehyde, phenylacetic acid, phenol, phenethyl

alcohol, 2-methoxyphenol, eugenol, ferulic acid and *p*-cumaric acid [4]

4) Flavonoid: Quercetin, taxifolin [2], kaempferol [4].

5) Fatty acids [6].

6) Iridoids: Ligustaloside A and B [7,8], ligustrosidic acid, oleuropeinic acid [9], neonuezhenide [9,10], oleuropein, 10-hydroxyligustroside, neuzhenin, acteoside, 10-hydroxyeulopein [2] and isonuezhenide [10], epikingiside [8].

7) Carbohydrates: Ligustrin A [11], cordycepic acid [2].

8) Others: Linalool and 3-hexen-1-ol [4], nonacosanol [3].

Literatures:

[1] Kung-tu, K. *et al.*: *Nippon Kagakukaishi* **1965**, 86, 323.

[2] Kikuchi, M. *et al.*: *Annu. Rep. Tohoku Coll. Pharm.* **1983**, 30, 33.

[3] Takemoto, T. *et al.*: *Yakugaku Kenkyu* **1957**, 29, 877.

[4] Kikuchi, M. *et al.*: *Yakugaku Zasshi* **1981**, 101(6), 575.

[5] Kudo, K. *et al.*: *Planta Med.* **1980**, 40(3), 250.

[6] Kashimoto, T.: *Nippon Kagaku Kaishi*, **1958**, 79, 403.

[7] Inoue, K. *et al.*: *Phytochem.* **1982**, 21(9), 2305.

[8] Kuwajima, H. *et al.*: *Phytochem.* **1989**, 28(5), 1409.

[9] Kikuchi, M. *et al.*: *Yakugaku Zasshi* **1985**, 105(2), 142.

[10] Fukuyama, Y. *et al.*: *Planta. Med.* **1987**, 53(5), 427.

[11] Kikuchi, M. *et al.*: *Yakugaku Zasshi* **1982**, 102(6), 533.

[T. Kimura]

525.   *Gelsemium elegans* **Benth.**   (Loganiaceae)

Hu-man-teng (C), Woo-marn-teng (H)

Whole Plant

Local Drug Name: Duan-chang-cao (C), Duan-cheung-cho (H).

Processing: use in fresh or dry under the sun (C, H).

Method of Administration: Topical (macerated fresh herb: C, H).

Folk Medicinal Uses:

1) Eczema (C, H).

2) Tinea corporis or tinea pedis (C, H).

3) Ttraumatic injury, fracture (C, H).

4) Hemorrhoids (C, H).

5) Leprosy (C, H).

6) Boils and pyodermas (C, H).

7) Pretibial ulcer (C, H).

8) Myiasis (C).

9) Scrofula (H).

Remarks: Poisonous, not for oral consumption.

Scientific Research:

Chemistry

1) Alkaloids: koumicine, koumidine, koumine, kouminidine, gelsemine [1–2, 17, 21], 7-deoxygelsemide, 9-deoxygelsemide [3], 20-hydroxydihydrorankinidine, N-desmethoxyhumantenine, 15-hydroxyhumantenine, gelsemoxonine[4], 19-(R)-hydroxydihydrogelsevirine, gelsevirine, 19-(R)-acetyldihydrogelsevirine, 19-(R)-hydroxydihydrogelsemine, 19-(S)-hydroxydihydrogelsevirine [5], 19-(Z)-akuammidine, 16-epi-voacarpine [6], dihydrokoumine [7], gelselegine, 11-methoxy-19-(R)-hydroxygelselegine [8], 19-(R)-hydroxydihydrokoumine, 19-(S)-hydrodihydrokoumine [9], (19R)-kouminol, (19S)-kouminol [10], N-methoxyanhydrovobasinediol [11], gelsamydine [12], N-desmethoxyrankinidine, 11-

hydroxyrankinidine, 11-hydroxyhumantenine, 11-methoxyhumantenine, rankinidine, humantenine, humantenrine (humantenirine) [13,17, 19–20, 22], gelsemamide, 11-methoxygelsemamide [14], elegansamine [15], 16-epivoacarpine, 19-(Z)-taberpsychine, 19-hydroxydihydrogelsevirine, 14-hydroxygelsedine, koumine-N-oxide, gelsemine-N-oxide, 19-oxogelsenicine, N-oxide, akuammidine [16, 17, 21], gelsenicine, 14-hydroxygelsenicine, 19-oxogelsenicine [17], humantendine (humantenidine) [18, 20, 22–23], gelsedine [21], humantenmine [22].

2) Gelsemide, gelsemiol [3].

Pharmacology
1) Analgesic activity [22].
2) Antitumor activity [24].
3) Cardiovascular effect [25–26].
4) Spasmolytic effect [27].

Literature:

[1] Liu, C.T. *et al.*: *Hua Hsueh Hsueh Pao* **1961**, 27, 47.
[2] Chi, Y.F. *et al.*: *J. Am. Chem. Soc.* **1938**, 60, 1723.
[3] Hiromitsu, Y. *et al.*: *Nat. Prod. Lett.* **1994**, 5,15.
[4] Lin, L.Z. *et al.*: *Phytochemistry* **1991**, 30, 1311.
[5] Lin, L.Z. *et al.*: *Phytochemistry* **1991**, 30, 679.
[6] Lin, L.Z. *et al.*: *Phytochem. Anal.* **1990**, 1, 26.
[7] Zhang, Z.P. *et al.*: *Chin. Chem. Lett.* **1991**, 2, 365.
[8] Lin, L.Z. *et al.*: *Phytochemistry* **1990**, 29, 3013.
[9] Lin, L.Z. *et al.*: *Phytochemistry* **1990**, 29, 965.
[10] Sun, F. *et al.*: *J. Nat. Prod.* **1989**, 52, 1180.
[11] Lin, L.Z. *et al.*: *Phytochemistry* **1989**, 28, 2827.
[12] Lin, L.Z. *et al.*: *J. Org. Chem.* **1989**, 54, 3199.
[13] Lin, L.Z. *et al.*: *J. Nat. Prod.* **1989**, 52, 588.
[14] Lin, L.Z. *et al.*: *Tetrahedron Lett.* **1989**, 30, 1177.
[15] Ponglux, D. *et al.*: *Tetrahedron Lett.* **1988**, 29, 5395 .
[16] Ponglux, D. *et al.*: *Tetrahedron* **1988**, 44, 5075.
[17] Sakai, S. *et al.*: *Tennen Yuki Kagobotsu Toronkai Koen Yoshishu* **1987**, 29, 224.
[18] Yang, J.S. *et al.*: *Yaoxue Xuebao* **1984**, 19, 437.
[19] Yang, J.S. *et al.*: *Yaoxue Xuebao* **1984**, 19, 686.
[20] Yang, J.S. *et al.*: *Yaoxue Xuebao* **1983**, 18, 104.
[21] Jin, H.L. *et al.*: *Huaxue Xuebao* **1982**, 40, 1129.
[22] Yang, J.S. *et al.*: *Yaoxue Tongbao* **1982**, 17, 119.
[23] Yang, J.S. *et al.*: *Yaoxue Xuebao* **1982**, 17, 633.
[24] Dai, R.H. *et al.*: *Zhongcaoyao* **1993**, 24, 471.
[25] Cahen, R. *et al.*: *Compt. Rend. Soc. Biol.* **1939**, 131, 686.
[26] Moisset de Espanes, E. *et al.*: *Compt. Rend. Soc. Biol.* **1938**, 129, 386.
[27] Uhlenbroock K. *et al.*: *Arzneimittel-Forsch* **1959**, 9, 419.

[P.P.H. But]

526.　　　　　　*Strychnos nux-vomica* L.　(Loganiaceae)

Ma-qian (C), Mar-chin-gee (H), Homika (J), Ma-jeon-ja (K)

Seed (JP, KP)
Local Drug Name: Ma-qian-zi (C), Mar-chin-gee (H), Homika (J), Ma-jeon-ja (K).
Processing: (1) Dry under the sun (C, H, J, K).
　　　　　　(2) Scald the clean seeds until inflated and turns into brown or dark brown (C).
　　　　　　(3) Pulverize the processed seed to fine powder (C).

111

Method of Administration: Oral (pills or powder after being processed: C, K; extract or tincture: J).
Folk Medicinal Uses:
> 1) Anorexia (J, K).
> 2) Dyspepsia (J, K).
> 3) Protracted arthritis, rheumatoid arthralgia (C).
> 4) Numbness and paralysis (C).
> 5) Boils and sores (C).
> 6) Traumatic injury (C).
> 7) Sequela of poliomyelitis (C).
> 8) Rheumatism (H).
> 9) Fracture (H).

Contraindications: Toxic. Stimulating heart.

Scientific Researches:

Chemistry
> 1) Alkaloids: Strychnine, vomicine [1,2], brucine [2], α-, β-colubrine, pseudostrychnine, pseudo-brucine, struxine, novacine, icajine, brucine *N*-oxide, 12-hydroxystrychnine, cantleyine [4], isostrychnine [5] and protstrychnine [7], 15-hydroxystrychnine [8], 3-methoxyicajine [9]
> 2) Iridoids: Loganin [3], secologanin, dehydrologanin, 7-deoxyloganin [4] and loganic acid [6], ligustrinoside [15].
> 3) Phenolic compounds: Cuchiloside [14].
> 4) Polysaccharides [17]

Pharmacology
> 1) Analgesic effect (seed alkaloids) [10].
> 2) Cytotoxicity (B-16 melanoma) in vitro (strychnopentaine, usambrensine) [11], cytotoxicity on some tumor cell lines (alkaloids from processed drug) [18].
> 3) Antioxidant effect (alcoholic extract) [12].
> 4) Insecticide [13].
> 5) Processing and acute toxicity (alkaloids) [16].

Literatures:

[1] Bisset, N. G. *et al.: Phytochem.* **1973**, 12, 2049.
[2] Quirin, M. *et al.: Ann. Pharm. Franc.* **1965**, 23, 93.
[3] Merz, K. W. *et al.: Arch. d. Pharm.* **1957,** 290, 543.
[4] Bisset, N. G. *et al.: Phytochem.* **1974**, 13(1), 265.
[5] Galeffi, C. *et al.: J. Chromatogr.* **1974**, 88(2), 416.
[6] Guarnaccia, R. *et al.: J. Am. Chem. Soc.* **1974**, 96(22), 7079.
[7] Baser, K. H. C. *et al.: Phytochem.* **1979,** 18(3), 512.
[8] Galeffi, C. *et al.: Atti Accad. Naz. Lincei, Cl. Sci. Fis., Mat. Nat., Rend.* **1978**, 65(6), 297; *Tetrahedron* **1979**, 35(21), 2545.
[9] Rodriguez, F. *et al.:* Phytochem. 1979,18(12), 2065.
[10] Cai, B.-C. *et al.: Biol. Pharm. Bull.*, **1996**, 19(1), 127.
[11] Bonjean, K. *et al.: Anticancer Res.* **1996**, 16(3A), 1129.
[12] Tripathi, Y. B. *et al.: Phytomedicine*, **1996**, 3(2), 175.
[13] Suryakala, G. *et al.: J. Reprod. Biol. Comp. Endocrinol.* **1983**, 3(2), 33.
[14] Bisset, N. G. *et al.: Phytochem.* **1989**, 28(5), 1553.
[15] Mitsunaga, K. *et al.: Chem. Pharm. Bull.* **1991**, 39(10), 2737.
[16] Cai, B.-C. *et al.: Wakan Iyakugaku Zasshi* **1994**, 11(2), 134.
[17] Corsaro, M. M. *et al.: Phytochem.* **1995,** 39(6), 1377.
[18] Cai, B.-C. *et al.: Nat. Med.* **1995**, 49(1), 39.

[T. Kimura]

527.　　　　　　*Gentiana lutea* L.　(Gentianaceae)

Genchiana (J), Gen-chi-a-na (K)

Root (JP)
Local Drug Name: Genchiana (J), Gen-chi-a-na (K).
Processing: Dry under the sun (J, K).
Method of Administration: Decoction (J, K).
Folk Medicinal Uses:
　　　　　1) Gastritis (J, K).
　　　　　2) Anorexia (J, K).
　　　　　3) Dyspepsia (J, K).

Scientific Researches:
Chemistry
　　1) Iridoids: Gentiopicroside [1], amarogentin, swertiamarin [2].
　　2) Xanthones: Gentisin, isogentisin [3], hydroxymethoxyprimeverosylxanthone [4].
　　3) Phenolic compounds: gentisic acid, mangiferin, gentioside, isoorientin, isovitexin [5].
　　4) Glycosides: Isoorientin-4-*O*-glucoside, isovitexin-4'-*O*-glucoside and isogentisin [6], iso-
　　　　orientin-2"-O-glucoside and isovitexin-2"-O-glucoside [7].
　　5) Carbohydrates: L-(+)-Bornesitol and meso-inositol [8], gentiobiose [9].
　　6) Essential oil: Limonene and many monoterpenoids [10], sesquiterpenoids [11].
　　7) Others [12].
Pharmacology
　　1) Increasing reflex secretion of gastric juice (extract, gentiopicroside) [13].
　　2) Increasing reflex secretion of saliva (extract) [14].
　　3) Choleretic activity (extract) [15].

Literatures:
　[1] Kromeyer, A. *et al.*: *Arch. d. Pharm.* **1862**, 110, 27; Korte *et al.*: *Ber.* **1954,** 87, 512; 780; **1958**,
　　　91, 759; 780; Canonica, L. *et al.*: *Gazz. Chem. Ital.* **1951,** 87, 1251; *Tetrahedron Lett.* **1960**(24),
　　　7; *Tetrahedron* **1961**, 16, 192; Manitto, P. *et al.*: *Gazz. Chim. Ital.* **1964,** 94, 229; Inouye, H. *et*
　　　al.: *Tetrahedron Lett.* **1968,** 4429.
　[2] Kubota, T. *et al.*: *Chem. Pharm. Bull.* **1961**, 34, 1345; Inouye, H. *et al.*: *Chem. Pharm. Bull.*
　　　1970, 18, 1856; Inouye, H. *et al.*: *Tetrahedron Lett.* **1967,** 3221; Bricout, J.: *Phytochem.* **1974**,
　　　13(12), 2819.
　[3] Nikolaeva, G. G. *et al.*: *Khim. Prir. Soedin* **1983**, (1), 107.
　[4] Hayashi, T. *et al.*: *Phytochem.* **1988**, 27(11), 3696.
　[5] Bellman, G. *et al.*: *Helv. Chim. Acta* **1973**, 56, 284.
　[6] Hostettmann, K. *et al.*: *Helv.*, **1973**, 56, 3050.
　[7] Burret, F. *et al.*: *Planta Med.* **1979**, 36(2), 178.
　[8] Bellman, G. *et al.*: *Helv. Chim. Acta* **1973**, 56, 773.
　[9] Badenhuizen, R. J. *et al.*: *J. Org. Chem.* **1964**, 29, 2079.
　[10] Chialva, F. *et al.*: Z. Lebensm.-Unters. Forsch. 1986, 182(3), 212.
　[11] Arberas, I. *et al.*: *Dev. food Sci.* **1995**, 37A, 207.
　[12] Inouye, H.: *Farumashia* **1971**, 7(3), 172.
　[13] Carlson, A. J. *et al.*: *J. Pharmacol. Exp. Ther.* **1914-5**, 6, 209; Chiarva, F. *et al.*: *Z. Lebensm.-*
　　　Unters. Forsch. **1986**, 182, 212; Ivancevic, I. *et al.*: *Arch. Exp. Pathol. Pharmakol.* **1938**, 189,
　　　557; Schmid, W.: *Planta Med.* **1966**, 14, Suppl. 34; Moorhead, L. D.: *J. Pharmacol. Exp. Ther.*
　　　1915, 7, 577; Ikuta, M.: *Osaka Igakkai Zasshi* **1942**, 41, 649; Esaki, T.: *Nippon Yakurigaku*
　　　Zasshi **1954**, 50, 103; 1955, 51, 62; Okabe, S. *et al.*: *Ibid*, **1983**, 81, 285; Niiho, Y. *et al.*: *Wakan*
　　　Iyaku Gakkaishi **1988**, 5(3), 540; *Nippon Yakurigaku Zasshi* **1977**, 73, 45p; Suga, S.: *Osaka*
　　　Igakkai Zasshi **1942**, 41, 649.
　[14] Blumberger, W. *et al.*: *Planta Med.* **1966**, 14, Suppl. 52.

[15] Glatzel, H. *et al.*: *Planta Med.* **1967**, 15, 223.

[T. Kimura]

528.   *Melodinus suaveolens* **Champ. ex Benth.**   (Apocynaceae)

Shan-cheng (C), Sarn-tsarng (H),

Fruit
 Local Drug Name: Shan-cheng (C), Sarn-tsarng (H).
 Processing: Use in fresh or dry under the sun (C, H).
 Method of Administration: Oral (decoction: C, H); Topical (decoction for washing or powder: H).
 Folk Medicinal Uses:
   1) Hernia (C, H).
   2) Orchitis (C, H).
   3) Infantile malabsorption (C, H).
   4) Productive cough (C, H).
   5) Indigestion (C, H).
   6) Abdominal pain (C).
   7) Scrofula (H).
   8) Gastric distention (H).
   9) Stomachache (H).
   10) Skin infection (H).
   11) Ringworm infection (H).
 Contraindications: Slightly toxic, may cause vomiting.

Scientific Research:
 Chemistry
  1) Alkaloids: Δ^{14}-vincine, vindolinine, vincadifformine, hazuntine, cathovalinine, vincoline, tabersonine, 11-methoxytabersonine, 11-hydroxytabersonine, 11-methoxyvincadifformine, (19R)-hydroxytabersonine, 11-methoxy-(19R)-hydroxytabersonine, 11,19R-dihydroxytabersonine, suaveolenine [1], α-methylene indolines [2].
 Pharmacology
  1) Antibacterial activity [3]

Literature:
   [1] Ye, J. H. *et al.*: *Phytochemistry* **1991**, 30, 3168.
   [2] Lai, M. C. S. *et al.*: *Biochem. Pharmacol.* **1969**, 18, 1553.
   [3] Au, K. S. *et al.*: *Biochem. Pharmacol* **1969**, 18, 2673.

[P.P.H. But]

529.   *Cynanchum caudatum* **Maxim.**   (Asclepiadaceae)

Ikema (J)

Related plant: *C. wilfordii* : Keun-jo-rong (K); *C. chinense* R. Br.: E-rong-teng (C).

Root
 Local Drug Name: Gohishokon (J).
 Processing: Dry under the sun (J).
 Method of Administration: Decoction (J).

Folk Medicinal Uses:
  1) Weakness, anemia (J, K).
  2) Traumatic injury (J).
  3) Beriberi (J).
  4) White hair (J).

Scientific Researches:
Chemistry
  1) Cardiac glycoside: Cynanchotoxin [1].
  2) Aglycones of the glycosides: Cynanchogenin [1,2], penupogenin [3], deacylcynanchogenin, isodeacylcynanchogenin, sarcostin, and deacetylmetaplexigenin [4], ikemagenin, and isoikemagenin [6], glycocynanchogenin [7], glycosarcostin [9], glycocaudatin [10], glycopenupogenin[11], 20-O-cinnamoylsarcostin [12].
  3) Triterpenoids and steroids: Lupeol acetate and β-sitosterol [1], caudatin [5], 5α-,6α-epoxycaudatin [14].
  4) Steroid alkaloids: Gagaminin [8].
  5) Steroid glycosides: Cynanchoside C_1 and C_2 [13], [17].
  6) Carbohydrates: Glaucobioside [15].
Pharmacology
  1) Lipid peroxidation (alkaloid) [16].

Literatures:
  [1] Mitsuhashi, H. *et al.*: *Chem. Pharm. Bull.* **1960**, 8, 313; 318.
  [2] Mitsuhashi, H. *et al.*: *Chem. Pharm. Bull.* **1959**, 7, 749; *Ibid* **1960**, 738; *Ibid* **1962**, 719.
  [3] Mitsuhashi, H. *et al.*: *Chem. Pharm. Bull.* **1960**, 8, 565; *Ibid* **1962,** 10, 725.
  [4] Mitsuhashi, H. *et al.*: *Chem. Pharm. Bull,* **1962,** 10, 808; 811; *Ibid* **1963**, 11, 1198.
  [5] Yamagishi, T. *et al.*: *Chem. Pharm. Bull.* **1972**, 20(3), 625.
  [6] Yamagishi, T. *et al.*: *Chem. Pharm. Bull.* **1972**, 20(9), 2070.
  [7] Yamagishi, T. *et al.*: *Tetrahedron Lett.* **1972**, (39), 4005.
  [8] Yamagishi, T. *et al.*: *Chem. Pharm. Bull.* **1972**, 20(10), 2289.
  [9] Yamagishi, T. *et al.*: *Tetrahedron Lett.* **1973**, (48), 4735.
  [10] Yamagishi, T. *et al.*: *Chem. Pharm. Bull.* **1976**, 24(8), 1842.
  [11] Bando, H. *et al.*: *Chem. Pharm. Bull.* **1976**, 24(12), 3085.
  [12] Bando, H. *et al.*: *Chem. Pharm. Bull.* **1978**, 26(7), 2128.
  [13] Wada, K. *et al.*: *Chem. Pharm. Bull.* **1979**, 27(9), 2252; *Ibid* **1982**, 30(10), 3500; Zenyaku Kogyo Co. Ltd.: Japan Kokai Tokkyo Koho JP 80167300, 801226, Appl. JP 7974870, 790614; JP 8163997, 810530, Appl. JP 79140316, 791030.
  [14] Bando, H. *et al.*: *Chem. Pharm. Bull.* **1980**, 28(7), 2258.
  [15] Nakagawa, T. *et al.*: *Tetrahedron Lett.* **1982**, 23(51), 5431.
  [16] Lee, D.-U. *et al.*: *Yakhak Hoechi* **1994**, 38(6), 786.
  [17] Warashina, T. *et al.*: *Phytochemistry* **1995**, 39(1), 199; *Chem. Pharm. Bull.* **1995**, 43(6), 977; **1995**, 43(10), 1734; **1996**, 44(2), 358.
  [18] Warashina, T. *et al.*: *Phytochemistry* **1997**, 44(5), 917.

[T. Kimura]

530.   *Metaplexis japonica* **Makino**   (Asclepiadaceae)

Luo-mo (C), Gagaimo (J), Bak-ju-ga-ri (K)

Fruit
  Local Drug Name: Luo-mo (C), Ramashi (J), Na-ma-ja (K).
  Processing: Dry under the sun (C, J, K).
  Method of Administration: Decoction (C, J, K)

Folk Medicinal Uses:
  1) Weakness (C, J, K).
  2) Traumatic injury (C, J, K).
  3) Cough (C).
  4) Impotence (C).
  5) Emission (C).,
  6) Female diseases (K).
  7) Pain of the toe (K).

Leaf
Local Drug Name: Ramayo (J), Na-ma-yeop (K).
Processing: Dry under the sun (J, K).
Method of Administration: Decoction (J, K)
Folk Medicinal Uses:
  1) Traumatic injury (J, K).
  2) Insect bite (J).
  3) Breeding (J).

Scientific Researches:
Chemistry
  1) Aglycones of the steroid glycosides: Pergularin [1], metaplexigenin, benzoylramanone [2], sarcostin, deacylmetaplexigenin, deacylcynanchogenin, utendin [3,4], gagaimol [5], dibenzoylgagaimol, nicotinoyl-cinnamoyl-sarcostin [5], gagaimol -7-methylether, 7β-methoxysarcostin [6].

Literatures:
[1] Mitsuhashi, H. *et al.*: *Chem. Pharm. Bull. Tokyo* **1962**, 10, 811; **1964**, 12, 1523.
[2] Mitsuhashi, H. *et al.*: *Ibid* **1965**, 13, 267, 274, 1332.
[3] Mitsuhashi, H. *et al.*: *Ibid* **1966**, 14, 717.
[4] Nomura, T. *et al.*: *Planta Medica* **1981**, 41(2), 206.
[5] Nomura, T. *et al.*: *Chem. Pharm. Bull. Tokyo* **1972,** 20, 1344.
[6] Nomura, T. *et al.*: *Chem. Pharm. Bull. Tokyo* **1979**, 27(2), 508.

[T. Kimura]

531.   *Periploca sepium* **Bge.**   (Araliaceae)

Gang-liu (C), Heung-gar-pay (H), Deong-gul-go-mu-na-mu (K)

Root bark (CP)
Local Drug Name: Xiang-jia-pi (C), Heung-gar-pay (H), Hyang-ga-pi (K).
Processing: Eliminate foreign matter, wash clean, soften thoroughly, cut into thick slices, and dry in the sun
              (C).
Method of Administration: Oral (decoction: C, H).
Folk Medicinal Uses:
  1) Rheumatic arthritis with aching and weakness of the loins and knees (C, H, K).
  2) Cardiac palpitation (C, H).
  3) Shortness of breath (C, H).
  4). Edema of the lower extremities (C).

Scientific Researches:
Chemistry
  1) Aldehydes: 4-Methoxysalicylaldehyde [1].

2) Glycosides and genins: Pregnane glycoside I~V [2], glycoside E, G, K, H [3-6], H_2 [7], reridienone-A, periplocogenin [8], periplocoside A, B, C [9], D, E, M, N, L [10], periplocoside J, K, F, O [11], xysmalogenin [12].

3) Steroids: S-20 [10].

4) Sugars: Oligosaccharide C_1, D_2, F_1, F_2 [13].

5) Coumarins: Scopoletin [14].

Pharmacology

1) Antitumor activity [8].

2) Effect on heart [15,16].

Literatures:

[1] *"Zhongyao Zhi"* **1994,** Vol.5, 433.

[2] Itokawa, H. *et al.: Chem. Pharm. Bull.* **1988,** 27(4), 1173.

[3] Sakuma, S. *et al.: Chem. Pharm. Bull.* **1972,** 17, 2183.

[4] Sachiko, K. *et al.: Chem. Pharm. Bull.* **1972,** 20, 469.

[5] Kasai, R. *et al.: Chem. Pharm. Bull.* **1972,** 20, 1869.

[6] Hisoyuki, I. *et al.: Chem. Pharm. Bull.* **1972,** 20, 2402.

[7] Sakuma, S. *et al.: Chem. Pharm. Bull.* **1980,** 28(1), 163.

[8] Itokawa, H. *et al.: Chem. Pharm. Bull.* **1987,** 35(11), 4524.

[9] Itokawa, H. *et al.: Chem. Pharm. Bull.* **1988,** 36(3), 982.

[10]Itokawa, H. *et al.: Chem. Pharm. Bull.* **1988,** 36(6), 2084.

[11]Itokawa, H. *et al.: Chem. Pharm. Bull.* **1988,** 36(11), 4441.

[12]Xu, J.P. *et al.: Phytochemistry* **1990,** 29(1), 244.

[13]Sakuma, S. *et al.: Chem. Pharm. Bull.* **1977,** 25(8), 2055.

[14]Komissarenko, N.F. *et al.: Khim. Prir. Soedin.* **1983,** (1), 102.

[15]Li, Z.W. *et al.: Zhonghua Yixue Zazhi* **1956,** 7, 651.

[16]Qian, J.Q. *et al.: Wuhan Yixueyuan Xuebao* **1963,** 16, 5.

[J.X. Guo]

532.   *Cephaelis ipecacuanha* **A. Richard**   (Rubiaceae)
[= *Uragoga ipecacuanha* Baill.]

Tokon (J), To-geun (K)

Root (JP, KP)

Local Drug Name: Tokon (J), To-geun (K).

Processing: Dry under the sun (J, K).

Method of Administration: Powder (J, K).

Folk Medicinal Uses:

1) Cough (J, K).

2) Intractable phlegm (J, K).

Scientific Researches:

Chemistry

1) Alkaloids: Emetine, cephaeline, psychotrine, *O*-methylpsychotrine, ipecamine, hydroipecha-mine, emetamine, protoemetine [1].

2) Alkaloid glycosides: Ipecoside, neoipecoside, 7-methylneoipecoside [2].

Pharmacology

1) Stimulation of trachea secretion (powder or aq. extract) [3].

2) Anti-virus activity against influenza virus (aq. extract) [4].

3) Anti-amoebic activity (emetine) [5].

4) Inhibition of dopamine receptor D2 (alkaloid) [6].

Literatures:

[1] Pelletier, P. *et al.*: *Ann. Chim. Phys.* **1817**, 4, 172; Kunz, H.: *Arch. Pharm.* **1887**, 225, 461; Paul, B. H. *et al.*: *Pharm. J.* **1894/1895**, 25, 111; 690; Terashima, M. *et al.*: *Chem. Pharm. Bull.* **1960**, 8, 517; Battersby, A. R. *et al.*: *Chem. & Ind.* **1957**, 982; 983; *J. Chem. Soc.* **1965**, 7459; **1968**, 2467; *Chem. Commun.* **1967**, 219; *J. Chem. Soc.* **1961**, 3899.

[2] Itoh, A. *et al.*: *Chem. Pharm. Bull.* **1989**, 37(4), 1137; Bellet, M. P. *et al.*: *Ann. Pharm. Fr.* **1954**, 12, 466; Kennard, O. *et al.*: *Chem. Commun.* **1971**, 899.

[3] Perry, W. F. *et al.*: *J. Pharmacol. Exp. Ther.* **1941**, 73, 65; Akiba, K. *et al.*: *Ouyou Yakuri* **1981**, 22, 339; Kase, Y. *et al.*: *Nippon Yakuri Gakkai Zasshi* **1977**, 73, 605.

[4] May, G. *et al.*: *Arzneim. Forsch.* **1978**, 28, 1.

[5] Keenw, A. et al.: *Planta Med.* **1986**, 52, 278; **1987**, 53, 201; Csuka, I..: *Biochem. Pharmacol.* **1984**, 33, 2061.

[6] Sumita, T. et al.: *Yakugaku Zasshi*, **1988**, 108, 450.

[T. Kimura]

533.   *Morinda officinalis* **How**   (Rubiaceae)

Ba-ji-tian (C), Bar-gick-tin (H), Pa-geuk-cheon (K)

Root (CP)

Local Drug Name: Ba-ji-tian (C), Bar-gick-tin (H), Hagekiten (J), Pa-geuk-cheon (K).

Processing: 1) Eliminate foreign matter (C, K).

2) Steam the clean Radix Morindae Officinalis, remove the woody cores while hot, cut into sections, and dry (C).

3) Steam the clean Radix Marrndae Officinalis with salt-water, until it steamed thoroughly, remove the woody cores while hot, cut into sections, and dry (C).

Method of Administration: Oral (decoction: C, H, K).

Folk Medicinal Uses:

1) Impotence (C, H, K).

2) Rheumatic arthralgia (C, H, K).

3) Infertility (C, H, K).

4) Menstrual disorders (C, H, K).

5) Pain and cold feeling in the lower abdomen (C, H).

6) Seminal emission (C, H).

7) Limpness of the legs (C, H).

Scientific Researches:

Chemistry

1) Steroids: β-Sitosterol [1,2], 24-ethylcholesterol [3].

2) Hydrocarbons: Nonadecane [2].

3) Organic acids: Palmitic acid [2], succinic acid [4].

4) Sugars: Insulin-type hexasaccharide, heptasaccharide [4], glucose, mannose [5].

5) Glycosides: Monotropein, asperuloside tetraacetate [6].

6) Trace elements: Fe, Mn, Zn, et al [7].

7) Anthraquinones: Rubiadin, rubiadin 1-Me ether, 2-hydroxy-3-(hydroxymethyl)-anthraquinone, physcion [2], 2-methylanthraquinone [3], 1-hydroxyanthraquinone, 1-hydroxy-2-methylanthraquinone, 1,6-dihydroxy-2,4-dimethoxyanthraquinone, 1,6-dihydroxy-2-methoxyanthraquinone, 1-hydroxy-2-methoxyanthraquinone [8].

Pharmacology

1) Antidepressant effect [4].

2) Effect on sex and learning behaviors and tyrosine hydroxylase activity [9].

3) Adrenocorticotropic effect [10].

118

Literatures:

[1] *"Zhongyao Jianbie Shouce"* **1978,** Vol.2, 81.
[2] Zhou, F.X. *et al.*: *Zhongyao Tongbao* **1986,** 11(9), 554.
[3] Li, S. *et al.*: *Zhongguo Zhongyao Zazhi* **1991,** 16(11), 675.
[4] Cui, C.F. *et al.*: *Zhongguo Zhongyao Zazhi* **1995,** 20(1), 36.
[5] Wang, Y.F. *et al.*: *Zhiwu Xuebao* **1986,** 28(5), 566.
[6] Chen, Y.W. *et al.*: *Zhongyao Tongbao* **1987,** 12(10), 613.
[7] Li, S. *et al.*: *Zhongguo Yiyao Xuebao* **1987,** (4), 29.
[8] Yang, Y.J. *et al.*: *Yaoxue Xuebao* **1992,** 27(5), 358.
[9] Saito, H. *et al.*: *Proc. Int. Symp. 3rd* **1983** (Pub. **1984**), 1,467.
[10]Shen, D.X. *et al.*: *Zhongxiyi Jiehe Zazhi* **1985,** 5(3), 192.

[J.X. Guo]

534.   *Oldenlandia diffusa* **(Willd.) Roxb.**   (Rubiaceae)
[= *Hedyotis diffusa* Willd.]

Bai-hua-she-she-cao (C), Bark-far-sair-sit-cho (H), Baek-un-pul (K)

Herb
Local Drug Name: Bai-hua-she-she-cao (C), Bark-far-sair-sit-cho (H), Hakkadazetsuso (J), Baek-
hwa-sa-seol-cho (K).
Processing: Wash clean, and dry in the sun or use in fresh (C, K).
Method of Administration: Oral (decoction: C, H, K); Topical (paste: C).
Folk Medicinal Uses:
1) Toosillitis (C, H, K).
2) Boil (C, H, K).
3) Appendicitis (C, H, K).
4) Dysentery (C, H, K).
5) Infection of urethra (C, H).
6) Hepatitis (C, H).
7) Cancer (C, H).
8) Snake bite (K).

Scientific Researches:
Chemistry
1) Iridoids: 6-O-*p*-coumaroyl scandoside methyl ester, 6-O-*p*-methoxycinnamoyl scandoside
methyl ester, 6-O-feruloyl scandoside methyl ester [1], oldenlandoside I, II [2].
2) Lactones: asperuloside [1,2].
3) Polysaccharide [3].
Pharmacology
1) Anti-inflammatory effect [2].
2) Antitumor effect [2,3].

Literatures:
[1] Nishihama, Y. *et al.*: *Planta Med.* **1981,** 43(1), 28.
[2] Huang, J.T. *et al.*: *Arch. Pharm. (Weinheim. Ger.)* **1981,** 314(10), 831.
[3] Meng, Y.F. *et al.*: *Lanzhou Daxue Xuebao, Ziran Kexuebao* **1990,** 26(4), 113.

[J.X. Guo]

535.   *Psychotria rubra* **(Lour.) Poir.**   (Rubiaceae)

Jiu-jie (C), Sarn-die-doe (H)

Root or Leaf
Local Drug Name: Shan-da-yan (C), Sarn-die-doe (H)
Processing: Use in fresh or dry under the sun (C, H)
Method of Administration: Oral (decoction: C, H); Topical (crushed fresh leaves: C, H).
Folk Medicinal Uses:

        1) Diphtheria (C, H).
        2) Tonsillitis (C, H).
        3) Pharyntitis (C, H).
        4) Dysentery (C, H).
        5) Typhoid fever (C, H).
        6) Rheumatic bone pain (C, H).
        7) Leg ulcer (C, H).
        8) Traumatic injury (C, H).
        9) Wound bleeding (C, H).
        10) Snake bites (C, H).
        11) Stomachache (C).
        12) Sore ulcer (C).
        13) Fractures (H).
        14) Lumbago (H).
        15) Pyodermas (H).

Scientific Research:
Chemistry
  1) Naphthoquinone: Psychorubrin [1].
Pharmacology
  1) Cytotoxic effect [1].

Literature:
[1] Hayashi, T. *et al.*: *J. Med. Chem.* **1987,** 30, 2005.

                                      [P.P.H. But]

536.   *Uncaria gambir* **Roxb**.   (Rubiaceae)

Er-cha-gou-teng (C).

Leaf and stem (JP, KP)
Local Drug Name: Fang-er-cha (C), Asenyaku (J), A-seon-yak (K).
Processing: Extraction with water, concentrate and dry (J, K).
Method of Administration: Oral (powder or pill: J, decoction: C, J, K), topical (decoction: C).
Folk Medicinal Uses:

        1) Diarrhea (C, J, K).
        2) Gastrointestinal disorder (C, J, K).
        3) Tonsillitis (C).
        4) Cough due to lung-heat (C).
        5) Hemoptysis (C).
        6) Sore (C).
        7) Eczema (C).
        8) Aphtha (C).
        9) Hoarce voice (J).

Scientific Researches:
Chemistry
1) Tannins: (+)-catechin, (+)-epicatechin, quercetin, gambiriin and (-)-epicatechin [1].
2) Alkaloids: Roxburghine B, C and E [2], gambritanniine, oxogambirtannine [3], indol alkaloids [4].
Pharmacology
1) Skin lightening, melanin inhibitor (extract) [5].

Literatures:
[1] Zust, A. *et al.*: *Helv. Chim. Acta* **1960**, 43, 1274.
[2] Cistara, C. *et al.*: *Gazz. Chim. Ital.*, **1973**, 103, 153.
[3] Irie, H. *et al.*: *J. Chem. Soc., Chem. Commun.* **1975**,(2), 63.
[4] Merlini, L.: *Corsi Semin. Chim.* **1968**, 11, 96; *Phytochem.* **1972**, 11(4), 1525.
[5] Yokogawa, Y. *et al.*: *Japan Kokai Tokkyo Koho*, JP 9730949 A2, JP 0930949 19970204.

[T. Kimura]

537.   *Calystegia japonica* **Choisy**   (Convolvulaceae)

Xuan-hua(C), Hirugao(J), Me-ggot (K)

Flower
Local Drug Name: Xuan-hua(C), Senka(J), Seon-hwa(K)
Processing: Dry under the sun(C, K), topical(decoction: C, J)
Method of Administration: Oral(decoction, J, K)
Folk Medicinal Uses:
1) Wound dehiscence(C, J, K)
2) Hypertension(C)
3) Difficult urination(C)
4) Erysipelas(C)
5) Constipation(J)
6) Indigestion(K)
7) Diabetes(K)

Scientific Research:
Chemistry
1) Flavonoids: Afzelin, astragalin, kaempferol-3-O-α-L-galactoside, nicotiflorin[1], 3-hydroxy-4',5,7-trimethoxyflavone[2]
2) Steroids: β-Sitosterol[1]
3) Lipids: Linoleic acid, palmitic acid, stearic acid[1]
Phamacology
1) Toxic effect[3]

Literature:
[1] Takagi, S. *et al.*: *Yakugaku Zasshi* **1977**, 97, 1369.
[2] Hukuti, G.: *Yakugaku Zasshi* **1939**, 59, 258.
[3] Chang, I. M. *et al.*: *Korean J. Pharmacog.* **1982**, 13(2), 62.

[C. K. Sung]

538.   *Caryopteris incana* **Miq.**   (Verbenaceae)

Lan-xiang-cao (C), Larn-heung-cho (H), Cheung-ggot-na-mu (K)

Whole Plant
Local Drug Name: Lan-xiang-cao (C), Larn-heung-cho (H), Nan-hyang-cho (K).
Processing: Use in fresh or dry in shade (C, H, K).
Method of Administration: Oral (decoction: C, H, K); Topical (decoction or macerated fresh herbs: C, H).
Folk Medicinal Uses:

    1) Rheumatic arthralgia (C, H, K).
    2) Chronic bronchitis (C, H, K).
    3) Whooping cough (C, H, K).
    4) Colds and fever (H, K).
    5) Traumatic injury (C, H).
    6) Gastroenteritis (C, H).
    7) Pruritus (C, H).
    8) Postpartum pain (C, H).
    9) Boils and Pyodermas (H).
    10) Eczema (C, H).
    11) Snake bite (C).
    12) Wound bleeding (H).
    13) Dysmenorrhea (H).

Scientific Research:
Chemistry
    1) α-thujene, α-pinene, camphene, sabinene, β-pinene, β-myrcene, α-terpinene, p-cymene, limonene, β-ocimene, β-phellandrene, α-terpinolene, α-cubebene, α-copaene, α-cedrene, β-caryophyllene, γ-cadinene, *l*-aromadendrene, α-humulene, β-bisabolene, δ-cadinene [1].

Literature:
[1] Pu, Z. *et al.*: *Huaxue Xuebao* **1984**, 42, 1103.

[P.P.H. But]

539.   *Stachytarpheta jamaicensis* **(L.) Vahl**   (Verbenaceae)

Yu-long-bian (C), Yuk-lung-bin (H)

Whole Plant
Local Drug Name: Yu-long-bian (C), Yuk-lung-bin (H).
Processing: Slice, dry under the sun (C, H).
Method of Administration: Oral (decoction: C, H); Topical (macerated fresh herb: C, H).
Folk Medicinal Uses:

    1) Urinary tract infection, stones (C, H).
    2) Rheumatism (C, H).
    3) Acute conjunctivitis (C, H).
    4) Pharyngitis (C, H).
    5) Boils and Pyodermas (C, H).
    6) Traumatic injury (H).

Scientific Research:
Chemistry
    1) Iridoid glucoside: tarphetalin [1].
    2) Choline, phenolic acids, chlorogenic acid, catechuic tannins [2].

3) Flavonoids: 6-hydroxyluteolol 7-glucuronide, luteolol 7-glucuronide, apigenol 7-glucuronide [2].
4) n-$C_{29}H_{60}$, n-$C_{30}H_{62}$, n-$C_{32}H_{66}$, n-$C_{31}H_{64}$, n-$C_{33}H_{68}$, n-$C_{34}H_{70}$, n-$C_{35}H_{72}$, α-spinasterol, a satd. aliphatic ketone, a satd. aliphatic carboxylic acid and an unsatd. hydroxy carboxylic acid [3].

Literature:
[1] Jawad, F.H. *et al.: Egypt. J. Pharm. Sci.* **1977,** 18, 511.
[2] Duret, S. *et al.: Plant. Med. Phytother.* **1976,** 10, 96.
[3] Lin, S.R. *et al.: Chung-Kuo Nung Yeh Hua Hsueh Hui Chih* **1976,** 14, 151.

[P.P.H. But]

540.   *Vitex cannabifolia* **Sieb. et Zucc.**   (Verbenaceae)
[= *V. negundo* L. var. *cannabifolia* (Sieb. et Zucc.) Hand.-mazz.]

Mu-jing (C), Wong-ging (H), Ninjinboku (J)

Leaf
Local Drug Name: Huang-jing (C), Wong-ging (H), Bokeikon (J).
Processing: Dry in shade or use in fresh (C, H).
Method of Administration: Oral (decoction: C, H).
Folk Medicinal Uses:
                    1) Influenza (C, H).
                    2) Malaria (C, H).
                    3) Enteritis (C, H).
                    4) Dysentery (C, H).
                    5) Genitourinary tract infection (C, H).
                    6) Eczema (C, H).
                    7) Dermatitis (C, H).
                    8) Edema (J).

Fruit
Local Drug Name: Huang-jing (C), Wong-ging (H).
Processing: Dry under shade (C, H).
Method of Administration: Oral (decoction: H).
Folk Medicinal Uses:
                    1) Cough (C, H, J).
                    2) Asthma (C, H, J).
                    3) Epigastric pain (C, H, J).
                    4) Dyspepsia (C, H).
                    5) Enteritis (C, H).
                    6) Dysentery (C, H).

Root and Stem
Local Drug Name: Huang-jing (C), Wong-ging (H).
Processing: Dry under shade (C, H).
Method of Administration: Oral (decoction: H).
Folk Medicinal Uses:
                    1) Bronchitis (C, H).
                    2) Malaria (C, H).
                    3) Hepatitis (C, H).

Scientific Research:
Chemistry

1) Diterpenoids: Vitexilactone [1].
2) *p*-Hydroxybenzoic acid [1], methyl *p*-hydroxybenzoate [2].
3) Glycosides: Agnuside [1-2], aucubin, negundoside, maltoglucoside [2].
4) Flavonol: Artemetine [1].
5) Iridoids: Nishindaside, isonishindaside [3].

Literature:

[1] Taguchi, H. *et al.*: *Chem. Pharm. Bull.* **1976,** 24, 1668.
[2] Iwagawa, T. *et al.*: *Kagoshima Daigaku Rigakubu Kiyo, Sugaku, Butsurigaku, Kagaku* **1993**, 26, 57.
[3] Iwagawa, T. *et al.*: *Phytochemistry* **1993**, 32, 453.

[P.P.H. But]

541. *Clerodendranthus spicatus* (Thunb.) C.Y. Wu ex H.W. Li (Labiatae)
[= *Clerodendron spicatum* Thunb., *Orthosiphon stramineus* Benth.]

Mao-xu-cao (C), Mao-soe-cho (H)

Whole Plant
Local Drug Name: Mao-xu-cao (C), Mao-soe-cho (H).
Processing: Wash, chop, and dry under the sun (C, H).
Method of Administration: Oral (decoction: C, H).
Folk Medicinal Uses:

        1) Acute and chronic nephritis (C, H).
        2) Cystitis (C, H).
        3) Urinary tract stones (C, H).
        4) Rheumatic arthritis (C, H).
        5) Gallstones (C, H).

Scientific Research:
Chemistry
  1) Eupatrin, sinensetin, isosinensetin, 3'-hydroxy-5,6,7,4'-tetramethoxyflavone, 5-hydroxy-6,7,3',4'-tetramethoxyflavone, 4',5,6,7-tetramethoxyflavone [1-3, 6].
  2) α-amyrin, β-sitosterol, ursolic acid, daucosterol, salvigenin, 6-methoxygenkwanin, scutellarein tetramethylether, limonene, borneol, thymol, glucose, fructose, pentose, urea, inorganic salts [2–5].
Pharmacology
  1) Antibiotic [3].

Literature:

[1] Matsuura, S. *et al.*: *Yakugaku Zasshi* **1973,** 93, 1517.
[2] Zhong, J. Y. *et al.*: *Yunnan Zhiwu Yanjiu* **1984,** 6, 344.
[3] Schneider, G. *et al.*: *Deut. Apoth. Ztg.* **1973,** 113(6), 201.
[4] Schunck, De. Goldfiem *et al.*: *Presse Med.* **1938,** 52, 1039.
[5] Takemoto, T. *et al.*: *Yakugaku Kenyu*   **1957,** 29, 702.
[6] Bombardell, E. *et al.*: *Fitoterapia* **1972,** 43(2), 35.

[P.P.H. But]

542.   *Perilla frutescens Britton* var. *japonica* Hara   (Labiatae)

Egoma(J), Deul-ggae(K),

Seed
  Local Drug Name: Egoma(J), Baek-so-ja(K)
  Processing: Dry under the sun(K)
  Method of Administration: Oral(decoction, K)
  Folk Medicinal Uses:
                    1) Weakness(K)
                    2) Chronic gastritis(K)
                    3) Cough(K)
                    4) Poisoned dermatitis with lacquer(K)

Scientific Research:
  Chemistry
    1) Terpenenes: β-Caryophyllene[1], isoegomaketone, (-)-limonene, perilla ketone
    2) Phenylpropanoids: Myristicin[1]
    3) Alkaloids: 3-(3,4-Dihydroxy-phenyl) lactamide, 5-(3,4-dihydroxy-phenyl-methyl) oxazolidine-
       2,4-dione[2]
  Phamacology
    1) Uterine stimulant effect[3]
    2) Antihepatotoxic activity[4]

Literature:
  [1] Yuba, A. *et al.*: *Shoyakugaku Zasshi* **1992**, 46(3), 257.
  [2] Nagatsu, A. *et al.*: *Chem. Pharm. Bull.* **1995**, 43(5), 887.
  [3] Woo, W. S. and Lee, E. B.: *Korean J. Pharmacog.* **1979**, 10(1), 27.
  [4] Choi, S. Y. and Chang, I. M.: *Ann. Rep. Nat. Prod. Res. Inst. Seoul Natl. Univ.* **1982**, 21, 49.
                                                                    [C. K. Sung]

543.   *Salvia miltiorrhiza* **Bunge**   (Labiatae)

                    Dan-shen(C), Darn-sum(H), Dan-sam(K)

Root (CP)
  Local Drug Name: Dan-shen(C), Darn-sum(H), Tanjin(J), Dan-sam(K)
  Processing: 1) Remove foreign matter and remains of stems, wash clean, soften thoroughly, cut into
                    thick slices, and dry(C). 2) Stir-fry the slices with wine to dryness(C)
  Method of Administration: Oral(decoction, K,H)
  Folk Medicinal Uses:
                    1) Menorrhalgia(H, J, K)
                    2) Dysmenorrhea(H, J, K)
                    3) Cough(J, K)
                    4) Menoschesis(J, K)
                    5) Angina pectoris(C)
                    6) Menstrual disorders, amenorrhea, dysmenorrhea(C)
                    7) Mars formation in the abdomen(C)
                    8) Pricking pain in the chest and abdoma, pain in acute arthritis and
                       subcutaneous infections(C)
                    9) Fidgets and insomnia(C)
                    10) Hepatosplenomegaly(C)
                    11) Coronary disease(H)
                    12) Insomnia(H)
                    13) Abdominal pain(J)

                                    125

14) Hysterorrhea(K)
Contraindication: Incompatible with Rhizoma et Radix Veratri

Scientific Research:
Chemistry
1) Flavonoids: baicalin [1], 3',5-dihydroxy-4',7-dimethoxy flavanone [2], 3,3',5-trihydroxy-4',7-dimethoxy flavanone [3]
2) Diterpene: isocryptotoanshinone, danshenxinkun D, isotanshinone I, isotanshinone II, tanshinone II-B, 7-dehydrotanshinone, hydroxy tanshinone[3], 7β-hydroxy abieta-8-13-diene-11-12-dione, saliva tanshinone 31, saliva tanshinone 32, saliva tanshinone 33, saliva tanshinone 37, 1,2,5,6-tetrahydrotanshinone I, formyl tanshinone[4], arucadiol, salviolone, norsalvioxide[5], cryptanshinone, danshenxinkun B [6], cryptoacetalide, epi-cryptoacetalide[7], cryptotanshinone [8], neocryptotanshinone, danshenxinkun A , isotanshinone II-B[9], deoxy neocryptotanshinone, dan-shen spiroketallactone [10], danshenspiroketallactone, epidanshenspiroketallactone[11], danshenxinkun C, methyl tanshinate, hydroxy tanshinone II-A[13], ferruginol [14], miltionone I, miltionone II, isocryptotanshinone[15], miltiopolone [16], miltirone, 1-dehydro miltirone, 1-dehydrotanshinone[17], dehydromiltirone, tanshindiol A, tanshindiol B, tanshindiol C [18], przewanoic acid A, przewanoic acid B [19], salvinone [20], salvilenone [21], salviol [22], sugiol, nortanshinone [23], tanshinlactone [24], tanshinol I [25], tanshinol II [26], 1,2-dihydro tanshinone I[27], dihydro tanshinone I[28], dihydro isotanshinone I[29], tanshinone I-A [30], tanshinone II, dihydrotanshinone[31], 1-hydroxy tanshinone II, tanshinonic acid methyl ester [32], tanshinone II-A [33], 3α-hydroxy tanshinone II-A[34], tanshinone V, tanshinone VI[35], tanshinone II-B[36], cryptotanshinone[37], methyl dihydrotanshinone, nordihydrotanshinone[38], 1,2-dihydrotanshinquinone[39], methyl tanshinquinone, tanshinone I, methyl tanshiquinone[46], transhinone VI [47],tanshinaldehyde, 1,2,15,16-tetrahydrotanshiquinone [48]
3) Triterpenes: oleanolic acid, przewanoic acid A, przewanoic acid B [19]
4) Benzenoids: 3,4-dihydroxy benzaldehyde[40], catecholaldehyde [41], dan shen suan A, dan shen suan B, dan shen suan C [42], protocatechualdehyde [43], protocatechuic acid, protocatechuic aldehyde [44], salvianolic acid A [45]
5) Quinoids: 2-iso-propyl-8-methyl phenanthrene-3,4-dione[27]
6) Phenylpropanoids: isoferulic acid[50], rosmarinic acid, rosmarinic acid methyl ester [51], salvianolic acid D [52]
7) Lignans: lithospermic acid dimethyl ester, lithospermic acid monomethyl ester [51], ethyl lithospermate, salvianolic acid E [52], dihydrocaffeic acid tetramer[53], lithospermic acid [54], lithospermic acid B[55], lithospermic acid Mg salt [56], salvianolic acid B, salvianolic acid C [57], salvianolic acid G[58]
8) Steroids: daucosterol , β-sitosterol[1], stigmasterol [15]
9) Tannins[59]
Pharmacology
1) Platelet aggregation inhibition effect [27, 79, 80, 85, 89]
2) Antimutagenic activity [28, 73, 74, 83]
3) Antibacterial activity [46, 67]
4) Antiinflammatory activity [60, 88]
5) Antiviral activity [61]
6) CNS depressants activity [62, 87]
7) Cytotoxic activity [63]
8) Antihypertensive activity [64, 72]
9) Vasodilator activity [65, 72]
10) Diuretic activity [66]
11) Antihepatotoxic activity [68, 70, 71, 82]
12) Antianginal activity [69, 86]
13) Antitumor activity [75]
14) HMG-CoA reductase inhibition effect [76]

15) Immunosuppressant activity [77]
16) Phosophodiesterase inhibition effect [78, 79]
17) Anticoagulant activity [81]
18) Antioxidant activity(salvianolic acid)[88, 89]

Literature:
[1] Kong, D.Y. *et al.*: *Shang-Hai Ti I Hsueh Pao* **1983**, 10 (4), 313
[2] Hsu, H.Y. *et al.*: *Asian J. Pharm. Suppl.* **1986**, 6 (8), 127
[3] Gao, H. *et al.*: *Int. J. Orient. Med.* **1992**, 12 (2), 183
[4] Chang, H.M. *et al.*: *J. Prg. Chem.* **1990**, 55 (11), 3537
[5] Ginda, H. *et al.*: *Tetrahedron Lett.* **1988**, 29 (36), 4603
[6] Zhang, K.Q. *et al.*: *J. Agr. Food Chem.* **1990**, 38 (5), 1194
[7] Asari, F. *et al.*: *Chem. Lett.* **1990**, (10), 1885
[8] Hu, Z.B. *et al.*: *Phytochemistry* **1993**, 32 (3), 699
[9] Lee, A.R. *et al.*: *J. Nat. Prod.* **1987**, 50 (2), 157
[10] Kong, D.Y. *et al.*: *Yao Hsueh Hsueh Pao* **1985**, 20 (10), 747
[11] Luo, H.W. *et al.*: *Phytochemistry* **1988**, 27 (1), 270
[12] Luo, H.W. *et al.*: *Yao Hsueh Hsueh Pao* **1985**, 20 (7), 542
[13] Fang, C.N. *et al.*: *Hua Hsueh Hsueh Pao* **1976**, 34, 197
[14] Nakanishi, T. *et al.*: *Phytochemistry* **1983**, 22 (3), 721
[15] Ikeshiro, Y. *et al.*: *Phytochemistry* **1989**, 28 (11), 3139
[16] Haro, G. *et al.*: *Chem. Lett.* **1990**, (9), 1599
[17] Luo, H.W. *et al.*: *Yao Hsueh Hsueh Pao* **1988**, 23 (11), 830
[18] Yagi, A. *et al.*: *Planta Med.* **1991**, 57 (3), 288
[19] Luo, H.W. *et al.*: *Yao Hsueh Hsueh Pao* **1989**, 24 (5), 341
[20] Wang, N. *et al.*: *Planta Med.* **1989**, 55 (4), 390
[21] Kusumi, T. *et al.*: *Phytochemistry* **1985**, 24 (9), 2118
[22] Hayashi, T. *et al.*: *Chem. Commun.* **1971**, 1971, 541
[23] Lin, H.C. *et al.*: *Chin. Pharm. J.* **1991**, 43 (6), 501
[24] Luo, H.W. *et al.*: *Chem. Pharm. Bull.* **1986**, 34 (8), 3166
[25] Li, C.P.: *Book* **1974**
[26] Zhang, R. *et al.*: *Chung Ts 'Ao Yao* **1993**, 24 (10), 517
[27] Onitsuka, M. *et al.*: *Chem. Pharm. Bull.* **1983**, 31 (5), 1670
[28] Sato, M. *et al.*: *Mutat. Res.* **1992**, 265 (2), 149
[29] Kong, D.Y. *et al.*: *Yao Hsueh Hsueh Pao* **1984**, 19 (10), 755
[30] Zhang, G.Q. *et al.*: *Zhongguo Yaoke Daxue Xuebao* **1988**, 19 (3), 175
[31] Yagi, A. *et al.*: *Planta Med.* **1989**, 55 (1), 51
[32] Okamura, N. *et al.*: *Planta Med.* **1992**, 58 (6), 571
[33] Luo, S. *et al.*: *Yaowu Fenxi Zazhi* **1988**, 8 (3), 154
[34] Luo, H.W. *et al.*: *Phytochemistry* **1985**, 24 (4), 815
[35] Yagi, A. *et al.*: *Patent-Japan Kokai Tokkyo Koho* **1989**, 233 (215), 9pp-
[36] Hu, Z.B. *et al.*: *Planta Med. Suppl.* **1992**, 58 (1), A621
[37] Honda, G. *et al.*: *Chem. Pharm. Bull.* **1988**, 36 (1), 408
[38] Lin, H.C. *et al.*: *Chin. Pharm. J.* **1991**, 43 (1), 11
[39] Feng, B.S. *et al.*: *Tao Hsueh Hseuh Pao* **1980**, 15, 489
[40] Wen, T. *et al.*: *Sepu.* **1985**, 2 (5), 282
[41] Chen, W. *et al.*: *Chung Ts 'Ao Yao* **1980**, 11, 442
[42] Chen, Z. *et al.*: *Yao Hsueh T 'Ung Pao* **1981**, 16 (9), 24
[43] Gao, C.F. *et al.*: *Zhongguo Yaoke Daxue Xuebao* **1991**, 22 (6), 379
[44] Ni, K.Y. *et al.*: *Yao Hsueh Hsueh Pao* **1988**, 23 (4), 293
[45] Li, L.N. *et al.*: *Planta Med.* **1984**, (3), 227
[46] Cheng, S.Z. *et al.*: *Chung Ts 'Ao Yao* **1981**, 12 (3), 12
[47] Takeo, S. *et al.*: *Biochem. Pharmacol.* **1990**, 40 (5), 1137
[48] Li, Z.T. *et al.*: *Yao Hsueh Hsueh Pao* **1991**, 26 (3), 209
[49] Wang, C.G. *et al.*: *Chin Wu Hsueh Pao* **1982**, 24, 100

[50] Hu, T.M. *et al.*: *Yiyao Gongye* **1988**, 19 (12), 541

[51] Kohda, H. *et al.*: *Chem. Pharm. Bull.* **1989**, 37 (5), 1287

[52] Ai, C.B. *et al.*: *Planta Med.* **1992**, 58 (2), 197

[53] Yokozawa, T. *et al.*: *Chem. Pharm. Bull.* **1988**, 36 (1), 316

[54] Ora, H. *et al.*: *Patent-Japan Kokai Tokkyo Koho*-01 **1989**, 268 (682), 10pp-

[55] Fung, K.P. *et al.*: *Life Sci.* **1993**, 52 (22), PL239

[56] Ora, H. *et al.*: *Patent-Japan Kokai Tokkyo Koho*-01 **1989**, 268 (682), 10pp-

[57] Ai, C.B. *et al.*: *J. Nat. Prod.* **1988**, 51 (1), 145

[58] Ai, C.B. *et al.*: *Chin. Chem. Lett.* **1991**, 2 (1), 17

[59] Hu, G.S. *et al.*: *Chung Ts 'Ao Yao* **1991**, 22 (11), 491

[60] Wu, Z.H. *et al.*: *Chung-Hwa I Hsueh Tsh Chih (Engl Ed)* **1982**, 95 (1), 67

[61] Yu, L.A. *et al.*: *Phytother. Res.* **1989**, 3 (3), 13

[62] Zhang, H.Y. *et al.*: *Yao Hsueh Hsueh Pao* **1979**, 14, 288

[63] Lee, J.H. *et al.*: *Korean J. Pharmacog.* **1986**, 17 (4), 286

[64] Yokozawa, T. *et al.*: Chem. Pharm. Bull. **1987**, 35 (3), 1157

[65] Lei, X.L. *et al.*: *Amer. J. Chin. Med.* **1981**, 9, 193

[66] Chung, H.Y. *et al.*: *Chem. Pharm. Bull.* **1987**, 35 (6), 2465

[67] Namba, T. *et al.*: *Shoyakugaku Zasshi* **1981**, 35 (4), 295

[68] Choi, S.Y. *et al.*: *Ann. Rep. Nat. Prod. Re.s Inst. Seoul Nat'l Univ.* **1982**, 21, 49

[69] Fang, S.D. *et al.*: *Amer. J. Bot.* **1981**, 68, 300

[70] Han, J.H. *et al.*: *Nat'l Med. J. China* **1979**, 59, 577

[71] Han, J. *et al.*: *Nat'l Med. J. China* **1979**, 59, 584

[72] Zhao, Y.F. *et al.*: *Chin. Mad. J.* **1984**, 97 (7), 473

[73] Liu, D.X. *et al.*: *Chung-Kuo Chung Yao Tsa Chi Li* **1990**, 15 (10), 617

[74] Wall, M.E. *et al.*: *J. Nat. Prod.* **1988**, 51 (5), 866

[75] Xang, K.R. *et al.*: *Chin. Med. J.* **1982**, 95 (7), 527

[76] Han, G.Q. *et al.*: *Int. J. Chinese Med.* **1991**, 16 (1), 1

[77] Qin, W.Z: *J. Clin. Dermatology* **1988**, 17 (2), 91

[78] Chao, S.H. *et al.*: *Sheng Wu Hsueh Yu Sheng Wu Wu Li Hsueh Pao* **1980**, 12, 357

[79] Chen, K.: *Amer. J. Chin. Med.* **1981**, 9, 193

[80] Wang, H.F. *et al.*: *J. Ethnopharmacol.* **1991**, 34 (2/3), 215

[81] Kosuge, T. *et al.*: *Yakugaku Zasshi* **1984**, 104 (10), 1050

[82] Kumazawa, N. *et al.*: *Yakagaku Zasshi* **1990**, 110 (12), 950

[83] Choi, Y.U. *et al.*: *Yakhak Hoeji* **1994**, 38 (3), 332

[84] Eun, J.S. *et al.*: *Korean J. Pharmacog.* **1991**, 22 (2), 95

[85] Yun-Choi, H.S. *et al.*: *Korean J. Pharmacog.* **1986**, 17 (1), 19

[86] Chen, W.Z. *et al.*: *Yao Hsueh Hsueh Pao* **1979**, 14, 326

[87] Fan, S.F. *et al.*: *Yao Hsueh Hsueh Pao* **1979**, 14, 199

[88] Wu Y. J. *et al.*: *Arterioscler. Thromb. Vasc. Biol.* **1998**, 18(3), 481-486.

[89] Xing, Z. Q. *et al.*: *Chung Kuo Chung His I Chieh Ho Tsa Chih* **1996**, 16(5) 287-288.

[C. K. Sung]

544.   *Thymus quinquecostatus* **Celakovsay**   (Labiatae)

Wu-mai-di-jiao(C), Ibukijakoso(J), Baek-ri-hyang(K)

Whole plant
Local Drug Name: Bai-li-xiang(C), Ji-cho(K)
Processing: Dry under the sun(K) wash clear, cut into sections, use in fresh or dry in the sun(C)
Method of Administration: Oral(decoction, C, K)
Folk Medicinal Uses:

        1) Acute gastroenteritis(C)

        2) Hypertension(C)

3) Common cold(C)
4) Cough(C)
5) Toothache(C)
6) Indigestion(C)
7) Aneilema(K)
8) Headache(K)

Scientific Research:
Chemistry
1) Hydrocarbons: Hept-1-en-3-ol[1], oct-1-en-3-ol[2]
2) Terpenes: 1,8-Cineol[1], borneol, camphene, α-pinene, terpinen-4-ol[1,2], carvacrol, geraniol, linalool, thymohydraquinone, thymol, thymol methyl ether, β-bisabolene, γ-cadinene[2]

Literature:
[1] Pa, X. Q. *et al.*: *Chung Ts'ao Yao* **1980**, 11, 101-102.
[2] Annon: *Chih Wu Hsueh Pao* **1978**, 20(1), 31-36.

[C. K. Sung]

545.   *Thymus vulgaris* L.   (Labiatae)

Tachi-jakoso (J)

Related plant: *Thymus quinquecostatus* Celak.: Ibuki-jakoso (J), Baek-ri-hyang (K).

Herb with flower bud
Local Drug Name: Taimu (J).
Processing: Dry in the shade, steam distillation (J).
Method of Administration: Decoction, essential oil (J).
Folk Medicinal Uses:
1) Cough (J).
2) Gastroenteritis (J).
3) Traumatic Injury as bacteriocidal (J).

Scientific Researches:
Chemistry
1) Monoterpenes: Thymol, carvacrol, *p*-cymene, pinene, *l*-linalool, bornylacetate, α-terpineol, terpinyl acetate, γ-terpinene [1], trans-4-thujanol and 4-terpineol [8], thymol glycoside and carvacrol glycoside [9].
2) Flavonoid: Thymonin, cirsilineol [10], and eriodictyol [2].
3) Biphenyl compound: 3,4,3',4'-Tetrahydroxy-5,5'-diisopropyl-2,2'-dimethylbiphenyl [3].
4) Organic acids: Caffeic acid [15].
5) Carbohydrates: Planteose [16].
Pharmacology
1) Antiperoxidative activity (3,4,3',4'-tetrahydroxy-5,5'-diisopropyl-2,2'-dimethylbiphenyl) [3].
2) Strongest antioxidant activity (*p*-cymene-2,3-diol) [4], antioxidative activity (flavonoids, oil) [13].
3) Protein glycation inhibitor (flavonoid) [5].
4) Nervous system stimulant (essential oil) [6].
5) Cytostatic activity against human cancer cell line HEp-2 (essential oil) [7].
6) Deodorant activity (biphenyl compounds) [11].
7) Antimicrobial activity (thymol), antifungal activity [12].
8) Insecticidal effect (essential oil) [14].

Literatures:

[1] Gabel, E. *et al.*: *Deut. Apotheker-Ztg.* **1962**, 102, 293; Granger, R. *et al.*: *Compt. rend.* **1965**, 260, 2619; *Bull. Trav. Soc. Pharm. Lyon* **1965**, 9, 113; *Phytochem.* **1973**, 12, 1683; Dorman, H. J. *et al.*: *J. Essential Oil Res.*, **1995**, 7(6), 645.

[2] Zygadlo, J. A. *et al.*: *Grasas Aceibes* (Seville), **1995**, 46(4-5), 285.

[3] Haraguchi, H. *et al.*: *Planta Med.* **1996**, 62(3), 217.

[4] Schwarz, K. *et al.*: *J. Sci. Food Agric.* **1996**, 70(2), 217.

[5] Morimitsu, Y. *et al.*: *Biosci. Biotechnol. Biochem.*, **1995**, 59(11), 2018.

[6] Inoue, S. *et al.*: *Jpn. Kokai Tokkyo Koho*, JP 08218208 A2 (**1996**) Japan.

[7] Saenz, M. T. *et al.*: *Farmaco*, 1996, 51(7), 539; *C. A.* **1996**, 125, 237797.

[8] Granger, R. *et al.*: *C. R. Acad. Sci., Paris, Ser. D*, **1968,** 267(22), 1886.

[9] Skopp, K. *et al.*: *Planta Med.* **1976**, 29(3), 208.

[10] Van den Broucke, C. O. *et al.*: *Phytochem.* **1982**, 21(10), 2581.

[11] Nakatani, N. *et al.*: *Agric. Biol. Chem.* **1989**, 53(5), 1375; Miura, K. *et al.*: *Chem. Pharm. Bull.* **1989,** 37(7), 1816.

[12] Farag, R. S. *et al.*: *J. Food Prot.* **1989**, 52(9), 665; Panizzi, L. *et al.*: *J. Ethnopharmacol.* **1993**, 39,(3), 167; Perrucci, S. *et al.*: *Planta Med.* **1994**, 60(2), 184; El-Kady, I. A. *et al.*: Qatar Univ. Sci. J. 1993, 13(1), 63.

[13] Miura, K. *et al.*: *Agric. Biol. Chem.* **1989,** 53(11) 3043; Zygadlo, J. A. *et al.*: *Grassas Aceites (Seville)*, **1995**, 46(4-5), 285..

[14] Kurowska, A. *et al.*: *Pestycydy (Warsaw)* **1991**, 225.

[15] Awe, W. *et al.*: *Pharm. Zentralhalle* **1959**, 98, 356.

[16] French, D. *et al.*: *Arch. Biochem. Biophys.* **1959**, 85, 471.

[T. Kimura]

546. *Physochlaina infundibularis* **Kuang** (Solanaceae)

Lu-du-po-lan-cao (C)

Root (CP)

Local Drug Name: Hua-shan-shen (C), Kasanjin (J).

Processing: Eliminate foreign matter, wash clean, and dry. Break to pieces before use (C).

Method of Administration: Oral (decoction: C).

Folk Medicinal Uses:

       1) Cough and asthma with thin expectoration (C).

       2) Palpitation (C).

       3) Insomnia (C).

Contraindications: Contraindicated to patients with glaucoma. Used with caution in pregnancy and in patients with marked prostatomegaly. Overdosage may cause intoxication.

Scientific Researches:

Chemistry

  1) Hyoscypicrin [1].

  2) Steroids [1].

  3) Organic acids [1].

  4) Sugars: sucrose [1].

  5) Oils [1].

  6) Alkaloids: hyoscine (scopolamine) [1,2], 6(s)-hydroxyhyoscyamine, choline [1], hyoscyamine [1,2], anisodamine, anisodine. bellaradine [2], *dl*-anisodamine, atropine, aposcopolamine, scopoline [3].

  7) Coumarins: scopoletin [1], fabiatrin [3].

Pharmacology

  1) Antiasthmatic, antitussive and expectorant effects [1].

2) Tonic and sedative effects [3,4].

3) Effect on endings of parasympathetic nerves [5].

Literatures:

[1] *"Fangzhi Ganmao Ji Qiguanyan Zhongcaoyao Shouce"* **1976,** 120.

[2] Hsiao, P.K. *et al.: Chih Wu Hsueh Pao* **1973,** 15(2), 187.

[3] Chen, Z.A. *et al.: Zhongcaoyao* **1981,** 12(7), 1.

[4] Che, X.P. *et al.: Yaoxue Xuebao* **1965,** 12(6), 368.

[5] Ma, S.D. *et al.: Shanxi Xinyiyao* **1986,** (5), 36.

[J.X. Guo]

547.   *Scopolia japonica* **Maxim.**   (Solanaceae)

[= *S. parviflora* Nakai]

Hashiridokoro (J), Mi-chi-gwng-i-pul(K)

Rhyzome (JP, KP)

Local Drug Name: Routokon (J), Nang-tang-geun (K).

Processing: Dry under the sun (J, K).

Method of Administration: External (J, K). Materials for Atropine sulphate and Scopolamine
hydrobromide.

Folk Medicinal Uses:

         1) Scabies (J).

         2) Pleurisy (K).

Contraindication: Toxic.

Leaf

Local Drug Name: Routoyo (J), Nang-tang-yeop (K).

Processing: Dry under the sun (J, K).

Method of Administration: oral(decoction, J, K).

Folk Medicinal Uses:

         1) Stomach cramps (J, K).

         2) Gout (J, K).

         3) Convulsion (J, K).

         4) Headache (J, K).

         5) Epilepsy (J, K).

Contraindication: Toxic. Mydriatic, thirst, lethargic, headache, nausea, vomitting.

Scientific Researches:

Chemistry

     1) Alkaloids: *l*-Hyoscyamine, scopolamine [1], calystegine A3, A5, B1, B2, B3, B4, C1 [3].

     2) Coumarines: Scopoletin, scopolin [4].

     3) Steroid glycosides: Scoopoloside I and II, and scopologenin [5].

Pharmacology

     1) Parasympatholytic activity (hyoscyamine, scopolamine).

     2) Anticholinergic and rhinitis inhibitor (mequitazine) [2].

     3) Trehalase inhibitor (calystegine B4) [3].

     4) Anti-parkinsonism (scopolamine).

Literatures:

[1] Konoshima, M. *et al.: Shoyakugaku Zasshi* **1978,** 32(1), 43.

[2] Adachi, Y. *et al.: Jpn. Kokai Tokkyo Koho*, JP 08208483, A2, **1996,** (Japan).

[3] Asano, N. *et al.: Carbohydr. Res.* **1996,** 292(2), 195.

[4] Anetai, M. *et al.*: *Hokkaidoritsu Eisei Kenkyushoho* **1985**, 35, 52.
[5] Okamura, S. *et al.*: *Chem. Pharm. Bull.* **1992**, 40(11), 2981.

[T. Kimura]

548.   *Solanum melongena* **L.**   (Solanaceae)

Bai-qie (C), Ngai-gwar (H), Nasu (J), Ga-ji (K)

Fruit
  Local Drug Name: Ngai-gwar (H), Kashi (J), Ga-ji (K).
  Processing: Dry under the sun (J, K).
  Method of Administration: Decoction (J, K), soup (H).
  Folk Medicinal Uses:
                    1) Swelling (J, K).
                    2) Pain (J, K).
                    3) Melena (J, K).
                    4) Boils (H).

Calyx
  Local Drug Name: Katei (J), Ga-che (K).
  Processing: Dry under the sun (J, K).
  Method of Administration: Decoction (J, K).
  Folk Medicinal Uses:
                    1) Toothache (J).
                    2) Stomatitis (J).
                    3) Stomach cancer (K).
                    4) Stomach ulcer (K).
                    5) Melena (J).

Flower
  Local Drug Name: Kaka (J), Ga-hwa (K).
  Processing: Dry under the sun (J, K).
  Method of Administration: Decoction (J, K).
  Folk Medicinal Uses:
                    1) Toothache (J).
                    2) Traumatic injury (J).
                    3) Mastitis (K).

Whole herb and Root
  Local Drug Name: Qie-zi-gen (root: C), Kayo, Kakon (J), Ga-yeop, Ga-geun (K).
  Processing: Dry under the sun (C, J, K).
  Method of Administration: Oral (decoction: C, J, K), topical (decoction of root: C).
  Folk Medicinal Uses:
                    1) Frostbite (C, K).
                    2) Rheumatic arthritis (C).
                    3) Senile chronic tracheitis (C).
                    4) Emission (C).
                    5) Dysentery (C).
                    6) Leukorrhea (C).
                    7) Edema (C).
                    8) Cough (C).
                    9) Melena (J).
                    10) Myalgia (J).

11) Congelation (J).
12) Carbuncle (J).
13) Lumbago (K).
14) Burn, wart (K).

Scientific Researches:
Chemistry
1) Phenolic compounds: 4-Hydroxycinnamic acid glycosides [1], 3,4-dihydroxybenzoic acid, chlorogenic acid, caffeic acid, 3-(3,4-dihydroxyphenyl)propanoic acid, vanillin, ferlic acid, 4-aminobenzaldehyde [2].
2) Cumarins: Scopoletin [3] and isoscopoletin [2].
3) Anthocyanins: Delphinidin 3,5-diglucoside-p-cumarate, delphinidin 3,5-diglucoside and delphinidin 3-glucoside [4].
4) Alkaloids: A glyco-alkaloid [5], N-feruloyl tylamine, moupiamide [2].
5) Sesquiterpenoids: Lubimin [6].
6) Steroids and sapogenins: Diosgenin [7], 24(R)-ethyllophenol and 4-methylstigmast-7-en-3-ol [8].
7) Fatty acids [9].
8) Enzymes: Catechol oxidase [10].
Pharmacology
1) Strong inhibitory effect for the infiltration of HT-1080 cancer cells (ethanol extract) [11].

Literatures:
[1] Ramaswamy, S. *et al.*: *Acta Aliment. Acad. Sci. Hung.* **1975**, 4(4), 381.
[2] Yoshihara, T. *et al.*: *Nippon Nogei Kagaku Kaishi* **1978**, 52(2), 101; *Agric. Biol. Chem.* **1978,** 42(3), 623.
[3] Kala, H.: *Planta Med.* **1958**, 6, 186.
[4] Nagashima, Y. *et al.*: *Eiyo to Shokuryo* **1965**, 17, 50.
[5] Waal, H. L. *et al.*: *J. S. African Chem. Inst.* **1960**, 13, 45; Sakamura, S et al.: *Agr. Biol. Chem. Japan* **1961**, 25, 750.
[6] Stoessl, A. *et al.*: *J. Chem. Soc., Chem. Commun.* **1974**, 17, 709.
[7] Shabana, M. *et al.*: *Egypt. J. Pharm. Sci.* **1976**, 16(3), 359.
[8] Itoh, T. *et al.*: *Phytochem.* **1980**, 19(11), 2491.
[9] Kashimoto, T. *et al.*: *Nippon Kagaku Kaishi* **1958,** 79, 873.
[10] Sharma, R. C. *et al.*: *Phytochem.* **1980**, 19(8), 1597.
[11] Sato, T. *et al.*: *Igaku Oyo Kenkyu Zaidan Kenkyu Hokoku*, **1995**, 13, 198; *C. A.* **1996**, 124, 332157.

[T. Kimura]

549.   *Adenosma glutinosum* **(L.) Druce**   (Scrophulariaceae)

Mao-she-xiang (C), Moe-sair-heung (H)

Whole Plant
Local Drug Name: Mao-she-xiang (C), Moe-sair-heung (H).
Processing: Dry under shade (C, H)
Method of Administration: Oral (decoction: C, H); Topical (macerated fresh herb or decoction: C, H).
Folk Medicinal Uses:
   1) Early stage of poliomyelitis (C, H).
   2) Rheumatic arthralgia (C, H).
   3) Traumatic injury (C, H).
   4) Eczema (C, H).

5) Urticaria (C, H).
6) Boil and carbuncles (C).
7) Wasp sting (C).
8) Snake bite (H).
9) Stomachache (H).
10) Pyodermas (H).

Scientific Research:
Chemistry
1) Flavonooid glycoside [1].
2) Phenols [1].
3) Triterpenes [1].
4) Amino acids [1].
5) Volatile oil: α-thujene, α-pinene, sabinene, β-myrcene, carene-3, α-terpinene, m-cymene, 1,8-cineole, γ-terpinene, carene-2, linalool, safrole, copaene, β-elemene, β-caryophyllene, α-caryophyllene, α-guaiene, β-cubebene, α-selinene, β-bisabolene, nerolidol, selinenol [2].

Literature:
[1] Anonymous: *Nong Cun Zhong Cao Yao Zhi Ji Ji Shu* **1971,** 237.
[2] Zhu L.F. *et al.*: *Aromatic Plants and Essential Constituents (Supplement 1).* South China Institute of Botany, Chinese Academy of Sciences, Guangzhou, **1995**, 143.

[P.P.H. But]

550.   *Digitalis lanata* **Ehrh.** (Scrophulariaceae)

Mao-hua-yang-di-huang (C), Kejigitarisu (J), Teol-di-gi-ta-li-seu (K)

Leaf (JP)
Local Drug Name: Mao-hua-yang-di-huang (C), Kejigitarisu (J), Teol-di-gi-ta-li-seu (K).
Processing: Dry quickly under hot air stream below 60 °C(C, J, K).
Method of Administration: Extraction material for digoxin, lanatoside C, deslanoside (C, J, K).
Folk Medicinal Uses:
1) Congestive heart failure (J, K).
2) Myocardial infarction (J, K).
3) Angina (J, K).
4) Edema caused by cardiac insufficiency (J, K).

Scientific Researches:
Chemistry
1) Cardiac glycosides: Digoxin [1], lanatoside A, B, C [2], D [3], E [4], maxoside [5], glucodigifucoside, neoglucodigifucoside and digitoxigenin allomethyloside [6], neo-odorobioside G, neodigitalinum verum, digitoxigenin-glucosido-glucomethyloside, glucodigitoxigenin-bis-digitoxoside, neo-gluco-verodoxin, digitoxigenin-glucosido-acetylglucomethyloside, digoxigenin-digilanidobiose, digoxigenin-glucosido-bis-digitoxoside and gluconeodigoxin [7], gitorin (=gitoxigenin digilanidobioside) [8], diginatigenin [9], digitoxigenin glucomethyloside and gitaloxin [10], glucoevatromonoside (digitoxigenin digilanidobioside), glucogitroside (gitoxigenin digilanidobioside), glucolanadoxin (gitaloxigenin digilanido-bioside), odorobioside G and glucoverodoxin [11].
2) Steroids: Digifolein, lanafolein and their aglycone, digifologenin [12], digiprogenin [13].
3) Flavonoids: Scutelarein, luteolin and dinantin [14].
Pharmacology
1) Cardiotonic activity [15].

134

Literatures:
[1] Smith, *et al.*: *J. Chem. Soc.* **1930**, 508.
[2] Pekic, *et al.*: *Acta Pharm. Jugoslav.*, **1973**, 23, 161.
[3] Angliker, F. B. *et al.*: *Ann.* **1957,** 607, 131.
[4] Angliker, E. *et al.*: *Helv. Chim. Acta* **1958**, 41, 479.
[5] Brieger, D. *et al.*: *Pharmazie,* **1995**, 50(10), 707.
[6] Kaiser, F.: *Experientia* **1965**, 21, 575.
[7] Kaiser, F. *et al.*: *Naturwissenschaften* **1965**, 52,108; *Ann.* **1965**, 688, 216.
[8] Tschesche, R. *et al.*: *Chem. Ber.* **1952**, 85, 1103; Uchibayashi, M.: *Pharm. Bull. Jap.* **1958,** 6, 504; Sasakawa, Y.: *Yakugaku Zasshi* **1959**, 79, 825; *Chem. Pharm. Bull.* **1959,** 7 265.
[9] Murphy, J. E.: *J. Amer. Pharm. Assoc.* **1955**, 44, 719; Okada, M. *et al.*: *Chem. Pharm. Bull.* **1960**, 8, 535.
[10] Kaiser, F. *et al.*: *Naturwissenschaften* **1962**, 49, 468.
[11] Kaiser, F. *et al.*: *Ann.* **1964**, 678, 137.
[12] Tschesche, R. *et al.*: *Chem. Ber.* **1955**, 88, 1569.
[13] Tschesche, R. *et al.*: *Ann.* **1955**, 603, 59; **1957**, 615, 210.
[14] Rangswami, S. *et al.*: *Proc. Indian Acad. Sci.* **1961**, 54A, 51.
[15] Aronson, J. K.: *Clinical Pharmacokinet.* **1980**, 5, 137.

[T. Kimura]

551.   *Digitalis purpurea* L.   (Scrophulariaceae)

Zi-hua-yang-di-huang (C), Kitsunenotebukuro (J), Di-gi-ta-li-seu (K)

Leaf (JP, KP)
Local Drug Name: Yang-di-huang-ye (C), Jigitarisu (J), Di-gi-ta-li-seu (K).
Processing: Dry quickly under hot air below 60 °C(C, J, K).
Method of Administration: Powder after controling strength (J, K).
Folk Medicinal Uses:
     1) Congestive heart failure (J, K).
     2) Myocardial infarction (J, K).
     3) Angina (J, K).
     4) Edema caused by cardiac insufficiency (J, K).
     5) Used for the preparation of dosage forms only (C).
Contraindications: Cumlation of medicament.   Arrhithmia, nausea, vomiting, auriculoventricular
    and sinoatrial block.

Scientific Researches:
Chemistry
    1) Cardiac glycosides: Purpurea glucoside A, B [1,2], glucogitaloxin [1], digitoxin [1,3], gitoxin, gitaloxin, gitostin [1], gitroside [4], glucodigifucoside [5], neogitostin [6], glucogitaloxin[7], allo-neogitostin, perlanoside A, B, digitalinum verum monoacetate and acetylglucogitroside [8], odorobioside G [9], allo-digitalinum verum [10,11], digifuco cellobioside, glucogitoroside, and gitoxin cellobioside [10], digitalinum verum, 16-formyldigitalinum verum and 16-formylpurpurea glycoside [2].
    2) Steroid glycosides: Diginin [12,13], purpuronin, F-gitonin [12], desgalactotigonin [4], digitalonin [4,13], digifolein and lanafolein [13], digipronin [14,15], purpnin [14,16,17], digacetinin[18], glucogitaloxin [6], digipurpurogenin [19] and purpnigenin [17].
    3) Saponins and sapogenins: Digitonin, gitonin, desglucodigitonin, digalonin and digalogenin [20,21,22].
    4) Flavonoids: Luteolin.
    5) Others: 8-Oxabicyclo-(3,3,1)-5-hydroxy-4-oxo-non-2-ene and 2-hydroxy-2-(2-hydroxyethyl)-cyclohexanone [23], digiprolactone (= loliolide) [24].

135

Pharmacology
    1) Cardiotonic activity (digitoxin) [25,26].

Literatures:
[1] Miyatake, K. *et al.: Pharm. Bull. Japan* **1957**, 5, 157; 163.
[2] Lemli, J.: *Congr. Sci. Farm., Conf. Commun. 21, Pisa* **1961**, 641.
[3] Lichti, H. *et al.: Helv. Chim. Acta* **1962**, 45, 868.
[4] Satoh, D. *et al.: Pharm. Bull. Japan* **1956**, 4, 284.
[5] Satoh, D. *et al.: Pharm. Bull. Japan* **1957**, 5, 253.
[6] Okano, J.: *Pharm. Bull. Jap.* **1958**, 6, 173; 178
[7] Haack, R. *et al.: Chem. Ber.* **1958**, 91, 1758.
[8] Miyatake, K. *et al.: Chem. Pharm. Bull.* **1961,** 9, 591; Hoji, K.: *Ibid* **1961**, 9, 276; 291; 566.
[9] Hoji, K.: *Chem. Pharm. Bull.* **1961,** 9, 289.
[10] Okano, A. *et al.: Chem. Pharm. Bull.* **1959**, 7 212; 222; 226.
[11] Miyatake, K. *et al.: Chem. Pharm. Bull.* **1961,** 9, 375.
[12] Kawasaki, T. *et al.:* Tetrahedron **1965**, 21, 299.
[13] Shoppee, C. W. *et al.: Proc. Chem. Soc.* **1962**, 65; *J. Chem. Soc.* **1962**, 3610.
[14] Tschesche, G. L. *et al.: Ann*, **1957**, 606, 160.
[15] Satoh, D.: *Chem. Pharm. Bull.* **1960**, 8, 270; **1962**, 10, 43; Shoppee, C. W. *et al.: J. Chem. Soc.* **1964**, 3619; Satoh, D. *et al.: Chem. Pharm. Bull.* **1960, 8**, 270; **1962**, 10, 43; **1964**, 12, 981;
[16] Satoh, D.: *Chem. Pharm. Bull.* **1960**, 8, 657.
[17] Ishii, H.: *Chem. Pharm. Bull.* **1961**, 9, 411; **1962**, 10, 354.
[18] Tschesche, R. *et al.: Ann*, **1958**, 614, 136; Mitchell, H. I.: *Am. J. Pharm.* **1964**, 136, 71; Shoppee, C. W. *et al.: J. Chem. Soc.* **1964**, 3611.
[19] Tschesche, R. *et al: Ann*, **1961**, 648, 185; *Tetrahedron Lett.* **1964**, 473.
[20] Tschesche, R. *et al: Chem. Ber.* **1952**, 85, 1103; Sasakawa, Y.: *Yakugaku Zasshi* **1959**, 79, 825.
[21] Tschesche, R. *et al: Chem. Ber.* **1961**, 94, 2019.
[22] Kawasaki, T. *et al.: Chem. Pharm. Bull.* **1964**, 12, 1250; 1311.
[23] Raymakers, A. *et al.: Phytochem.,* **1973**, 12, 2287.
[24] Wada, T.: *Chem. Pharm. Bull.* **1965**, 13, 43; Sato, D. *et al.: ibid* **1956**, 4, 284; Wada, T. *et al.: ibid* **1964,** 12, 118; 752; 1117.
[25] Akera, T. *et al.: Pharmacol. Rev.* **1978**, 29, 187; Langer, G. A.: *Biochem. Pharmacol.* **1981**, 30, 3261; Dwenger, A.: *Arzneim.-Forsch.* **1973**, 23, 1439.
[26] Jackoviljevic, I. M.: *"Analytical Profiles of Drug Substances" Vol. 3*, Flory, K. ed. Academic Press, N. Y. **1974**.; Foerster, *et al.: Arch. Int. Pharmacodyn. Ther.* **1966**, 159, 1.

[T. Kimura]

552.   *Picrorhiza kurroa* **Royle**   (Scrophulariaceae)

Koouren(J), Ho-hwang-ryeon(K)

Root
  Local Drug Name: Koouren(J), Ho-hwang-ryeon(K)
  Processing: Dry under the sun(K)
  Method of Administration: Oral(decoction, K)
  Folk Medicinal Uses:
            1) Convulsion(J, K)
            2) Haemorrhoid(J, K)
            3) Hematemesis(J, K)
            4) Diarrhea(J)
            5) Acute conjunctivitis(K)
            6) Rhinorrhagia(K)

Scientific Research:
Chemistry
1) Monoterpenes: Amphicoside[1, 2, 3, 6, 7, 10, 11], 6-trans-feruloyl catalpol, minecoside [1], catalpol, 6-feruloyl catalpol[3], kutkoside [4, 12, 13, 14, 15, 16], picroside [5], picroside I [1, 4, 6], picroside III [2, 3, 5, 7, 10, 11, 13, 14, 15, 16], veronicoside [1, 3, 5]
2) Triterpenes: 25-acetoxy-3-16-20-trihydroxy-9-methyl-19-norlanosta-5-24-diene-3-11-22-trione 2-O-β-glucoside, 25-acetoxy-3-16-20-trihydroxy-9-methyl-19-norlanosta-trans-23-dien-22-one 2-O-beta-D-glucoside[1], 3β,16α,20(R),25-tetrahydroxy-10α-cucurbit-5-en-22-one 2-β-D-glucoside[2], 25-acetoxy-3,16,20-trihydroxy-9-methyl-19-norlanosta-5-23-dien-22-one 2-O-β-D-glucoside [6], arvenin III, 2-β-glucosyl-oxycucurbitacin O, 16,20,22-trihydroxy-9-methyl-19-nor-lanosta-5-24-diene-3-11-dione 2-β-O-glucoside[8], cucurbitacin B, 23,24-dihydrocucurbitacin B, deacetoxy cucurbitacin B 2-O-β-D-glucoside, cucurbitacin Q 2-O-β-D-glucoside[9]
3) Benzenoids: androsin [1, 3, 17, 18], picein [1,3], apocycin [19]
4) Phenylpropanoids: cinnamic acid 6-β-D-glucoside [2], kutkin [12, 15, 20, 21]
Pharmacology
2) Antioxidant effect(picroside III)[14]
8) Antiaggression effect [23]
9) Anticholestatic activity [24, 36, 46, 51]
11) Antihepatotoxic activity(picroside I, kutkoside)[4][23, 27, 30, 32-34, 37, 38, 39-42, 46, 48, 52]
12) Antistress activity [23]
14) Antiulcer activity [23]
16) Bronchodilator activity [5, 25, 44, 45]
17) Choleretic activity [22, 24, 36]
21) Histamine release inhibition effect [5, 19, 45]
26) Immunostimulant activity [26, 54]
28) Antiinflammatory activity [28, 53, 59]
29) Diuretic activity [29]
35) Antibacterial activity [31]
38) Anti-allergy activity [35]
47) Antihypercholesterolemic activity [37, 47, 49]
48) Antihyperlipemic activity [43, 49]
68) Antiasthmatic activity [50]
74) Liver regeneration stimulation effect [55]
81) Pyretic activity [56]

Literature:
[1] Stuppner, H. et al.: Sci. Pharm. **1992,** 60, 73
[2] Weinges, K. et al.: Liebigs Ann. Chem. **1989,** 1989 (11), 1113
[3] Stuppner, H. et al.: Planta Med. **1989,** 55 (5), 467
[4] Aswal, R. S. et al.: Patent-Us **1992,** 5 (145, 955), 6pp-
[5] Dorsch, W. et al.: Int. Arch. Allergy Appl. Immunol. **1991,** 94 (1/2), 262
[6] Laurie, W. A. et al.: Phytochemistry **1985,** 24 (11), 2659
[7] Weinges, K. et al.: Justus Liebigs Ann. Chem. **1977,** 1977, 1053
[8] Stuppner, H. et al: Phytochemistry **1990,** 29 (5), 1633
[9] Stuppner, H. et al.: Planta Med. **1989,** 55 (6), 559
[10] Vanhaelen, M. et al.: J. Chromatoger. **1984,** 312, 497
[11] Vanhaelen, M. et al.: J. Chromatoger. **1984,** 312, 497
[12] Das, P. K. et al.: Indian J. Exp. Biol. **1976,** 14, 456
[13] Dwivedi, A. K. et al.: Indian J Pharm. Sci. **1989,** 51 (6), 274
[14] Chander, R. et al.: Biochem. Pharmacol. **1992,** 44 (1), 180
[15] Singh, B. et al.: Int. J. Cancer **1972,** 10, 29
[16] Floersheim, G. L et al.: Agents Actions **1990,** 29 (3/4), 386
[17] Dorsch, W. et al.: Int. Arch. Allerg. Appl. Immunol. **1991,** 95 (2/3), 128

[18] Dorch, W. *et al.*: *Int. Arch. Allergy Immunol.* **1992**, 99 (2/3/4), 493

[19] Engels, F. *et al.*: *FEBS Lett.* **1992,** 305 (3), 254

[20] Trivedi, V. P. *et al.*: *Q J Crude Drug Res.* **1972,** 12, 1988

[21] Ansari, R. A. *et al.*: *Indian J. Med. Res.* **1988,** 87 (4), 401

[22] Visen, P. K. S. *et al.*: *Planta Med.* **1993,** 59 (1), 37

[23] Singh, N. *et al.*: *Abstr. Internat Res. Cong. Nat. Prod. Coll. Pharm. Univ. N Carolina Chapel Hill Nc,* **1985,** July 7-12, Abestr-202

[24] Saraswat, B. *et al.*: *Ind. J. Exp. Biol.* **1993,** 31 (4), 316

[25] Mahajani, S. S. *et al.*: *Aspects Allergy Appl. Immunol* **1979,** 12, 205

[26] Sharma, M. L. *et al.*: *J. Ethnopharmacol.* **1994,** 41 (1/2), 185

[27] Vaishwanar, I. *et al.*: Indian J. Exp. Biol. **1976,** 14, 58

[28] Paney, B. L. *et al.*: *Indian J. Physiol. Pharmacol.* **1989,** 33 (1), 28

[29] Dhar, M. L. *et al.*: *Indian J. Exp. Biol.* **1973,** 11, 43

[30] Ansari, R. A. *et al.*: *J. Ethnopharmacol.* **1991,** 34 (1), 61

[31] Namba, T. *et al.*: *Shoyakugaku Zasshi* **1981,** 35 (4), 295

[32] Choi, S. Y. *et al.*: *Ann. Rep. Nat. Prod. Res. Inst. Seoul Nat'l Univ.* **1982,** 21, 49

[33] Yun, H. S. *et al.*: *Korean J. Pharmacog.* **1980,** 11, 149

[34] Chang, I. M. *et al.*: *Advances In Chinese Medicinal Materials Research*, H M Chang H W Yeung W W Tso And A Koo (EDS), World Scientific press Philadelphia Pa **1984,** 269

[35] Mokkhasmit, M. *et al.*: *J. Med. Ass. Thailand* **1971**, 54 (7), 490

[36] Shukla, B. *et al.*: *Planta Med.* **1991,** 57 (1), 29

[37] Dwivedi, Y. *et al.*: *Pharmacol. Res.* **1993,** 27 (2), 189

[38] Visen, P. K. S. *et al.*: *Phytother. Res.* **1991,** 5 (5), 224

[39] Saksena, S. *et al.*: *Drug Dev. Res.* **1994,** 33 (1), 46

[40] Dwivedi, Y. *et al.*: *Phytother. Res.* **1991,** 5 (3), 115

[41] Tripathi, S. C. *et al.*: *Indian J. Pharmacy* **1991,** 23 (3), 143

[42] Dwivedi, Y. *et al.*: *Planta Med.* **1993,** 59 (5), 418

[43] Khanna, A. K. *et al.*: *Phytother Res.* **1994,** 8 (7), 403

[44] Mahajani, S. S. *et al.*: *Int. Arch. Allergy Appl. Immunol.* **1976,** 53, 137

[45] Dorsch, W. *et al.*: *Int. Arch. Allergy Appl. Immunol.* **1991,** 95 (2/3), 128

[46] Chander, R. *et al.*: *Indian J. Med. Res.* **1990,** 92 (1), 34

[47] Dwivedi, Y. *et al.*: *Pharmacol. Toxic.* **1992,** 71 (5), 383

[48] Dwivedi, Y. *et al.*: *Pharmacol. Res.* **1991,** 23 (4), 399

[49] Singh, V. *et al..*: *Indian J. Biochem. Biophys.* **1992,** 29 (5), 428

[50] Yegnanarayan, R. *et al.*: *Boybay Hosp. J.* **1982,** 24 (2), 15

[51] Shukula, B. *et al.*: *Phytother. Res.* **1992,** 6 (1), 53

[52] Antarkar, D. S. *et al.*: *Indian J. Med. Res.* **1980,** 72, 588

[53] Pandey, B. L. *et al.*: *Indian J. Physiol. Pharmacol.* **1988,** 32 (4), 289

[54] Atal, C. K. *et al.*: *J. Ethnopharmacol.* **1986,** 18 (2), 133

[55] Srivastava, S. *et al.*: *Ind. J. Pharmacology* **1994,** 26 (1), 19

[56] Debelmas, A. M. *et al.*: *Plant Med. Phytother.* **1976,** 10, 128

[57] Simons, J. M. *et al.*: *Pharm. Weekbl.* **1987,** 9 (2), 157

[58] Chongsiri, A. *et al.*: *J. Pharm. Ass. Siam* **1949,** 2 (4), 165

[59] Pandey, B. L. *et al.*: *Indian J. Physiol. Pharmacol.* **1988,** 32 (2), 120

[C. K. Sung]

553.   *Picrorhiza scrophulariiflora* **Pennell**   (Scrophulasiaceae)

Hu-huang-lian (C), Woo-wong-lin (H), Seo-jang-ho-hwang-ryun (K)

Rhizome (CP)
Local Drug Name: Hu-huang-lian (C), Woo-wong-lin (H), Ko-oren (J), Ho-hwang-ryun (K).
Processing: Eliminate foreign matter, and cut into slices, or break to pieces before use (C, K).

Method of Administration: Oral (decoction: C, H, K).
Folk Medicinal Uses:

       1) Dysentery or jaundice cauced by damp-heat (C, H, J, K).

       2) Hemorrhoids (C, H).

       3) Consumptive fever and fever in infantile malnutrition due to digestive disturhance (C, H).

Scientific Researches:
Chemistry

  1) Iridoid glycosides: picroside I, II [1], III [2,3], catalpol, aucubin [4].

  2) Glucosides: cinnamoyl-α-D-glucopyranose, 6-cinnamoyl-D-glucopyranose [2].

  3) Organic acids: vanillic acid, cinnamic acid, ferulic acid [3].

  4) Phenolic glycosides: androsin [4].

  5) Cucurbitacin glycosides: 2β-glucopyranosyloxy-3,16,20,22-tetrahydroxy-9-methyl-19-norlanosta-5,24-diene [4].

Pharmacology

  1) Inhibitive effect on dermatomyces [5].

Literatures:
[1] Weinges, K. et al.: *Justus Liebigs Ann. Chem.* **1972,** 759, 173.

[2] Weinges, K. et al.: *Justus Liebigs Ann. Chem.* **1977,** (6), 1053.

[3] Xie, P.S.: *Zhongcaoyao* **1980,** 14(8), 341.

[4] Wang, D.Q. et al.: *Yunnan Zhiwu Yanjiu* **1993,** 15(1), 83.

[5] Cao, R.L. et al.: *Zhonghau Pifuke Zazhi* **1957,** (4), 286.

                                           [J.X. Guo]

554.   *Scoparia dulcis* L.   (Scrophulariaceae)

Ye-gan-cao (C), Yair-gum-cho (H)

Whole Plant
Local Drug Name: Bing-tang-cao (C), Yair-gum-cho (H).
Processing: Use in fresh or dry under the sun (C, H).
Method of Administration: Oral (decoction: C, H); Topical (juice squeezed from fresh herb: C, H).
Folk Medicinal Uses:

       1) Colds (C, H).

       2) Fever (C, H).

       3) Cough (C, H).

       4) Bacillary dysentery (C, H).

       5) Oliguria (C, H).

       6) Eczema (C, H).

       7) Enteritis (C).

       8) Sudamen (C).

       9) Beri-beri (H).

      10) Edema (H).

      11) Heat rash (H).

Scientific Research:
Chemistry

  1) Flavonoids [1–2]: Acacetin (flavone) [2–3], hymenoxin (flavone) [4], 5,7,8,3',4',5'-hexahydroxyflavone glucuronide (flavone glucoside) [5], isovitexin (flavone) [5].

  2) Triterpenoids: Glutinol [1, 3, 6], betulinic acid [6, 18], friedelin, α-amyrin, ifflaionic acid [6].

3) Diterpenoids: Scopadulcic acids A–B [3, 7–9, 11, 21], scoparic acids A–C [11–13], scopadulin [14], scopadulciol [3, 15], scopadiol [15], scoparinol, dulcinol [16].

4) 6-Methoxybenzoxazolinone [3, 17].

5) Hydrocarbons: D-Mannitol [18].

6) Amides: Coixol [18].

7) Glut-5(6)-en-3β-ol [19].

Pharmacology

1) Analgesic effect [1].

2) Antiinflammatory effect [1].

3) Sedative effect [1].

4) Hypertensive effect [1].

3) Antiviral activity [2, 7, 9, 14].

4) Cytotoxic effect [4].

5) β-Glucuronidase inhibitory effect [5, 12].

6) Inhibiting of Na⁺, K⁺-ATPase [3, 8].

6) Inhibiting of Na^+, K^+-ATPase [3, 8].

7) Sympathomimetic activity [20].

8) Muscle-relaxant effect [20].

9) Antitumor effect [21].

Literature:

[1] De Farias Freire, S.M. *et al.*: *Phytother. Res.* **1993,** 7, 408.

[2] Hayashi, K. *et al.*: *Antiviral Chem. Chemother.* **1993**, 4, 49.

[3] Hayashi, T. *et al.*: *J. Nat. Prod.* **1991**, 54, 802.

[4] Hayashi, T. *et al.*: *Chem. Pharm. Bull.* **1988**, 36, 4849.

[5] Kawasaki, M. *et al.*: *Phytochemistry* **1988**, 27, 3709.

[6] Mahato, S.B. *et al.*: *Phytochemistry* **1981**, 20, 171.

[7] Hayashi, K. *et al.*: *Antiviral Res.* **1988**, 9, 345.

[8] Hayashi, T. *et al.*: *Chem. Pharm. Bull.* **1990**, 38, 2740.

[9] Hayashi, T. *et al.*: *Tetrahedron Lett.* **1987**, 28, 3693.

[10] Hayashi, T. *et al.*: *J. Nat. Prod.* **1988**, 51, 360.

[11] Hayashi, T. *et al.*: *Tennen Yuki Kagobutsu Toronkai Koen Yoshishu* **1987**, 29, 544.

[12] Hayashi, T. *et al.*: *J. Nat. Prod.* **1992**, 55, 1748.

[13] Kawasaki, M. *et al.*: *Chem. Pharm. Bull.* **1987**, 35, 3963.

[14] Hayashi, T. *et al.*: *Chem. Pharmm. Bull.* **1990**, 38, 945.

[15] Hayashi, T. *et al.*: *Phytochemistry* **1993**, 32, 349.

[16] Ahmed, M. *et al.*: *Phytochemistry* **1990**, 29, 3035.

[17] Hayashi, T. *et al.*: *Phytochemistry* **1994**, 37, 1611.

[18] Li, J.X. *et al.*: *Yunnan Zhiwu Yanjiu* **1981**, 3, 475.

[19] Ferous, A.J. *et al.*: *Fitoterapia* **1993**, 64, 469.

[20] Freire, S.M. *et al.*: *J. Pharm. Pharmacol.* **1996**, 48, 624.

[21] Nishino, H. *et al.*: *Oncology* **1993**, 50, 100.

[P.P.H. But]

555. *Acanthus ilicifolius* **Linnaeus** (Acanthaceae)

Lao-shu-le (C), Loe-xue-luck (H)

Root

Local Drug Name: Lao-shu-le (C), Loe-xue-luck (H).

Processing: Wash, slice and dry under the sun (C, H).

Method of Administration: Oral (decoction: C, H).

Folk Medicinal Uses:

1) Hepatitis (C, H).

2) Hepatosplenomegaly (C, H).
3) Lymphadenopathy (C, H).
4) Asthma (C, H).
5) Gastric pain (C, H).
6) Cough (C).
7) Malignancy (H).

Scientific Research:
Chemistry
1) 2-Benzoxazolinone [1–2].
2) Alkaloid: Acanthicifoline [3], trigonellin [5].
3) Triterpenoid: Saponin [4], oleanolic acid, lupeol [5].
4) Flavonoids: Quercetin, quercetin 3-O-β-D-glucopyranoside [5].
5) Steroid: β-Sitosterol[5]
Pharmacology
1) Leishmanicidal effect [1].
2) Analgesic effect [6].
3) Anti-inflammatory effect [6].

Literature:
[1] Kapil, A. *et al.*: *Planta Med.* **1994**, 60, 187.
[2] Murty, M.S.R. *et al.*: *Indian J. Pharm. Sci.* **1984**, 46, 218.
[3] Tiwari, K.P. *et al.*: *Pol. J. Chem.* **1980**, 54, 857.
[4] Minocha, P.K. *et al.*: *Phytochemistry* **1981**, 20, 135.
[5] Minocha, P.K. *et al.*: *Pol. J. Chem.* **1980**, 54, 2089.
[6] Agshikar, N.V. *et al.*: *Indian J. Exp. Biol.* **1979**, 17, 1257.
[7] Untawale, A.G. *et al.*: *Mahasagar* **1978**, 11, 105.
[8] Untawale, A.G. *et al.*: *Mahasagar* **1980**, 13, 215.

[P.P.H. But]

556. *Rostellularia procumbens* **(L.) Nees von Esenbeck**   (Acanthaceae)
[= *Justicia procumbens* L.]

Jue-chuang (C), Jerk-chong (H), Kitsunenomago (J)

Related species: *Justicia hayatai* Yanmamoto var. *decumbens* Yamamoto.

Whole plant
Local Drug Name: Jue-chuang (C), Jerk-chong (H).
Processing: Dry under the sun (C, H).
Method of Administration: Oral (decoction: C, H); Topical (C, H).
Folk Medicinal Uses:
      1) Colds, fever (C, H).
      2) Sorethroat (C, H).
      3) Infantile malabsorption and malnutrition (C, H).
      4) Dysentery, enteritis (C, H).
      5) Nephritis (C, H).
      6) Bois, pyodermas (C, H).
      7) Hepatitis (C, H).
      8) Malaria (C, H).
      9) Traumatic injury (C, H).
     10) Cervical lumph gland tuberculosis (C, H).

11) Edema (H).

12) Urinary tract infection, chyluria (H).

Scientific Research:

Chemistry

1) Lignans: justicidins A–D [1–3, 7, 9], diphyllin [4–5, 7, 9], neojusticins A–B [6, 9], diphyllin apioside, diphyllin apioside-5-acetate [8], taiwanin E, taiwanin E methyl ether, 4'-demethylchinensinaphthol methyl ether, chinensinaphthol, chinensinaphthaol methyl ether [9].

2) Calcium [2].

3) Glucosides: justicidinosides A–C [8].

Pharmacology

1) Fish killing effect [1].

2) Antitumor effect [7].

3) Antiviral effect [8].

4) Antiplatelet effect [9].

Literature:

[1] Munakata, K. et al.: Tetrahedron. Lett. **1965**, 4167.

[2] Munakata, K. et al.: Tetrahedron. Lett. **1967**, 3821.

[3] Ohta, K. et al.: Tetrahedron Lett. **1970**, 923.

[4] Murakami, T.: Yakugaku Zasshi **1961**, 81, 1596.

[5] Horii, Z. et al.: Chem. Comm. **1968**, 653.

[6] Okigawa, M. et al.: Chem. Pharm. Bull. **1970**, 18, 862.

[7] Fukamiya, N. et al.: J. Nat. Prod. **1986**, 49, 348.

[8] Asano, J. et al.: Phytochemistry **1996**, 42, 713.

[9] Chen, C.C. et al.: J. Nat. Prod. **1996**, 59, 1149.

[P.P.H. But]

557.   *Nardostachys chinensis* **Batal.**   (Valerianaceae)

Gan-song (C), Gum-chung (H), Gam-song-hyang (K)

Related Plant: *N. jatamansi* DC.: Chi-ye-gan-song (C), Gwan-yeop-gam-song-hyang (K).

Root and Rhizome (CP)

Local Drug Name: Gan-song (C), Gum-chung (H), Kanshoko (J), Gam-song (K).

Processing: Eliminate foreign matter, and dry in the sun or in the shade (C, K).

Method of Administration: Oral (decoction: C, H); Topical (infusion, decoction or powder: C, H, K).

Folk Medicinal Uses:

1) Epigastric and abdominal distension (C, H, J, K).

2) Anorexia (C, H, J, K).

3) Vomiting (C, H, K).

4) Toothache (external use) (C, H).

5) Swelling of the foot (external use) (C, H).

Scientific Researches:

Chemistry

1) Steroids: β-sitosterol [1].

2) Glycosides: Et β-D-glucopyranoside [1].

3) Sesquiterpenoids: gansongone, nardosinonediol [1], nardosinone [2,3], valeranone, $\Delta^{1,10}$-aristolene, $\Delta^{9,10}$-aristolene, macliol, β-macliene [3], 1(10)-aristolen-2-one, nardostachone [4], dibelon [5], 1,2,9,10-tetradehydroaristolane, 9-aristolen-1-α-ol [6], desoxonarchinol A [7],

narchinol A [8], patchouli, β-patchoulene [9], nardonoxide [10], kanshone A, B [11], C [12], D, E, isonardosinone, nardofuran [13], eudesm-11-en-2,4α-diol [14], nardostachnol [15].

4) Triterpenoids: oleanolic acid [1], arsolic acid [16].

5) Iridoids: nardostachin [16].

6) Trace elements: Sr, Zn, Cu, Ni, Fe, Mn, Ti, Cr, Pb, Ca, K [17].

Pharmacology

1) Cytotoxic effect [18].

2) Sedative effect [19].

3) Antagonistic effect on electric shock [20] and antiarrhythmic effect [20,21].

Literatures:
[1] Shide, L. *et al.*: *Planta Med.* **1987,** 53(6), 556.
[2] Schulte, K. E.: *Tetrahedron Letters* **1965,** (35), 3083.
[3] Schulte, K. E.: *Planta Med.* **1967,** 15(3), 274.
[4] Ruecker *et al.*: *Justus Liebigs Ann. Chem.* **1968,** 717, 221.
[5] Ruecker *et al.*: *Planta Med.* **1971,** 19(1), 16.
[6]Ruecker *et al.*: *Justus Liebigs Ann. Chem.* **1971,** 748, 214.
[7] Ruecker *et al.*: *Phytochemistry* **1974,** 13(9), 1907.
[8] Hikino, H. *et al.*: *Phytochemistry* **1972,** 11(6), 2097.
[9] Ruecker, G. *et al.*: *Planta Med.* **1972,** 21(1), 1.
[10] Shide, L. *et al.*: *Planta Med.* **1987,** 53(4), 332.
[11] Bagchi, A. *et al.*: *Phytochemistry* **1988,** 27(4), 1199.
[12] Bagchi, A. *et al.*: *Phytochemistry* **1988,** 27(9), 2877.
[13] Bagchi, A. *et al.*: *Phytochemistry* **1988,** 27(11), 3667.
[14] Masuyama, K. *et al.*: *Phytochemistry* **1993,** 34(2), 567.
[15] Sun, H. D. *et al.*: *Yunnan Chih Wu Yen Chiu* **1980,** 2(2), 213.
[16] Bagchi, A. *et al.*: *Planta Med.* **1988,** 54(1), 87.
[17] Qin, J. F. *et al.*: *Zhongcaoyao* **1983,** 14(11), 492.
[18] Itokawa, H. *et al.*: *Chem. Pharm. Bull.* **1993,** 41(6), 1183.
[19] Pan, D. F.: *Zhongguo Yaoxuehui Dierjie Quanguo Huiyuan Daibiao Dahui Lunwen Zhaiyaoji* **1956,** (1), 133.
[20] *"Zhongyao Dacidian"* **1977,** 566.
[21] Ma, C. G. *et al.*: *Anyi Xuebao* **1980,** 15(4), 9.

[J.X. Guo]

558.   *Nardostachys jatamansi* **DC.**   (Valerianaceae)

Chi-ye-gan-song (C), Gum-chung (H), Kanshoko (J), Gwan-yeop-gam-song (K)

Related plant: *Nardostachys chinensis* Batal.: Gan-song (C).

Rhyzome

Local Drug Name: Gum-chung (H), Kanshoko (J), Gam-song-hyang (K).

Processing: Dry under in the shade (C, J, K).

Method of Administration: Oral (decoction: C, H, J, K).

Folk Medicinal Uses:

1) Abdominal pain (H, J, K).

2) Convulsion (J, K).

3) External use for toothache and swelling of the foot (C).

4) Epigastric and abdominal distension with anorexia and vomiting (C).

5) Flaturent (J).

Scientific Researches:

Chemistry

1) Sesquiterpenes: Valeranone (= jatamansone) [2], jatamansic acid [3], calarenol [4], calarene [5], nardol [5,6,7], nardostachone [4], elemol, β-eudesmol [7], β-maaliene [8] and aristolone [9].

2) Cumarins: Lomatin (= jatamansinol), selinidin (=jatamansin) and angelicin [7].

3) Steroids: β-Sitosterol [7].

Pharmacology

1) Bone sorption inhibitor for treatment of osteoporosis and hypercalcemia (sesquiterpene BR606) [1].

Literatures:

[1] Kawashima, A. *et al.*: *Japan Kokai Tokkyo Koho* JP 08041068 A2, **1996,** (Japan).
[2] Govindachari T. R. *et al.*: *Chem. Ber.* **1958**, 91, 908; *Tetrahedron Lett.* **1959,** 5; *Chem. & Ind.* **1960,** 1059; *Tetrahedron* **1961**, 12, 105; Krepinsky, J. *et al.*: *Tetrahedron Lett.* **1960,** 9; 11; Djerassi, C.: Tetrahedron Lett. 1961, 226; Klyne, W. *et al.*: *Tetrahedron Lett.* **1964,** 1443; Banerjee, D. K.: *J. Indian Chem. Soc.* **1972**, 49, 1; Seshadri, T. R. *et al.*: *Phytochem.* **1967**, 6, 445.
[3] Rucker, G. *et al.*: *Arch. Pharm.* **1974**, 307, 791.
[4] Sastry, S. D. *et al.*: *Tetrahedron* **1967**, 23, 1997; 2491.
[5] Buchi, G. *et al.*: *Tetrahedron Lett.* **1962**, 827; Sorm, F. *et al.*: *Coll. Czech. Chem. Comm.* **1953**, 18, 512.
[6] Sastry, S. D. *et al.*: *Tetrahedron Lett.* **1966,** 1035.
[7] Shabhag, S. N. *et al.*: *Tetrahedron Lett.* **1965**, 2605.
[8] Bates, R. B. *et al.*: *J. Am. Chem. Soc.* **1960**, 82, 2327; Buchi, G. *et al.*: *Tetrahedron Lett.* **1962**, 827.
[9] Furukawa, S. *et al.*: *Yakkugaku Zasshi* **1961**, 81, 559; 565; 570.

[T. Kimura]

559.   *Valeriana fauriei Briquet*   (Valerianaceae)

Zhi-zhu-qi(C), Kanokoso(J), Jwi-o-jum-pul(K)

Root

Local Drug Name: Zhu-zhi-qi(C), Kissokon(J), Gil-cho-geun(K),
Processing: Dry under the sun(C, J, K)
Method of Administration: Oral(decoction, C, J, K)
Folk Medicinal Uses:

1) Insomnia(C, J, K)
2) Neurasthenia(C, J, K)
3) Hysteria(J, K)
4) Prolapsus anus(K)

Scientific Research:

Chemistry

1) Monoterpenes: 2-iso-propyl-4-methyl anisole, borneol, borneol acetate, camphene, *p*-cymene, limonene, myrtenol iso-valerate, α-pinene, β-pinene, tertpineol acetate [1], kanokoside A [2, 3, 6], kanokoside C[2, 3], kanokoside D[2, 5], patrinoside [2, 3, 6]

2) Sesquiterpenes: cryptofauronol, faurinone, fauronol acetate, β-gurjunene, α-kessyl acetate, ledol, nardol, valeranone [1], kanokonol acetate [1, 3], kessyl glycol diacetate [1, 5], 2(R)-β-bisabolol, 2-acetoxy β-bisabolol[2], caryophyllene oxide, maaliol[3], cyclokessol acetate[3, 4, 5], kanokanol [5], patcouli alchol, 8-acetoxy patcouli alchol, 8-hydroxy patcouli alchol [6]

Phamacology

1) Antidepressant activity [5]

144

2) Antispasmodic activity [6]

Literature:
[1] Hikino, H. *et al.* : *Yakugaku. Zasshi.* **1971**, 91, 766
[2] Nishiya, K. *et al.*: *Phytochemistry.* **1994**, 36, 1547.
[3] Nishiya, K. *et al.*: *Phytochemistry.* **1992**, 31, 3511.
[4] Oshima, Y. *et al.*: *Tetrahedron lett.* **1986**, 27, 1829.
[5] Oshima, Y. *et al.*: *Chem. Pharm. Bull.* **1995**, 43, 169.
[6] Nishiya, K. *et al.*: *Phytochemistry.* **1995**, 39, 713.
[7] Itogawa, H.: *Shoyakugaku Zasshi* **1983**, 37, 223.

[C. K. Sung]

560.   *Dipsacus asper* **Wallich**   (Dipsacaceae)

Juk-duan (H), Tou-nabeba (J), Cheon-sok-dan (K).

Root
Local Drug Name: Juk-duan (H), Zokudan (J), Cheon-sok-dan(K)
Processing: Dry under the sun (J, K).
Method of Administration: Decoction (H, J, K).
Folk Medicinal Uses:
        1) Fracture (H, J, K).
        2) Traumatic injury (H, J).
        3) Lumbago (H).
        4) Nocturnal emission (H).

Scientific Researches:
Chemistry
   1) Saponins and triterpenoids: Tauroside St-G01 [1], akebia saponin D [2], saponin IX and X, XI, XII, and XIII [3], dipsacus saponin A, B and C [4].
   2) Iridoids: sweroside, loganin, loganic acid 6'-O-β-D-glucoside [1].
Pharmacology
   1) Antinociceptive (dipsacus saponin C) [5].

Literatures:
[1] Kouno, I. *et al.*: *Phytochem.* **1990**, 29(1), 338.
[2] Zhang, Y. W. *et al.*: *Yaoxue Xuebao* **1991**, 26(9), 676; 911.
[3] Zhang, Y. W. *et al.*: *Yaoxue Xuebao* **1992**, 27(12), 912; **1993**, 28(58), 358.
[4] Jung, K. Y. *et al.*: *Arch. Pharmacal Res.* **1993**, 16,(1), 32; *J. Nat. Prod.* **1993**, 56(11), 1912.
[5] Suh, H.-W., *et al.*: *Gen. Pharmacol.*, **1996**, 27(7), 1167.

[T. Kimura]

561.   *Adenophora remotiflora* **Miq.**   (Campanulaceae)

Sobana (J), Mo-si-dae (K)

Root
Local Drug Name: Seini (J), Je-ni (K).
Processing: Dry under the sun (J, K).
Method of Administration: Decoction (J, K).

Folk Medicinal Uses:
> 1) Snakebite (J).
> 2) Insectbite (J).
> 3) Swelling (J).
> 4) Poisoning (K).
> 5) Sputum (K).

Scientific Researches:
Chemistry
> 1) Polysaccharides [1].
> 2) Anthocyanidins: distribution in the flowers [2].

Literatures:
[1] Tu, Pengfei *et al.: Zhongcaoyao*, **1992**, 23,(7) 355.
[2] Kim, K. W. *et al.: Han'guk Wonye Hokhoechi*, **1996**, 37(4), 582.

[T. Kimura]

562.   *Achillea sibirica* **Ledeb.**   (Compositae)

Nokogiriso(J), Top-pul(K)

Whole plant
Local Drug Name: Giso(J), Il-ji-ho(K)
Processing: Dry under the sun(J, K)
Method of Administration: Oral(decoction, J, K), external(ointment, J)
Folk Medicinal Uses:
> 1) Scabies(J, K)
> 2) Weakness(J, K)
> 3) Stomach cramps(J, K)
> 4) Amenorrhea(J, K)
> 5) Hemorrhoid(K)
> 6) Panaris(J)
> 7) Eczema(J)
> 8) Contusion(K)
> 9) Stomach ulcers(K)
> 10) Breeding(K)

Contraindications: in pregnacy

Scientific Research:
Chemistry
> 1) Phenylpropanoids: Chlorogenic acid, iso-chlorogenic acid A[1]
> 2) Flavonoids: Quercetin-rhamno-glucoside, iso-orientin, vicenine[1]
> 3) Alkaloids[2]
> 4) Sterols and triterpenes[2]

Literature:
[1] Valant, K.: *Naturwissenschaften* **1978**, 65(8), 437.
[2] Woo, W. S. *et al.: Korean J. Pharmacog.* **1977**, 8, 103.
[3] Ishii, R. *et al.: Agr. Biol. Chem.* **1984**, 48(10), 2587.

[C. K. Sung]

563.   *Emilia sonchifolia* **(Linn.) DC.**   (Compositae)

Yi-dian-hong (C), Yut-dim-hung (H)

Whole Plant
Local Drug Name: Yi-dian-hong (C), Yut-dim-hung (H).
Processing: Wash and dry or use when fresh (C, H).
Method of Administration: Oral (decoction: C, H); Topical (decoction for washing or mashed herb
                            as poultice: C, H).
Folk Medicinal Uses:
                  1) Gastroenteritis (C, H).
                  2) Dysentery (C, H).
                  3) Furuncles and carbuncles (C, H).
                  4) Mastitis (C, H).
                  5) Stomatocace (C).
                  6) Pheumonia (C).
                  7) Orchitis (C).
                  8) Eczema (C).
                  9) Traumatic injury (C).
                  10) Upper respiratory tract infection (C).
                  11) Sore throat (C).
                  12) Colds (H).
                  13) Fever (H).
                  14) Infantile malabsorption (H).
                  15) Rheumatic arthralgia (H).
                  16) Snake bites (H).
Contraindication: Pregnancy.

Scientific Research:
  Chemistry
  1) Simiaral, β-sitosterol, stignasterol, palmitic acid, triacontanoic acid [1], n-hexacosanol,
     triacontane [3].
  2) Pyrrolizidine alkaloids: senkirkine, doronine [2].
  3) Flavonoids: kaempferol 3-β-D-gaalactoside, quercitrin, rutin, quercetin [3].

Literature:
  [1] Gao, J. Y. *et al.*: *Zhongguo Zhongyao Zazhi* **1993,** 18, 102.
  [2] Cheng, D. L. *et al.*: *Planta Med.* **1986,** 86, 484.
  [3] Srinivasan, K. K. *et al.*: *Fitoterapia* **1980,** 51, 241.

[P.P.H. But]

564.   *Farfugium japonicum* **(L.) Kitam.**   (Compositae)
[= *Senecio kaempferi*]

Da-wu-feng-cao (C), Tock-ng (H), Tsuwabuki (J), Teol-meo-wi (K)

Whole Plant or Rhizome
Local Drug Name: Ba-jiao-wu (C), Tock-ng (H), Takugo (J), Yeon-bong-cho (K).
Processing: Use when fresh or dry under the sun (C, H, J, K).
Method of Administration: Oral (decoction: C, H, J, K); Topical (crushed fresh herb: C, H, J, K).
Folk Medicinal Uses:
                  1) Boils, pyodermas (C, H, K).

2) Traumatic injury (C, H, K).
3) Mastitis (C, H).
4) Irregula menses (C, H).
5) Cough and hemoptysis (C, H).
6) Eczema (H, J).
7) Influenza (H, K).
8) Pharyngitis (H, K).
9) Tonsillitis (H, K).
10) Colds (H, K).
11) Hematochezia (C).
12) Hematemesis (H).
13) Melena (H).
14) Hematuria (H).
15) Scalds (H).
16) Snake bites (H).
17) Amenorrhea (H).
18) Diarrhea (J).
19) Gastroenteritis (J).
20) Suppuration (J).

Side effect: hepatotoxic.

Scientific Research:
Chemistry
1) α,α-bis(3β-angeloyloxyfuranoeremophilane), 3β-angeloyloxy-8β-hydroxy-9β-senecioyloxyere-mophilenolide[1], 3β-angeloyloxy-9-en-8-epi-eremophilenolide, 3β-angeloyloxy-8-epi-eremo-philenolide[2], 8β-hydroxyeremophilenolide, 3β-angeloyloxy-8β,10β-dihydroxyeremophileno-lide, 3β-angeloyloxy-6β-hydroxy-8-epieremophilenolide[3], farformolide A (3β-angeloyloxy-10β-hydroxyeremophilenolide), farformolide B (6β,8β-dimethoxy-10β-hydroxyeremophile-nolid) [4], 3β-angeloyloxy-10β-hydroxy-9β-senecioyloxyfuranoeremophilane, 3β-angeloyl-oxy-10β-hydroxyfuranoeremophilane [5].
2) Benzofuranosesquiterpenes: farfugin A and B [6-7].
3) Pyrrolizidine alkaloid: senkirkine [8].
4) Triterpenoids: α-amyrin, bakkenolide A, brein[1, 4].
5) Steroids: campesterol, stigmasterol, β-sitosterol [1].
6) Acids: linoleic acid, linolenic acid, palmitic acid[1].
Pharmacology
1) Carcinogenic effect [9].

Literature:
[1] Kurihara, T. et al.: Yakugaku Zasshi **1981,** 101, 35.
[2] Kurihara, T. et al.: Yakugaku Zasshi **1980,** 100, 681.
[3] Ito, K. et al.: Yakugaku Zasshi **1980,** 100, 69.
[4] Ito, K. et al.: Yakugaku Zasshi **1978,** 98, 1592.
[5] Nagano, H. et al.: Bull. Chem. Soc. Jpn. **1978,** 51, 3335.
[6] Nagano, H. et al.: Bull. Chem. Soc. Jpn. **1974,** 47, 1994.
[7] Nagano, H. et al.: Chem. Lett. **1972,** (1), 13.
[8] Furuya, T. et al.: Phytochemistry. **1971,** 10, 3306.
[9] Hirono, I. et al.: Cancer Letters **1983,** 20, 191.

[P.P.H. But]

565.   *Gynura bicolor* DC.   (Compositae)

Sam-chil-cho(K)

Related plant: *G. japonica* Juel: Sanshichiso(J)

Herb
  Local Drug Name: To-sam-chil(K)
  Processing: Dry under the sun(K)
  Method of Administration: Oral(decoction, K)
  Folk Medicinal Uses:
                  1) Styptic(K)

Scientific Researches:
  Pharmacology
      1) Hemostatic effect[1]

Literatures:
  [1] Li, C. Z.: *Chung Yao Tung Pao* **1985**, 10(9), 42.

                                                [C. K. Sung]

566.   *Gynura japonica* **Juel**   (Compositae)

                  Ju-ye-shan-qi (C), Sanshichiso (J)

Leaf
  Local Drug Name: Tu-shan-qi (C), Sanshichi (J).
  Processing: Fresh (C), Dry under the sun (C, J).
  Method of Administration: Decoction (C, J), external (paste: C, J).
  Folk Medicinal Uses:
          1) Bleeding (C, J).
          2) Traumatic injury (C, J).
          3) Hematemesis (C, J).
          4) Kaschin-Beck disease (C).

Scientific Researches:
  Chemistry
      1) Steroids and saponins: 3-epi-diosgenin, 3-epi-sceptumgenin, 3-epi-ruscogenin and 3-epi-
         neoruscogenin [1].

Literatures:
  [1] Takahira, M. *et al.*: *Tetrahedron Letters*, **1977**(41), 3647.

                                                [T. Kimura]

567.   *Helianthus annuus* **L.**   (Compositae)

              Xiang-ri-kui (C), Himawari (J), Hae-ba-ra-gi (K)

Fruit
  Local Drug Name: Xiang-ri-kui (C), Himawari (J), Hyang-il-gyu-ja (K).
  Processing: Dry under the sun (C, J, K).
  Method of Administration: Oral (decoction: C, K).
  Folk Medicinal Uses:
          1) Anorexia (C).

2) Serve intermittent headache (C).
3) Measles without adequate eruption (C).
4) Acute gastritis (K).
5) Apepsia (K).
6) Fever (K).

Scientific Researches:
Chemistry
  1) Sesquiterpenes: Annuolide F, annuolide G, heliangolide, helvypolide A and B [1].
  2) Diterpenoids: trachyloban-19-oic acid [15].
  3) Triterpenes and saponins: Helianol from the flower [2, 3], two oleanolic acid glycosides [11], taraxanthin (=lutein epoxide) [13], helianthoside C [14], lupeol, taraxasterol, pseudotaraxasterol, α-amyrin, calenduladiol diacetate, faradiol diacetate, brein diacetate and erythrodiol diacetate [16].
  4) Steroids: Stigmasterol, β-sitosterol [7], campesterol, stigmastadienol, stigmastatrienol [5], tocopherol and strols [8], Δ^7-stigmasterol, $\Delta^{7,24(25)}$-stigmastadienol and $\Delta^{7,9(11),24(28)}$-stigmastatrienol [17].
  5) Saccharides: Pectin [6].
  6) Polyacetylenes: Dehydrofalcarinone [9].
  7) Phenolic compounds: Chlorogenic acid, isochlorogenic acid, neochlorogenic acid and 3-*O*-feruloyl quinic acid [10].
  8) Fatty acids [12].
Pharmacology
  1) Allelopathic effect (annuolide F, G, heliangolide) [1].
  2) Antiinflammatory effect (triterpene alcohol in the flower) [3].
  3) Cytotoxicity and hemolytic index (saponins) [4].

Literatures:
[1]Macias, F. *et al.*: *Phytochem.* **1996**, 43(6), 1205.
[2]Akihisa, T. *et al.*: *Chem. Pharm. Bull.* **1996**, 44(6), 1255.
[3] Akihisa, T. *et al.*: *Phytochem.* **1996**, 43(6), 1255.
[4] Bader, G. *et al.*: *Pharmazie,* **1996**, 51(6), 414.
[5] Homberg, E. E. *et al.*: *Phytochem.* **1973**, 12, 1767.
[6] Zitko, V. *et al.*: *Canad. J. Chem.* **1965**, 43, 3206.
[7] Kozin, N. I. *et al.*: *Maslob.-Zhir. Prom.* **1964,** 30,11.
[8] Malysheva, A. G.: *Masloboino-Zhirovaya Prom.* **1961**, 27(9), 7.
[9] Bohlmann, F. *et al.*: *Chem. Ber.* **1962**, 95, 1320.
[10] Rice, E. L.: *Physiol. Plantarum* **1965,** 18, 255; Corse, J. W.: *Nature* **1953**, 172, 771; *Tetrahedron* **1962**, 1202; Scarpati, M. L. *et al.*: *Tetrahedron Lett.* **1963**, 1147; Zane, A. *et al.*: *Nature,* **1966**, 209, 81.
[11] Kasprzyk, Z. *et al.*: *Bull. Acad. Pol. Sci. Ser. Sci. Biol.* **1966**, 14, 747.
[12] Cummins, D. G. *et al.*: *J. Amer. Oil Chem. Soc.* **1967**, 44, 581.
[13] Egger, K.: *Planta* **1968**, 80, 65.
[14] Cheban, P. L. *et al.*: *Khim. Prir. Soedin.* **1969**, 129.
[15] Achmatowicz, O. Jr. *et al.*: *J. Chem. Soc. (D)* **1971**, 98.
[16] Kasprzyk, Z. *et al.*: *Phytochem.* **1971**, 10, 1946.
[17] Homberg, E. E. *et al.*: *Phytochem.* **1973**, 12, 1767.

[T. Kimura]

568.   *Inula britannica* Thunb. var. *chinensis* Regel   (Compositae)

Xuan-fu-hua(C), Geum-bul-cho(K)

Related plant: *I. britannica* L., *I. japonica* Thunb: Oguruma(J)

Flower(CP)
Local Drug Name: Xuan-fa-hua(C), Senpukuka(J), Seon-bok-hwa(K)
Processing: Dry under the sun(K)
      1) Eliminate pedicels, leaves, and other foreign matter(C).
      2) Stir-fry the clear Flos Inulae with honey until it is no longer sticky to fingers(C).
Method of Administration: Oral(decoction, C, J, K)
Folk Medicinal Uses:
      1) Emesis(J, K)
      2) Cough in common cold(C).
      3) Belching, nausea and vomiting with stuffiness sensation in the epigastric
        region(C).
      4) Cough with dyspnea and copious expectoration due to accumulation of
        phlegm(C).
      5) Swelling(K)

Scientific Research
Chemistry
  1) Sesquiterpenes: Inuchinenolide A - C, tomentosin, gaillardin, 4-epi-isoinuviscolide, ivalin, gaillardin[1], britannilactone, 1-O-acetyl britannilactone, 1,6-O-diacetyl britannilactone[2],

Literature
[1] Ito, K. *et al.*: *Phytochemistry 1981*, 20, 271.
[2] Zhou, B. N. *et al.*: *Phytochemistry* 1993, 34(1), 249.

[C. K. Sung]

569.   *Inula racemosa* **Hook. f.** (Compositae)

Zong-zhuang-tu-mu-xiang (C), Toh-muk-heung (H)

Related plant: *I. helenium* L.: Tu-mu-xiang (C), Mok-hyang (K).

Root (CP)
Local Drug Name: Tu-mu-xiang (C), Toh-muk-heung (H), To-mok-hyang (K).
Processing : Eliminate foreign matter, wash clean, moisten thoroughly, cut into slices, dry in the sun (C, K).
Method of Administration: Oral (pills or powder: C, H, decoction: K).
Folk Medicinal Uses:
      1) Distending pain in the chest, hypochondrium and epigastrium, vomiting and
        diarrhea(C, H).
      2) Bruise or sudden sprain of the chest with pain during breathing (C, H).
      3) Threatened abortion (C).
      4) Stomachic (K).
      5) Apepsia (K).

Scientific Researches:
Chemistry
  1) Terpenoids: alantolactone, iso-alantolactone [1-6], dihydro-alantolactone, dihydro-iso-alantolactone, alantolic acid, alantol [3-6], dammaradienyl acetate, friedelin, lupeol [7], *l*-dammara-20,24-dien-3β-yl acetate [8], alloalantolactone [9], inunal, isoalloalantolactone[10], aplotaxene, phenylacetonitrile [11], isoinunal I, II, III, telekin [12], alantodiene, isoalantodiene

[13], 4(-15)-α-epoxyisotelekin I, II [14].
2) Steroids: β-sitosterol, β-sitosterol-β-D-glucoside [1], γ-sitosterol-glucoside [7].
3) Alkanes [7].
4) Sugars: inulin [15], D-mannitol [16].
5) Organic acids: octadecanoic acid [16].

Pharmacology
1) Antidermatophytic effect [1].
2) Antifungal effect [1].
3) Antibacterial effect [17-20].
4) Antiscolic effect [21-23].

Literatures:
[1] Tripathi, V. D. *et al.*: *Indian J. Pharm. Sci.* **1978,** 40(4), 129.
[2] Arora, R. K. *et al.*: *Econ. Bot.* **1980,** 34(2), 175.
[3] Liu, G. S. *et al.*: *Zhongguo Yixue Kexueyuan Lunwen Zhaiyao* **1965,** 1, 20.
[4] Marshall, J. A. *et al.*: *J. Org. Chem.* **1964,** 29, 3727.
[5] Chunoshin, V. *et al.*: *J. Pharm. Soc. Japan* **1951,** 71, 859.
[6] Liu, Q. S.: *Zhongcaoyao Chengfen Huaxue* **1977,** 582.
[7] Olechnowicz, S. W. *et al.*: *Diss. Pharm. Pharmacol.* **1969,** 21(4), 337.
[8] Paknikar, S. K. *et al.*: *Idian J. Chem., Sect. B* **1982,** 22B(9), 894.
[9] Bhandari, P. *et al.*: *Indian J. Chem. Sect. B* **1983,** 22B(3), 286.
[10]Kaur, B. *et al.*: *Phytochemistry* **1986,** 24(9), 2007.
[11]Bokadia, M. M. *et al.*: *Phytochemistry* **1988,** 25(12), 2887.
[12]Kalsi, P. S. *et al.*: *Phytochemistry* **1988,** 27(7), 2079.
[13]Kalsi, P. S. *et al.*: *Phytochemistry* **1989,** 28(8), 2093.
[14]Goyal, R. *et al.*: *Phytochemistry* **1990,** 29(7), 2341.
[15]*"Zhongyao Zhi"* **1979,** Vol.1, 86.
[16]Purushothaman, K. K. *et al.*: *J. Res. Indian Med.* **1974,** 9(3), 30.
[17]Wahab, S. *et al.*: *J. Indian Bot. Soc.* **1981,** 60(3-4), 278.
[18]Lin, Q. S.: *Zhiwu Yaopin Huaxue* **1955,** 456.
[19]Yan, G. H. *et al.*: *Yaoxue Tongbao* **1960,** 8(2), 57.
[20]Olechnowicz, S. W. *et al.*: *Dissertationes Pharm.* **1963,** 15(1), 17.
[21]Semmler, F. W.: *Ber. Dtsch. Chem. Ges.* **1931,** 64(4), 943.
[22]*Jap. J. Med. S. Pharmacol.* **1941,** 13(3), 75.
[23]Auster, F. *et al.*: *Arzneipflanzen* **1955,** 21.

[J.X. Guo]

570.   *Laggera alata* **(D.Don) Sch.-Bip. ex Oliv.**   (Compositae)

Liu-leng-ju (C), Luk-ling-guk (H)

Whole Plant
Local Drug Name: Liu-leng-ju (C), Luk-ling-guk (H).
Processing: Use in fresh or dry under the sun (C, H).
Method of Administration: Oral (decoction: C, H); Topical (crushed fresh herb or decoction: C, H).
Folk Medicinal Uses:
1) Carbunculosis or furunculosis (C, H).
2) Burns (C, H).
3) Rheumatic arthralgia (C, H).
4) Eczema (C, H).
5) Nephritis (C, H).
6) Edema (C, H).
7) Amenorrhea (C, H).

8) Snake bites (C, H).
9) Multiple abscesses (H).
10) Colds (H).
11) Cellulitis (H).
12) Scrofula (H).
13) Tuberculosis of bones (H).
14) Productive cough (H).
15) Loin pain (H).
16) Postpartum abdominal pain (H).

Research:
Chemistry
  1) Mono- and sesquiterpenoids [1, 4]
  2) Eudesmanes [2]
  3) Artemetin [3]

Literature:
[1] Ekundayo, O. *et al.*: *Planta Med.* **1989,** 55, 573.
[2] Zdero, C. *et al.*: *Phytochemistry* **1989,** 28, 3097.
[3] Lee, T. J. *et al.*: *Tetrahedron Lett.* **1974,** (24), 2081.
[4] Onayade, O. A. *et al.*: *Flavour Fragrance J.* **1990,** 5, 165.

[P.P.H. But]

571. *Petasites japonicus* **Maxim.** (Compositae)

Feng-dou-cai (C), Fuki (J), Meo-wi (K)

Whole herb with flower bud
Local Drug Name: Feng-dou-cai (C), Ganto (J), Bong-du-chae (K).,
Processing: Dry under the sun (C, J, K).
Method of Administration: Oral (decoction; C, J, K, fresh juice; K), topical (paste: C).
Folk Medicinal Uses:
  1) Edema (J, K).
  2) Snake bite (C).
  3) Carbuncle (C).
  4) Trauma (C).
  5) Purgation of embryonic poison (J).
  6) Cough (J).
  7) Stomach ache (J).
  8) Contusion (K).
  9) Testis wound (K).
  10) Tonsilitis (K).

Scientific Researches:
Chemistry
  1) Sesquiterpenes: Petasitolone [1], furoeremophillane, petasalbin methylether, furanofukinol, furanopetasitin and furanojaponin [2], 6β-angeloyloxy-3β-hydroxyeremophil-7(11)-en-12,8β-olide, 3β-hydroxy-6β-tigloyloxyeremophil-7(11)-en-12,8β-olide, 3β,6β-diangeloyloxyeremophil-7(11)-en-12,8β-olide [3], 3β-hydroxyeremophil-7(11)-en-12,8β-olide, 3β-hydroxy-6β-methoxyeremophil-7(11)-en-12,8β-olide, 3β-hydroxy-6β,8α-dimethoxyeremophil-7(11)-en-12,8β-olide, 3β,8α-dihydroxy-6β-tigloyloxyeremophil-7(11)-en-12,8β-olide, 3β,8β-dihydroxy-6β-tigloyloxyeremophil-7(11)-en-12,8α-olide, 6β-angeloyloxy-8β-hydroxy-3-oxoeremo-

153

phil-7(11)-en-12,8β-olide [4], 6β-angeloyloxy-3β,9α-dihydroxyeremophil-7(11)-en-12,8β-
olide, 6β-angeloyl-oxy-3β, 9β-dihydroxy-eremophil-7(11)-en-12,8β-olide, 6β-angeloyloxy-
3β,8β,9α-trihydroxy-eremophil-7(11)-en-12,8α-olide, 6β-(3'chloro-2'-hydroxy-2'-methyl-
butyloyloxy)-3β-hydroxy-eremophil-7(11)-en-12,8β-olide, 6β-epoxyangeloyloxy-3β-hydr-
oxyeremophil-7(11)-en-12,8β-olide, 3β-hydroxy-6α-methoxyeremophil-7(11)-en-12,8β-olide,
6β-epoxy-angeloyloxy-3β-hydroxy-eremo-phil-7(11)-en-12,8α-olide, 8β-hydroxy-3-oxoere-
mophil-7(11)-en-12,8α-olide, 6β-hydroxy-8-oxo-eremophil-6-en-12-oic acid methyl ester [5],
(15R)-6β-angeloyloxy-3β,15-epoxy-9β,15-dihydroxyeremophil-7(11)-en-12,8α-olide, 6β-
(3'chloro-2'-hydroxy-2'-methyl-butyryloxy)-3β,8β-dihydroxyeremophil-7(11)-en-12,8α-
olide, 3β,6β-dihydroxyeremophil-7(11)-en-12,8α-olide, 6β,8β-dihydroxy-3-oxoeremophil-
7(11)-en-12,8α-olide [6], eremopetasinorone A, B, eremopetasinorlol, epoxyeremopetasinorol,
eremo-sulfoxynolide A, B, 3β,8α-dihydroxy-6β-methoxyeremo-phil-7(11)-en-12,8β-olide,
2β-hydroxyeremophil-7(11)-en-12,8α-olide [7], secoeremopetasitolide A and B from the
rhizomes [8], eremopetasidione [9], β-elemene, β-bisabolene, β-caryophylene [11].
  2) Flavonoids: Quercetin, kaempferol [13].
  3) Phenolic compounds: Fukinolic acid and fukliic acid [10], petasiphenone [9].
  4) Others: Isopentanol, 3-hexen-1-ol, 1-nonen-3-ol, 1-linalool, veratrole, 1-undecene, 1-
    tridecene, 3-acetoxy-1-nonene [11], β-sitosterol [13]
Pharmacology
  1) Anti-allergic and anti-histaminic activity (sesquiterpenoids) [12].

Literatures:
[1] Naya, K. *et al.: Tetrahedron Lett.* **1971,** 31, 2961.
[2] Naya, K. *et al.: Bull. Chem. Soc. Jap.* **1971,** 44(11), 3165.
[3] Yaoita, Y. *et al.: Chem. Pharm Bull.* **1992,** 40(12), 3277.
[4] Yaoita, Y. *et al.: Phytochem.,* **1994,** 37(6), 1773.
[5] Yaoita, Y. *et al.: Chem. Pharm Bull.,* **1995,** 43(10), 1738.
[6] Yaoita, Y. *et al.: Nat. Med.,* **1996,** 50(1), 49.
[7] Yaoita Y. *et al.: Chem. Pharm. Bull.,* **1996,** 44(9), 1731.
[8] Yaoita, Y. *et al.: Phytochem.,* **1996,** 42(3), 751.
[9] Yaoita, Y. *et al.: Phytochem.,* **1994,** 37(6), 1765.
[10] Sakamura, S. *et al.: Agr. Biol. Chem. Japan,* **1973,** 37, 1915.
[11] Kikuchi, M. *et al.: Yakugaku Zasshi* **1973,** 93, 123.
[12] Tobinaga, S. *et al.: Chem. Pharm Bull.* **1983,** 31, 745.
[13] Kurihara, T. *et al.: Tohoku Yakudai* **1957,** 4, 149; **1959,** 6,51.

[T. Kimura]

572.   *Piloselloides hirsuta* **(Forsk.) C. Jeffrey**   (Compositae)
              [= *Gerbera piloselloides* Cass.]

Mao-da-ding-cao (C), Moe-die-ding-cho (H)

Whole Plant
  Local Drug Name: Mao-da-ding-cao (C), Moe-die-ding-cho (H).
  Processing: Use in fresh or dry under the sun (C, H).
  Method of Administration: Oral (decoction: C, H), Topical (crushed fresh herb or decoction: C, H).
  Folk Medicinal Uses:
          1) Colds and fever (C, H).
          2) Cough (C, H).
          3) Infantile malabsorption (C, H).
          4) Dysentery (C, H).
          5) Traumatic injury (C, H).

154

6) Snake bites (C, H).
7) Gastroenteritis (H).
8) Nephritis (H).
9) Edema (H).
10) Pulmonary tuberculosis hemoptysis (H).
11) Pharyngitis (H).
12) Tonsillitis (H).
13) Gastric and duodenal ulcer (H).
14) Boils and pyodermas (H).
15) Trichomonal vaginitis (H).

Scientific Research:
Chemistry
1) Piloselloidal, acetophenones, chromenes [1]

Literature:
[1] Bohlmann, F. *et al.*: *Chem. Ber.* **1975,** 108, 26.

[P.P.H. But]

573.   *Pluchea indica* **(L.) Less.**   (Compositae)

Kuo-bao-ju (C), Yin-sight (H)

Whole Plant
Local Drug Name: Luan-xi (C), Yin-sight (H).
Processing: Use in fresh or dried (H).
Method of Administration: Oral (decoction: C, H).
Folk Medicinal Uses:
            1) Infantile indigestion (C, H).
            2) Cervical tuberculous lymphadenitis (H).
            3) Rheumatic bone pain (H).
            4) Lumbago (H).

Scientific Research:
Chemistry
1) Thiophene derivatives: 2-(prop-1-inyl)-5-(5,6-dihydroxyhexa-1,3-diinyl)-thiophene, 2-(prop-a-inyl)-5-(6-acetoxy-5-hydroxyhexa-1,3-iinyl)-thiophene [1].
2) Glycoside: linaloyl glucoside, linaloyl apiosyl glucoside, 9-hydroxylinaloyl glucoside, plucheosides A and B [2], plucheoside C, plucheosides D_1, D_2, D_3 [3].
3) Sesquiterpenes: plucheols A and B, plucheoside E [3].
4) Triterpenoids: hop-17(21)-en-3β-yl acetate, boehmeryl acetate [1].
4) 3-(2',3'-diacetoxy-2'-methylbutyryl) cuauhtemone [4].
Pharmacology
1) Sedative effect [5].
2) Decreased locomotor activity [5].
3) Suppressed social isolation-induced aggressive behavior [5].
4) Anti-inflammatory effect [6-9, 12].
5) Protective effect against gastric ulcer [6].
6) Diuretic effect [10–11].
7) Hypothermic effect [9].

Literature:

[1] Chakravarty, A. K. *et al.*: *Indian J. Chem., Sect. B. Org. Chem. Incl. Med. Chem.* **1994,** 33B, 978.
[2] Uchiyama, T. *et al.*: *Phytochemistry* **1989**, 28, 3369.
[3] Uchiyama, T. *et al.*: *Phytochemistry* **1991**, 30, 655.
[4] Mukhopadhyay, S. *et al.*: *J. Nat. Prod.* **1983**, 46, 671.
[5] Thongpraditchote, S. *et al.*: *Biol. Pharm. Bull.* **1996**, 19, 379.
[6] Sen, T. *et al.*: *Life Sc.* **1993**, 52, 737.
[7] Sen, T. *et al.*: *J. Ethnopharm.* **1991**, 33, 135.
[8] Sen, T. *et al.*: *Planta Med.* **1990**, 56, 661.
[9] Sen, T. *et al.*: *Phytother. Res.* **1992**, 6, 175.
[10] Nilvises, N. *et al.*: *Thai J. Pharmacol.* **1989**, 11, 1.
[11] Pal, S. *et al.*: *Phytother. Res.* **1989**, 3, 156.
[12] Chaudhuri, A. K. N. *et al.*: *Med. Sci. Res.* **1987**, 15, 487.

[P.P.H. But]

574. *Sonchus oleraceus* **L.** (Compositae)

Ku-ju-cai (C), Foo-gui-choi (H), Bang-ga-ji-ddong (K)

Whole Plant
Local Drug Name: Dian-ku-cau (C), Foo-gui-choi (H), Go-chae (K).
Processing: use in fresh or dried (C, H, K).
Method of Administration: Oral (decoction: C, H, K); Topical (juice or mashed fresh herb: C, H, K)
Folk Medicinal Uses:
        1) Infectious hepatitis (C, H, K).
        2) Dysentery (C, H, K).
        3) Enteritis (C, H).
        4) Otitis media (C, H).
        5) Appendicitis (C, H).
        6) Mastitis (C, H).
        7) Stomatitis (C, H).
        8) Pharyngitis (C, H).
        9) Tonsillitis (C, H).
        10) Hematemesis (C, H).
        11) Epistaxis (C, H).
        12) Hemoptysis (C, H).
        13) Boils and carbuncles (C, H).
        14) Massive uterine bleeding (H).
        15) Hepatic cirrhosis (H).
        16) Pyodermas (H).
        17) Melena (H).

Scientific Research:
Chemistry
  1) Monoterpenes: γ-terpineol, geraniol, bornyl acetate, anethole, geranial, butanol [1].
  2) Triterpenoids: 3β-25-epoxy-3-hydroxyolean-18-en-28-oic acid [1], α-amyrin [2].
  3) Disaccharide [3].
  4) Lutein, violaxanthin, β-carotene, neoxanthin, zeaxanthin, α-cryptoxanthin, provitamin A [4], vernolic acid [7].
  5) IAA, abscisic acid, dihydrozeatin, ribosylzeatin, gibberellin A$_3$, gibberellins GA$_4$+GA$_7$ [5].
  6) Glycosides: sonchusides A, B, C and D, glucozaluzanin C, macroliniside A, crepidiaside A, picrisides B and C [6], luteolin 7-β-D-glucuronidopyranoside [9].

7) Steroids: β-sitosterol [2].
8) Coumarins: scopoletin, aesculetin [2, 8].
9) Flavonoids: luteolin, quercetin, quercimetrin, cynaroside, isocynaroside [9].
10) Acids: heptonic acid, hexanoic acid [1].

Literature:
[1] Ahmed, A. F. *et al.*: *Egypt. J. Pharm. Sci.* **1992,** 33, 689.
[2] Dl-Khrisy, E. M. *et al.*: *Aswan Sci. Technol. Bull.* **1992,** 13, 15.
[3] Mousa, A. A. *et al.*: *Orient. J. Chem.* **1990,** 6, 205.
[4] Mercadante, A. Z. *et al.*: *Int. J. Food Sci. Technol.* **1990,** 25, 213.
[5] Shang, H. C. *et al.*: *Zhiwu Shenglixue Tongxun* **1988,** (5), 35.
[6] Miyase, T. *et al.*: *Chem. Pharm. Bull.* **1987,** 35, 2869.
[7] Ahmad, R. *et al.*: *Fette, Seifen, Anstrichm.* **1986,** 88, 490.
[8] Mansour, R. M. A. *et al.*: *Phytochemistry* **1983,** 22, 489.
[9] Bondarenko, V. G. *et al.*: *Khim. Prir. Soedin.* **1983,** (2), 234.

[P.P.H. But]

575.   *Synurus deltoides* (Ait.) Nakai   (Compositae)

Su-ri-chwi(K)

Whole plant
Local Drug Name: Su-ri-chwi(K)
Processing: dry under the sun(K)
Method of Administration: oral(decoction, K)
Folk Medicinal Uses:
　　　　　　　1) Diabetes(K)

Scientific Research:
Pharmacology
1) Antigenotoxic effect(methanol ext.)[1]

Literature:
[1] Ham, S.-S. et al.: *J. Food Sci. Nutr.* **1997,** 2(2), 162.

[C. K. Sung]

576.   *Wedelia chinensis* (Osb.) Merr.   (Compositae)

Peng-qi-ju (C), Parng-kay-guk (H)

Whole Plant
Local Drug Name: Peng-qi-ju (C), Parng-kay-guk (H)
Processing: Use in fresh or dried (C, H).
Method of Administration: Oral (decoction: C, H); Topical (mashed fresh herb: C, H).
Folk Medicinal Uses:
　　　　　　　1) Prevention of measles (C, H).
　　　　　　　2) Influenza (C, H).
　　　　　　　3) Common colds (C, H).
　　　　　　　4) Diphtheria (C, H).
　　　　　　　5) Pharyngitis (C, H).

6) Tonsillitis (C, H).
7) Bronchitis (C, H).
8) Pheumonitis (C, H).
9) Whooping cough (C, H).
10) Hemoptysis (C, H).
11) Hypertension (C, H).
12) Furuncles and boils (C, H).
13) Pyodermas (H).

Scientific Research:
Chemistry
1) (-)-Kaur-16-en-19-oic acid, stigmasteryl glucoside, stigmasterol, lignoceric acid, melissic acid
[1]
Pharmacology
1) Hepatoprotective effect [1–2].

Literature:
[1] Yang, L.L. *et al.*: *Planta Med.* **1986,** (6), 499.
[2] Lin, S.C. *et al.*: *Amer. J. Chin. Med.* **1994,** 22, 155.

[P.P.H. But]

577.   *Aloe arborescens* **Mill. var.** *natalensis* **Bergel.**   (Liliaceae)

Kidachi-aroe(J), Al-ro-e(K)

Related plants: *Aloe arborescens* Mill.

Leaf sap
Local Drug Name: Aroe(J), Al-ro-e(K)
Processing: Fresh juice or heat the juice to dryness (J, K)
Method of Administration: Oral(fresh juice, J, K), topical(fresh juice, J, K)
Folk Medicinal Uses:
                    1) Burns(J, K)
                    2) Stomach ulcer(J, K)
                    3) Trauma(J, K)
                    4) Insect bites(J, K)
                    5) Cathartic(J, K)
                    6) Gastrointestinal disturbances(J, K)
                    7) Hang over(K)
                    8) Emmeniopathy(K)
                    9) Athlete's foot(K)

Scientific Research:
Chemistry
1) Alkanes: C-23 to 33-primarily[1], dotriacontane, dotriacontan-1-ol, heneicosane, hentriacontane,
heptacosane, hepadecane, hexacosane, hexadecane[6], eicosane[7]
2) Quinoids: aloe emodin, barbaloin[2, 10], aloe emodin anthrone[3], aloechrysone[4], aloin A,
B[5]
3) Chromones: aloesin[6,10], 22"-O-feruloyl-aloesin, 2"-O-*p*-coumaroyl-aloesin[8]
4) Misc. lactones: aloenin[6,9,10]
5) Carbohydrates: aloe arborescens mannan[11]
6) Proteid: aloctin A[11]
Phamacology

158

1) Antifungal activity[12]
2) Laxative effect[13]
3) Carcinogenesis inhibition[14]
4) Antitumor activity[15]
5) Agglutinin activity[16]
6) Antihyperglycemic activity[17]
7) Antiulcer activity[18]
8) Bradykinin antagonist activity[19]
9) Antiradiation effect[20]
10) Antibacterial activity[15]

Literature:
[1] Herbins, G. A. and Robins, P. A.: *Phytochemistry* **1968**, 7, 239.
[2] Adamski, R. and Dodym, A.: *Herba Pol.* **1974**, 20, 26.
[3] Janik, J.: *Sb. Pr. Pedagog. Fak. Ostrave Rada E.* **1973** E3, 13.
[4] Dagne, E. *et al.*: *Phytochemistry* **1994**, 35(2), 401.
[5] Grun, M. and Franz, G.: *Arch. Pharm.(Weinheim)* **1982**, 315, 231.
[6] Hirata, T. and Suga, T.: *Z. Naturforsch. Ser. C* **1977**, 32, 731.
[7] Kameoka, H. *et al.*: *Nippon Nogei Kagaku Kaishi* **1981**, 55, 997.
[8] Kodym, A.: *Pharmazie* **1991**, 3, 217.
[9] Hirata, T. and Suga, T.: *Bull. Chem. Soc. Japan* **1978**, 51, 842.
[10] Yagi, A. *et al.*: *Planta Med.* **1987**, 53(6), 515.
[11] Yagi, A. *et al.*: *Planta Med.* **1977**, 31, 17.
[12] Fujita, K. *et al.*: *Antibicrob. Agents Chemother.* **1978**, 14, 132.
[13] Ishii, Y. *et al.*: *Yakugaku Zasshi* **1981**, 101, 254.
[14] Tsuda, H. *et al.*: *Phytother. Res.* **1993**, 7, 543.
[15] Suga, T. and Hirata, T.: *Cosmet. Toiletries* **1983**, 98(6), 105.
[16] Fujita, K. *et al.*: *Experientia* **1978**, 34, 523.
[17] Beppu, H. *et al.*: *Phytother. Res.* **1993**, 7, S37.
[18] Teradaira, R. *et al.*: *Phytother. Res.* **1993**, 7, 534.
[19] Yagi, A. *et al.*: *Planta Med.* **1987**, 53(1), 19.
[20] Sato, Y. *et al.*: *Yakugaku Zasshi* **1990**, 110(11), 876.

[C. K. Sung]

578.   *Dianella ensifolia* **(L.) DC**   (Liliaceae)

Shan-jian-lan (C), Sarn-garn-larn (H)

Rhizome
Local Drug Name: Shan-jian-lan (C), Sarn-garn-larn (H).
Processing: Wash, slice and dry under the sun (C, H).
Method of Administration: Topical(dry powder bledned with vinegar: C, H).
Folk Medicinal Uses:
        1) Furunculosis and abscesses (C, H).
        2) Lymphangitis (C, H).
        3) Tuberculous lymphadenitis (C, H).
        4) Tinea (C, H).
        5) Traumatic injury (H).
Remark: Not for oral consumption.

Scientific Research:
Chemistry
1) Benzenoids: Musizin(dianellidin), methyl 2,4-dihydroxy-3,5,6-trimethylbenzoate, methyl 2,4-

dihydroxy-3,6-dimethylbenzoate, methyl 2,4-dihydroxy-6-methylbenzoate (methyl orsellinate), 2,4-dihydroxy-6-methoxy-3-methylacetophenone[1]

2) Chromones: 5,7-dihydroxy-2,6,8-trimethylchromone, 5,7-dihydroxy-2,8-dimethylchromone (isoeugenitol)[1]

Literature:
[1] Lojanapiwatna, V. *et al.: J. Sci. Soc. Thailand* **1982,** 8(2), 95.

[P.P.H. But]

579.   *Erythronium japonicum* **Decne.**   (Liliaceae)

Katakuri (J), Eol-re-ji (K)

Bulb
  Local Drug Name: Katakuri (K), Eol-re-ji (K).
  Processing: fresh (J), dry under the sun (K).
  Method of Administration: Boil as food (J). Decoction or powder (K).
  Folk Medicinal Uses:
                1) Enterogastritis (J, K).
                2) Diarrhea (J, K).
                3) Vomitting (K).
                4) Burning (K).

Bulb starch
  Local Drug Name: Katakuri-ko (J).
  Processing: Grind, refine and precipitate (J).
  Method of Administration: Boil (J).
  Folk Medicinal Uses:
                1) General weakness (J).

Scientific Researches:
  Chemistry
    1) Steroids: β-Sitosterol, stigmasterol, daucosterol, campesterol [4], typhasterol, teasterone and catasterone[1].
    2) Aliphatic compounds: Heptacosanol and nonacosanol [2], palmitic acid, stearic acid, oleic acid, arachidic acid, behenic acid, lignoceric acid and tricosanoic acid [4].
    3) Anthocyanins [3, 5].

Literatures:
[1] Yasuta, E. *et al.: Biosci. Biotechnol. Biochem.,* **1995,** 59(11), 2156.
[2] Isono, H.: *Yakugaku Zasshi* **1976,** 96(8), 957.
[3] Yoshitama, K. *et al.: J. Fac. Sci., Shinshu Univ.* **1980,** 15(1), 19.
[4] Moon, Y. H. *et al.: Saengyak Hakhoechi* **1992,** 23(2), 115.
[5] Lee, M. S. *et al.: Saengyak Hakhoechi* **1993,** 24(3), 251.

[T. Kimura]

580.   *Paris polyphylla* **Smith var.** *chinensis* **(Franch.) Hara**   (Liliaceae)

Qi-ye-yi-zhi-hua (C), Chut-yip-yud-gee-far (H)

Related Plant: *P. polyphylla* Smith var. *yunnanensis* (Franch.) Hand.-Mazz.: Yun-nan-chong-bu (C).
　　　　　　P. rerticillata M. V. Bieb.: Sat-gat-na-mul (K).

Rhizome (CP)
Local Drug Name: Chong-lou (C), Chung-lou (H), Jurou (J), Jo-hyu (K).
Processing: Eliminate foreign matter, wash clean, soften thoroughly, cut into thin slices, and dry in
　　　　　　the sun (C, H, K).
Method of Administration: Oral (decoction: C, H, K); Topical (paste: C).
Folk Medicinal Uses:

　　　　　　　　1) Mastitis (C, H).
　　　　　　　　2) Appendicitis (C, H).
　　　　　　　　3) Encephalitis B (C, H).
　　　　　　　　4) Venomous snake bite (C, H).
　　　　　　　　5) Boils (C, K).
　　　　　　　　6) Carbuncles (C, K).
　　　　　　　　7) Sore throat (C, K).
　　　　　　　　8) Traumatic pain (C).
　　　　　　　　9) Convulsion (C).
　　　　　　　　10) Tonsillitis (H).
　　　　　　　　11) Pyodermas (H).
　　　　　　　　12) Tubeculous meningitis (H).
　　　　　　　　13) On trial in cancer therapy (H).

Scientific Researches:
Chemistry
　　1) Steroids: Diosgenin 3-O-α-L-rhamnopyranosyl-(1→2)-[α-L-arabinofuranosyl-(1→4)]-β-D-glucophyranoside, diosqenin 3-O-α-rhannopyranosyl-(1→4)-α-L-rhamnopyranosyl-(1→4)-[α-L-rhamnopyranosyl-(1→2)]-β-D-glucopyranoside, dioscin, pregna-5,16-dien-3β-ol-20-one 3-O-β-charotrioside [1], pariphyllin A, B [2], polyphyllin A, B, C, D, E, F, G, H [3], paristerone [4], diosqenin 3-O-α-L-rhamnosyl-(1→2)-β-D-glucopyranoside, diosqenin 3-O-α-L-arabinofuranosyl-(1→4)-[α-L-rhamnosyl (1→2)]-β-D-glucopyranoside, diosqenin 3-O-[α-L-rhamnopyranosyl-(1→4)-α-L-rhamnopyranosyl-(1→4)-[α-L-rhamnopyranosyl-(1→2)]-β-D-glucopyranoside [5].
　　2) Organic acids: Citric acid, Zn lactate [6].
Pharmacology
　　1) Antiinflammatory effect [5].
　　2) Spermicidal effect [6].
　　3) Hemostatic effect [5,9].
　　4) Antibacterial effect [7-9].
　　5) Sedative effect [10].
　　6) Analgesic effect [10].
　　7) Inhibition of protein synthesis [11].
　　8) Antiasthmatic and antitussive effects [12].
　　9) Antitumor effect [12].

Literatures:
[1] Nohara, T. *et al.*: *Chem. Pharm. Bull.* **1973**, 21, 1240.
[2] Khanna, I. *et al.*: *Indian J. Chem.* **1975**, 13(8), 781.
[3] Singh, S. B. *et al.*: *Planta Med.* **1980**, 40(3), 301; *Phytochemistry* **1982**, 21(8), 2079; *ibid* **1982**, 21(12), 2925.
[4] Singh, S.B. *et al.*: *Tetrahedron* **1982**, 38(14), 2189.
[5] Xu, X.M., *et al.*: *Zhongcaoyao* **1988**, 19(5), 194.
[6] Cao, L. *et al.*: *Zhongcaoyao* **1987**, 18(10), 451.
[7] Dai, H.S. *et al.*: *Zhonghua Yixue Zazhi* **1966**, 52, 57.

[8] "Quanguo Zhongcaoyao Huibian" **1973,** Vol.1, 4.
[9] Wang, Q. et al.: Zhongguo Yaoke Daxue Xuebao **1989,** 29(4), 251.
[10] Wang, Q. et al.: Zhongguo Yaoke Daxue Xuebao **1990,** 15(2), 109.
[11] Wang, R, et al.: Shengwu Huaxue Zazhi **1992,** 8(4), 395.
[12] Nanjing College of Pharmacy: "Zhongcaoyao Xue" **1980,** Vol.3, 1313.

[J.X. Guo]

581.   *Polygonatum cyrtonema* **Hua**   (Liliaceae)

Duo-hua-huang-jing (C).

Related Plant: *P. kingianum* Coll. et Hemsl.: Dian-huang-jing (C); *P. sibiricum* Red.: Huang-jing (C),
Kagikuromabanarukoyuri(J), Won-hwang-jeong(K); *P. falcatum* A. Gray: Jin-hwang-jeong(K).

Rhizome (CP)
Local Drug Name: Huang-jing (C), Wong-jing (H), Ousei (J), Hwang-jeong (K).
Processing: 1) Eliminate foreign matter, wash clean, slightly soften, cut into thick slices and dry
(C, K).
2) Stew or steam the clean Rhizoma Polygonati thoroughly with wine, dry briefly in the
air, cut into thick slices and dry (C).
Method of Administration: Oral (decoction: C, H, J, K).
Folk Medicinal Uses:
1) Weakness of the spleen and the stomach marked by lassitude, dryness in the
mouth and anorexia (C, H, J, K).
2) Deficiency of vital essence and blood (C, H, J, K).
3) Dry cough due to deficiency of yin of the lung (C, H, J).
4) Diabetes caused by internal heat (C, H, J).
5) Contusion of loin (K).
Scientific Researches:
Chemistry
1) Lectins: Polygonatum cyrtonema lectin(PCL II)[1]
Pharmacology
1) Hemagglutination(PCL II)[1, 2]

Literatures:
[1] Bao, J.-K. et al.: *Shengwu Huaxue Zazhi* **1996,** 12(2), 165.
[2] Bao, J.-K. et al.: *Shengwu Huaxue Zazhi* **1996,** 12(6), 747.

[J.X. Guo]

582.   *Rhodea japonica* **Roth.**   (Liliaceae)

Omoto (J), Man-nyun-cheong (K)

Whole Herb
Local Drug Name: Mannensei (J), Man-nyun-chong (K).
Processing: Dry under the sun (J, K).
Method of Administration: Decoction (J, K).
Folk Medicinal Uses:
1) Edema (J, K).

2) Hemorrhoidal diseases (J, K).
Contraindications: Toxic in overdose.

Scientific Researches:
Chemistry
   1) Cardiac glycoside: Rhodexin A, B, C [1, 5], rhodexin V, S [2], rhodexoside [8].
   2) Saponins and sapogenins: Rhodeasapogenin [6] and isorhodeasapogenin [4], periprogenin [5], spirost-25(27)-ene-1,2,3,4,5,6,7-heptol and 1β,2β,3β,4β,7α-hexahydroxyspirost-25(27)-en-6-one [7].
   3) Cumarins: Scopoletin, umbelliferone [3].
   4) Flavonoids: Kaempferol, quercetin, astragalin and isoquercetin [3].
Pharmacology
   1) Cardiac activity [9].

Literatures:
[1] Nawa, H. *et al.*: *Pharm. Bull. Jap.* **1958**, 6, 508; *Chem. & Ind.* **1958**, 653.
[2] Kuchukhidze, D. K. *et al.*: *Soobshch. Akad. Nauk Gruz. SSR*, **1973**, 70, 361.
[3] Kuchukhidze, D. K. *et al.*: *Khim. Prir. Soedin.*, **1973**, 9, 552.
[4] Nawa, H.: *Pharm. Bull. Jap.* **1958**, 6, 255.
[5] Kuchukhidze, D. K. *et al.*: *Khim. Prir. Soedin.*, **1977**(2), 286; "Khromatogr. Metody Farm." 1977, 175, Tbilis. Gos. Med. Inst., Tiflis, USSR.
[6] Kudo, K. *et al.*: *Chem. Pharm. Bull.* **1984**, 32(10), 4229.
[7] Miyahara, K. *et al.*: *Tetrahedron Lett.* **1980,** 83; *Tennen Yuki Kagobutsu Toronkai Yoshishu* **1979**, 22, 1.
[8] Kuchukhidze, D. K. *et al.*: *Izv. Akad. Nauk. Gruz. SSR., Ser. Khim.* **1982**, 8(2), 157.
[9] Kudo, K. *et al.*: *Oyo Yakuri* **1985,** 29(2), 253.

[T. Kimura]

583.   *Trillium smallii* **Maxim.**   (Liliaceae)

Enreiso (J)

Related plant: *T. tschonoskii* Maxim.: Yan-ling-cao (C),   Miyama- enreiso (J), Keun-yeon-ryung-cho,
          T. kamtschaticum Pallas: Bai-hua-yan-ling-cao (C),   Oobanano-enreiso (J),
          Yeon-ryung-cho (K).

Rhizome
   Local Drug Name: Yu-er-qi (C), Enreiso-kon (J).
   Processing: Dry under the sun (J).
   Method of Administration: Decoction (J).
   Folk Medicinal Uses:
                    1) Hypertension (C, J).
                    2) Low back pain (C, J).
                    3) Traumatic injury (C, J).
                    4) Headache (C).
                    5) Gastroenteritis(J).

Scientific Researches:
Chemistry
   1) Saponins and sapogenins: Dioscin and diosgenin [2], trillenoside A and trillenogenin [3], pennogenin-3-*O*-α-L-rhamnopyranosyl-(1→4)-α-L-rhamnopyranosyl-(1→2)-β-D-glucoside [5].
   2) Anthocyanins [4].

163

Pharmacology
   1) Active ingredients for massage to promote circulation (acidic heteropolysaccharides)[1].

Literatures:
[1] Minami, T. *et al.*: *Jpn Kokai Tokkyo Koho*, JP 08291038 A2 5, **1996**, Japan.
[2] Okanishi, T. *et al.*: *Chem. Pharm. Bull.* **1975**, 23(3), 575.
[3] Kawasaki, T.: *Jpn Kokai Tokkyo Koho*, JP 7751011 770423; Appl. Japan JP 75127727 751022.
[4] Yoshitama, K. *et al.*: *J. Fac. Sci., Shinshu Univ.* **1980**, 15(1), 19.
[5] Wang, Q. *et al.*: *Shoyakugaku Zasshi* **1988**, 42(1), 58.

[T. Kimura]

584.   *Stemona tuberosa* **Lour.**   (Stemonaceae)

Dai-ye-bai-bu (C), Bark-boe (K), Tsurubyakubu (J), Ma-ju-ip-baek-bu (K)

Related plants: *Stemona sessilifolia* (Miq.) Miq.: Zhi-li-bai-bu (C), *S. japonica* (Bl.) Miq.:
               Man-sheng-bai-bu (C).

Root-tuber (CP)
Local Drug Name: Bai-bu (C), Bark-boe (H), Byakubu (J).
Processing: Discard the rootlets, scald in boiling water, dry under the sun (C, H, J).
Method of Administration: Oral (decoction: C, H, J); Topical (decoction or powder: C, H).
Folk Medicinal Uses:
                    1) Skin itchiness (C, H, J, K).
                    2) Bronchitis (H, J, K).
                    3) Pertussis (C, H).
                    4) Oxyuriasis (C, H).
                    5) Cough (C, H).
                    6) Ascariasis (H, K).
                    7) Amebic dysentery (H, K).
                    8) Pulmonary tuberculosis (H, K).
                    9) Dermatitis (H, K).
                    10) Hookworm infestation (H).
                    11) Eczema (H).

Scientific Research:
   Chemistry
      1) Alkaloids [1]: Tuberostemonine [2–3], stenine [2, 4], tuberostemonone [3, 5], tuberostemonol,
         stemoamide, tuberostemospironine, didehydrotuberostemonine[3], stemonine LG[6],
         tuberostemoninol, stemoninoamide, tuberostemoamide[7–8], stemotinine, isostemotinine,
         stemonidine[9], bisdehydroneotuberostemonine, neotuberostemonine [10].
      2) Bibenzyls: 3,5-dihydroxy-4-methylbibenzyl, 3,5-dihydroxy-2'-methoxy-4-methylbibenzyl, 3-
         hydroxy 2',5'-dimethoxy-2-methylbibenzyl [11].
   Pharmacology
      1) Antimicrobial and antifungal effect [12–16].
      2) Insecticidal effect [17–18].
      3) Anthelmintic effect [19].
      4) Antitussive effect [20].
      5) Relaxant effect on the bronchial smooth muscles [21].

Literature:
[1] Cong, X.D. *et al.*: *Yaoxue Xuebao* **1992,** 27, 556.
[2] Pfeifer, S. *et al.*: *Pharmazie* **1968,** 23, 342.

[3] Lin, W.H. *et al.*: *J. Nat. Prod.* **1992,** 55, 571.

[4] Shojiro, U. *et al.*: *Chem. Pharm. Bull.* **1967,** 15, 768.

[5] Lin, W.H. *et al.*: *J. Crystallogr. Spectrosc. Res.* **1991,** 21, 189.

[6] Pham, T.K. *et al.*: *Tap Chi Duoc Hoc* **1991,** (5), 4.

[7] Lin, W.H. *et al.*: *Phytochemistry* **1994,** 36, 1333.

[8] Lin, W.H. *et al.*: *Chin. Chem. Lett.* **1993,** 4, 1067.

[9] Xu, R.S. *et al.*: *Tetrahedron* **1982,** 38, 2667.

[10] Ye, Y. *et al.*: *Phytochemistry* **1994,** 37, 1201.

[11] Zhao, W.M. *et al.*: *Phytochemistry* **1995,** 38, 711.

[12] Wang, W. *et al.*: *Yaoxue Tongbao* **1959,** 7, 522.

[13] Liu, G. *et al.*: *Zhonghua Xinyi Xuebao* **1950,** 1, 95.

[14] Wang, Y. *et al.*: *Zhiwu Xuebao* **1954,** 3, 121.

[15] Wang, Y. *et al.*: *Zhiwu Xuebao* **1953,** 2, 312.

[16] Cao, R. *et al.*: *Zhonghua Pifuke Zazhi* **1957,** (4), 286.

[17] Wang, L. *et al.*: *Chin. Med. J.* **1938,** 54, 151.

[18] Li, X. *et al.*: *Zhonghua Xinyi Xuebao***1952,** 3(1), 9.

[19] Feng, Y. *et al.*: *Shandong Daxue Xuebao* **1956,** 2(3), 102.

[20] Wang, Y. *et al.*: *Zhongyao Yaoli Yu Yingyong* **1983,** 420.

[21] Coordinating Research Unit on Bronchitis Prevention and Treatment : *Information on MedicalScience and* Technology **1973,** (4), 14.

[P.P.H. But]

585.   *Dioscorea tokoro* **Makino**   (Dioscoreaceae)

Shan-bei-ye (C), Pay-gie (H), Onidokoro (J), Do-ggo-ro-ma (K)

Rhizome

Local Drug Name: Bei-ye (C), Pay-gie (H), Hikai (J), Bi-hae (K).

Processing: Cut into slices and dry under the sun (C, H, J, K).

Method of Administration: Oral (decoction: C, H, J, K).

Folk Medicinal Uses:

                1) Arthritis and rheumatism (C, H, J, K).

                2) Snake bite (C).

                3) Lumbago (C).

                4) Urinary infection (C).

                5) Leukorrhea (C).

                6) Nocturnal emission (H).

                7) Fish poison (J).

Scientific Researches:

Chemistry

1) Saponins and sapogenins: Saponins [1, 2], dioscin, diosgenin, yamogenin [1,8], prosapogenin A and B of dioscin [4], gracillin, trillin, dioscorea sapotoxin A, B, okoronin [7], tokorogenin [9], tokorogenin glucopyranoside [6], protokoronin [10], yonogenin [9], protoyonogenin and protoneoyonogenin [12], igagenin [3], isodiotigenin [5,8,9], 19-hydroxy-yonogenin [11], $\Delta^{3,5}$-desoxytigogenin [13], kogagenin [14] and anhydrokogagenin[15].

Literatures:

[1] Tsukamoto, T. *et al.*: *Yakugaku Zasshi*, **1957,** 77, 1225; Akahori, A.: *Phytochem.* **1965,** 4, 97

[2] Tang, S. *et al.*: *Yaoxue Xuebao* **1964,** 11, 787; *Zhiwu Xuebao* **1987,** 29(2), 193.

[3] Akahori, A. *et al.*: *Chem. Pharm. Bull.* **1968,** 16(10), 1994; Yasuda, F. et al.: *Tetrahedron*, **1968,** 24(22), 6535.

[4] Kawasaki, T. *et al.*: *Chem. Pharm. Bull.* **1968,** 16(6), 1070.

[5] Akahori, A. *et al.*: *Phytochem.* **1969**, 8(1), 45.
[6] Miyahara, K. *et al.*: *Chem. Pharm. Bull.* **1969**, 17(8), 1735.
[7] Miyahara, K. *et al.*: *Chem. Pharm. Bull.* **1969**, 17(7), 1369.
[8] Akahori, A. *et al.*: *Phytochem.* **1969**, 8(11), 2213.
[9] Nishikawa, M. *et al.*: *Yakugaku Zasshi*, **1954**, 74, 1165; Morita, K.: *Pharm. Bull. Japan* **1957**, 5, 494; Takeda, K. *et al.*: *Yakugaku Zasshi* **1957**, 77, 822; *Pharm. Bull. Jap.* **1958**, 6, 532; Akahori, A *et al.*: *Chem. Pharm. Bull.* **1970,** 18(3), 436.
[10] Tomita, Y. *et al.*: *Phytochem.* **1974**, 13(4), 729.
[11] Miyahara, K. *et al.*: *Chem. Pharm. Bull.* **1975**, 23(11), 2550.
[12] Uomori, A. *et al.*: *Phytochem.* **1983**, 22(1), 203.
[13] Tsukamoto, T. *et al.*: *Pharm. Bull. Japan* **1957**, 5, 494.
[14] Akahori, A.: *Shionogi Kenkyusho Nenho* **1960**, 10, 1411.
[15] Takeda, K. *et al.*: *Tetrahedron* **1959**, 7, 62.

[T. Kimura]

586.   *Rhoeo discolor* **Hance**   (Commelinaceae)

Zi-wan-liang-qin (C), Pong-far (H), Murasaki-omoto (J), Ja-ju-man-nyun-cho (K)

Leaf and Flower
Local Drug Name: Ban-hua (C), Pong-far (H), Murasaki-omoto (J), Bang-ran-yeop (K).
Processing: Fresh leaf. (C, J). Fresh or dry (H). Dry under the sun (K).
Method of Administration: Oral (decoction: C, H, K), Extract (J).
Folk Medicinal Uses:
         1) Diarrhea (C, J, K).
         2) Enteritis, catarrhal enteritis (J, K).
         3) Cough (C).
         4) Bacillary dysentery (H).
         5) Melena (H).
         6) Acute and chronic bronchitis (H).
         7) Pertussis (H).
         8) Lymphatic tuberclosis (H).
         9) Epistaxis (H).
         10) Common cold (K).
         11) Sputum (K).

Scientific Researches:
Chemistry
     1) Flavonoid glycoside [1].
     2) Organic acids [1].
     3) Polysaccharides [2].
Pharmacology
     1) Aflatoxin formation inhibitor against the producing fungi (extract) [3].

Literatures:
[1] Anenymous: *Nong Cun Zhong Cao Yao Zhi Ji Ji Shu*, **1971**, 243.
[2] Albertini, L. *et al.*: *Actual. Bot.*, **1978**, (1-2), 45: *Acta Soc. Bot. Pol.*, **1981**, 50(1-2), 21.
[3] Sinha, K. K.: *J. Food Sci. Technol.*, **1985**, 22(3), 225.

[T. Kimura]

587. *Coix lachryma-jobi* L. (Gramineae)

Juzudama (J), Yeom-ju (K)

Related plant: *Coix lachryma-jobi* L. var. *ma-yuen* Stapf: Hatomugi (J), Yul-mu (K)

Fruit
Local Drug Name: Juzudama (J).
Processing: Dry under the sun.
Method of Administration: Decoction (J).
Folk Medicinal Uses:
1) Neuralgia (J).
2) Edema (J).
3) Pain (J).

Root
Local Drug Name: Senkoku-kon (J).
Processing: Dry under the sun (J).
Method of Administration: Decoction (J).
Folk Medical Uses:
1) Neuralgia (J).
2) Pain (J).

Scientific Researches:
Chemistry
1) Fatty oil and fatty acids: Coixenolide, cis-octadecenoic acid and fatty acids [1].
2) Benzoxazolinone, benzoxazinone [2].
Pharmacology
1) Seed coat toxin [3].

Literatures:
[1] Gray, J. R. *et al.*: *Phytochem.* **1972,** 11, 1192.
[2] Shigematsu, N. *et al.*: *Yakugaku Zasshi* **1981**, 101(12), 1156.
[3] Yasuda, K. *et al.*: *Tokyo Joshi Ika Daigaku Zasshi* **1982**, 53(2), 127.

[T. Kimura]

588. *Hordeum vulgare* L. (Gramineae)

Da-mai (C), Tai-mug (H), Omugi (J)

Related plant: *H. rulgare* L. var. *hexastichon*: Bo-ri (K).
H. rulgare L. var. *nudum*: Ssal-bo-ri (K).

Germinated ripe fruit (CP)
Local Drug Name: Mai-ya (C), Mug-gar (H), Bakuga (J), Maek-a (K).
Processing: 1) Eliminate foreign matter (unprocessed fruit) (C, K).
2) Stir-fry the clean Fructus Hordei Germinatus until its outer part becomes brown, cool
and sift (stir-fried fruit) (C, K). Stir-fry the clean Fructus Hordei Germinatus
until its outer part becomes dark brown (charred fruit) (C, K).
Method of Administration: Oral (decoction: C, H, K)
Folk Medicinal Uses:
1) Anorexia due to diminshed function of the spleen; galactostasis (unprocessed
fruit, C, H, J).

2) Indigestion; weaning a baby (stir-fried fruit, C, H, K).
3) Retention of undigested food with epigastic distension and pain
(charred fruit, C, H, K).
4) Bronchitis (J).
5) Headache (J).
6) Acute gastritis (K).
7) Venter disease (K).
8) Common cold (K).

Seed
Local Drug Name: Bo-ri-ssal (K).
Processing: Remove pill and dry (K).
Method of Administration: Oral (steamed: K).
Folk Medicinal Uses:
1) Beri-beri (K).
2) Measles (K).
3) Jaundice (K).
4) Acute gastritis (K).

Scientific Researches:
Chemistry
1) Enzymes: starch hydrolase, proteolytic enzyme [1].
2) Sugars: starch, maltose [1].
3) Proteins [1].
4) Vitamins: vitamin B [1].
5) Quinone compounds: α-tocopheryl quinone [1].
6) Phenols: α-tocotrienol [1].
7) Glycosides: saponarin, lutonarin [1].
8) Phytochromes: leucoanthocyanin [1].
9) Alkaloids: herdenine [1], hordatine A, B and glucosides [2].
Pharmacology
1) Effect on the secretion of gastric juice, starch hydrolase and proteolytic enzyme [1].

Literatures:
[1] *"Quanguo Zhongcaoyao Huibian"* **1978,** Vol.2, 311.
[2] Lin, Q. S.: *Zhongcaoyao Chengfen Huaxue* **1977,** 182, 689.

[J.X. Guo]

589. *Imperata cylindrica* Beaur. var. *major* (Nees) C. E. Hubb.   (Gramineae)

Bai-mao (C), Chigaya (J)

Related plant: *I. cylindrica* var. *koenigii* (Retz.) Durand et Schinz: Ddui (K).

Rhizome (CP, JP)
Local Drug Name: Bae-mao-gen (C), Bokon (J), Baek-mo-geun (K).
Processing: 1) Wash clean, soften briefly, cut into sections, dry , and sift (C, K).
2) Stir-fry the sections of Rhizoma Imperatae until it becomes brown (C).
Method of Administration: Oral (decoction: C, J, K).
Folk Medicinal Uses:
1) Edema in acute nephritis (C, J).
2) Spitting of blood, epistaxis and hematuria due to heat in the blood (C, K).
3) Jaundice (C).

4) Urinary infection with difficult painful urination (C).
5) Febrile diseases with thirst (C).
6) Hemorrhage (K).

Scientific Researches:
Chemistry
1) Carbohydrates.
2) Triterpenes: arundoin, cylindrin, fernenol, siminarenol [1-3].
3) Tannins: catechol [4].
4) Coumarins: scopolin, scopoletin [4].
5) Organic acids: chlorogenic acid, isochlorogenic acid, *p*-coumaric acid, neochlorogenic acid [4].
6) Aldehydes: *p*-hydroxybenzaldehyde [4].
7) Sesquiterpenoids: cylindrene [5].
8) Biphenyl ethers: cylindol A, B [6].
Pharmacology
1) Diuretic effect [3].
2) Antibacerial effect [3].
3) Inhibitory effect on contractions of vascular smooth muscle [5].
4) 5-lipoxygenase inhibitory activity [6].

Literatures:
[1] Ohomoto, T. *et al.*: *Chem. Pharm. Bull.* **1965,** 13, 224.
[2] Ohomoto, T. *et al.*: *Chem. Pharm. Bull.* **1966,** 14, 97.
[3] *"Zhongyao Dacidian"* **1977,** Vol.1, 721.
[4] Khalil, A. I. *et al.*: *Iraqi J. Sci.* **1979,** 20(1), 15.
[5] Matsunaga, K. *et al.*: *J. Nat. Prod.* **1994,** 57(8), 1183.
[6] Matsunaga, K. *et al.*: *J. Nat. Prod.* **1994,** 57(9), 1290.

[J.X. Guo]

590.   *Cocos nucifera* **L.**   (Palmae)

Yair-shh(H), Kokoyashi(J), Ya-ja-na-mu(K)

Fruit
Local Drug Name: Yair-gee(H), Kokonattsa(J), Ya-ja(K)
Processing: Dry under the sun(K)
Method of Administration: Oral(decoction, H, K)
Folk Medicinal Uses:
                    1) Hemorrhage(K)
                    2) Syphilis(K)
                    3) Poisoning(K)

Scientific Research:
Chemistry
1) Inorganics: Al[1], Mn, Cu and Co ions[2]
2) Alkanes: n-Docosane, n-dotriacontane, n-eicosane, n-heneicosane, n-hentriacontane, n-hexacosane, n-heptacosane, n-heptadecane, n-nonacosane, n-nonadecane, n-octacosane, n-octadecane, n-pentacosane, n-tetracosane, n-triacontane, n-tricosane, heptan-2-ol[4], butyloin[3]
3) Terpenes: Limonene, menthol, α-terpineol[3], dihydrophaeseic acid, hydroxy phaseic acid[5], α-, β-amyrin, cycloartenol, cycloartenol 24-methylene[4], squalene[4, 6]
4) Benzenoids: Gentisic acid[7]
5) Steroids: Campesterol, stigmasterol[4]

169

6) Lipids: Caproic acid, decanoic acid, lauric acid, octanoic acid[8], myristic acid[9]
7) Carbohydrates: Sucrose[10], fructose, glucose[10, 11], lactose, raffinose[11], galactitol, sorbitol[12]
8) Proteids: Hydroxyproline[13], alanine, phenylalanine, arginine, aspartic acid, glutamic acid, glycine, isoleucine. Lysine, methionine, serine, valine[13, 14], histidine, leucine, proline, threonine, tyrosine[14], linamarase[15]
9) Alkaloids: Ligustrazine, 2,3,5-trimethylpyrazine[8], 2-(3-methyl-but-2-enyl-amino) purin-6-one[16], 14-O-(3-O-[β-D-galactopyranosyl-(1->2)-α-galactopyranosyl-(1->3)-α-L-arabinofuranosyl]-4-O-(α-L-arabinofuranosyl)-β-D-galactopyranosyl)-trans-zeatin riboside[17, 18]
10) Tannins[19]

Phamacology
1) Diuretic activity[20, 22]
2) Hyperglycemic activity[21]
3) Hypotensive activity[21, 23]
4) Repiratory stimulant activity[21]
5) Plant growth promotion[16, 17, 18]
6) Desensitization effect[24]
7) Cytotoxic activity[25]
8) Estrogen effect[26]
9) Antifungal activity[27, 29]
10) Hypercholesterolemic activity[28]

Literature:
[1] Lancaster, L. A. and Rajakurai, B.: *J. Sci. Food Agr.* **1974**, 25, 381.
[2] Biddappa, C. C. and Cecil, S. R.: *Plant Soil* **1984**, 79(3), 445.
[3] Stalcup, A. M. *et al.*: *J. Agr. Food Chem.* **1993**, 41(10), 1684.
[4] Mourafe, J. A. *et al.*: *J. Sci. Food Agr.* **1975**, 26, 523.
[5] Hoae, G. V. and Gaskin, P.: *Planta* **1980**, 150, 347.
[6] Fitelson, J.: *J. Ass. Offic. Agr. Chem.* **1943**, 26, 506.
[7] Griffiths, L. A.: *J. Exp. Biol.* **1959**, 10, 437.
[8] Kinerlerer, J. L. and Kellard, B.: *Chem. Ind.(London)* **1987**, 16, 567.
[9] Bibicheva, A. I. *et al.*: *Maslo-Zhir Prom-St* **1987**, 4, 26.
[10] Dang, K. K. *et al.*: *Rev. Pharm.* **1984**, 1984, 27.
[11] Bopaiah, B. M. *et al.*: *Curr. Sci.* **1987**, 56(16), 832.
[12] Saittagaroon, S. *et al.*: *J. Food Sci.* **1985**, 50(3), 757.
[13] Atakeuchi, K.: *Chiba Daigaku Buurii Gakuba Kiyo Shizen Kagaku* **1961**, 3, 321.
[14] Yeoh, H. H. *et al.*: *Biocheml Syst. Ecol.* **1986**, 14(1), 91.
[15] Jansz, E. R. *et al.*: *J. Natl. Sci. Counc. Sri Lanka* **1974**, 2, 57.
[16] Letham. D. S.: *Plant Sci. Lett.* **1982**, 26, 241.
[17] Kobayashi, H. *et al.*: *Chem. Pharm. Bull.* **1997**, 45(2), 260.
[18] Kobayashi, H. *et al.*: *Experientia* **1995**, 51(11), 1081.
[19] Wall, M. E. *et al.*: *J. Pharm. Sci.* **1969**, 58, 839.
[20] Caceres, A. *et al.*: *J. Ethnopharmacol.* **1987**, 19(3), 233.
[21] Ketusinh, O.: *J. Med. Ass. Thailant* **1954**, 37(5), 249.
[22] Dhawan, B, N. *et al.*: *Indian J. Exp. Biol.* **1977**, 15, 208.
[23] Feng, P. C. *et al.*: *J. Pharm. Pharmacol.* **1962**, 14, 556.
[24] Karmakar, P. R. and Chatterjee, B. P.: *Int. Arch Allergy Immunol.* **1994**, 103(2), 194.
[25] Salerno, J. W. and Smith, D. E.: *Anticancer Res.* **1991**, 11(1), 209.
[26] Booth, A. N. *et al.*: *Science* **1960**, 131, 1807.
[27] Jain, S. K. and Agrawal. S. C.: *Indian J. Med. Sci.* **1992**, 46(1), 1.
[28] Chindavanig, A.: *Master Thesis, Department of Biochemistry, Faculty of Science, Mahidol Univ.*, Bangkok, Thailand, **1971**, 58p, 58.
[29] Venkataraman, S. *et al.*: *J. Ethnopharmacol.* **1980**, 2(3), 291.

[C. K. Sung]

591.   *Pandanus tectorius* **Soland.**   (Pandanaceae)

Lou-dou-le (C), Low-dau-luck (H)

Root
Local Drug Name: Lou-dou-le (C), Low-dau-luck (H).
Processing: Use in fresh or dry under the sun (C, H).
Method of Administration: Oral (decoction: C, H).
Folk Medicinal Uses:
        1) Colds, fever (C, H).
        2) Nephritis (C, H).
        3) Edema (C, H).
        4) Urinary tract infection or stones (C, H).
        5) Hepatitis (C, H).
        6) Ascites (C, H).
        7) Hepatic cirrhosis (C, H).
        8) Conjunctivitis (C, H).
        9) Infantile summer heat (C).

Fruit
Local Drug Name: Lou-dou-le (C), Low-dau-luck (H).
Processing: Use in fresh or dry under the sun (C, H).
Method of Administration: Oral (decoction: C, H).
Folk Medicinal Uses:
        1) Dysentery (C, H).
        2) Cough (C, H).

Seed
Local Drug Name: Lou-dou-le (C).
Processing: Use in fresh or dry under the sun (C).
Method of Administration: Oral (decoction: C).
Folk Medicinal Uses:
        1) Orchitis (C).
        2) Hemorrhoids (C).
Contraindication: Pregnancy.

Scientific Research:
Chemistry
  1) Steroids: β-sitosterol, stigmasterol [1-2], β-sitostenone, stigmast-4-en-3,6-dione [1].
  2) Physcion, cirsilineol, palmitic acid, stearic acid, triacontanol-1, campesterol, daucosterol [2].
  3) Essential oil: α-pinene, 3-methyl-2(5H)-furanone, *p*-cymene, limonene, 1,8-cineole, methyl benzoate, camphor, naphthalene [3].

Literature:
[1] Qu, W. H. *et al.*: *Zhongguo Yaoke Daxue Xuebao* **1990,** 21(1), 51.
[2] Wu, L. Z. *et al.*: *Zhongcaoyao* **1987,** 18, 391.
[3] Zhu L. F. *et al.*: *Aromatic Plants and Essential Constituents (Supplement 1)*. South China Institute of Botany, Chinese Academy of Sciences, Guangzhou, **1995**, 70.

[P.P.H. But]

592.   *Sparganium stoloniferum* **Buch.-Ham.**   (Sparganiaceae)

Hui-san-leng (C), Sarm-ling (H), Mikuri (J), Heuk-sam-reung (K)

Related plants: *Sparganium stenophylum* Maxim.: Ezomikuri (J).

　　　　　S. longifolium Turcz., *Scirpus yagara* Ohwi: Ukiyagara (Cyperaceae) (J).

Rhyzome

Local Drug Name: San-leng (C), Sarm-ling (H), Keisanryo (J), Sam-reung (K).

Processing: (1) Cut and dry under the sun (C, J, K). (2) Stir-fry the sliced drug with vinegar until a
　　　　deep color is produced (C).

Method of Administration: Oral (decoction: C, H, J, K).

Folk Medicinal Uses:

　　　　　1) Menstrual disorder (H, J, K).

　　　　　2) Lactation deficiency (J, K).

　　　　　3) Blood stasis (H, J, K).

　　　　　4) Mass in the abdomen (C, J).

　　　　　5) Amenorrhea due to blood stasis (C, J).

　　　　　6) Abdominal distension and pain caused by retention of undigested food (C).

Contraindication: Caution in pregnancy (C, H), qi-deficiency (H).

Scientific Researches:

Chemistry

　　1) Steroids: β-sitosterol, daucosterol [1].

　　2) Organic acids: succinic acid and fatty acids [1].

　　3) Phenypropanoids: 1,3-*O*-di-*p*-coumaroylglycerol, 1,3-*O*-diferuloylglycerol, 1-*O*-feruloyl-3-*O*-
　　　　p-coumaroylglycerol,　β-D-(1-*O*-acetyl-3,6-*O*-diferuloyl)-fructofuranosyl　α-D-3',4',6'-*O*-
　　　　triacetyl-glucopyranoside, β-D-(1-*O*-acetyl-3,6-*O*-diferuloyl)-fructofuranosyl α-D-2',4',6'-*O*-
　　　　triacetyl-glucopyranoside, β-D-(1-*O*-acetyl-3,6-*O*-diferuloyl)-fructofuranosyl α-D-2',3',6'-*O*-
　　　　triacetyl-glucopyranoside [2].

　　4) Flavonoids: Kaempferol and a glycoside [3].

Literatures:

[1] Zhang, S.: *Zhongguo Zhongyao Zazhi*, **1995,** 20(8), 356; 486.

[2] Shirota, O. *et al.*: *J. Nat. Prod.* **1996**, 59(3), 242.

[3] Zhang, S.: *Zhongguo Zhongyao Zazhi*, **1996,** 21(9), 550.

[T. Kimura]

593.　　　　　　　*Amomum cardamomum* L.　(Zingiberaceae)

　　　　　　　　[= *Elettaria cardamomum* Maton.]

Ziao-dou-kou(C), Bark-dou-kou(H), Byakuzuku(J), Baek-du-gu(K)

Fruit

Local Drug Name: Xiao-dou-kou(C), Bark-dou-kou(H), Byakuzuku(J), Baek-du-gu(K)

Processing: Dry under the sun(C, K)

Method of Administration: Oral(decoction, C, J, K)

Folk Medicinal Uses:

　　　　　1) Indigestion(C, J, K)

　　　　　2) Emesis(C, K)

　　　　　3) Malaria(K)

Scientific Research:

Phamacology

　　1) Improvement of skin permeation of drug[1]

2) Reduction of side effect of anticancer drug[2]

Literature:
[1] Huang, Y. B. et al.: Kao Hsiung I Hsueh Ko Hsueh Tsa Chih **1993**, 9(7), 392.
[2] Liu, J. Q. and Wu, D. W.: Chung Kuo Chung His I Chieh Ho Tsa Chih **1993**, 13(3), 150.

[C. K. Sung]

594.   *Amomum xanthioides* **Wall.**   (Zingiberaceae)

Suo-sha(C), Sar-yun(H), Shukusha, Shajin(J), Chuk-sa(K)

Fruit
Local Drug Name: Suo-sha(C), Sar-yun(H), Shukusha, Shajin(J), Sa-in(K)
Processing: Dry under the sun(K)
Method of Administration: Oral(decoction, H, J, K)
Folk Medicinal Uses:
                   1) Stomachache(H, J, K)
                   2) Dyspepsia(J)
                   3) Meteorism(J)
                   4) Emmeniopathy(K)
                   5) Cough(K)
                   6) Thirsty throat(K)
                   7) Fever(K)

Scientific Research:
Chemistry
   1) Monoterpenes: borneol, iso-borneol, iso-borneol acetate, camphor, D-carvone, 1,4-cineol,1,8-
      cineol[1], D-limonene, linalool[2]
   2) Sequiterpenes: aromadendrene, β-bisabolene, γ-cadinene, caryophyllene, β-chamigrene,
      humulene[1], nerokidol[2]
Phamacology
   1) Antioxytocic effect[3]
   2) Antitumor activity[4]
   3) Spasmolytic activity[3]
   4) Histaminergic effect[5]
   5) Gastric secretory inhibition effect[6]
   6) Antihepatotoxic activity[7]
   7) Anticholesterolemic activity[7]

Literature:
[1] Okugawa, H. et al.: Shoyakugaku Zasshi **1987**, 41(2), 108.
[2] Nguyen, XD et al.: Tap Chi Duoc Hoc **1990**, 1, 17.
[3] Lee, E. B.: Korean J. Pharmacog. **1991**, 22(4), 246.
[4] Chang, I. M.: Arch. Pharm. Res. **1980**, 3(2), 75.
[5] Mokkhasmit, M. et al.: J. Med. Ass. Thailand **1971**, 54(7), 490.
[6] Sakai, K. et al.: Chem. Pharm. Bull. **1989**, 37(1), 215.
[7] Hong, N. D. et al.: Korean J. Pharmacog. **1982**, 13, 33.

[C. K. Sung]

595.   *Zingiber mioga* **Rosc.**   (Zingiberaceae)

Xiang-he(C), Sheung-hor(H), Myoga(J), Yang-ha(K)

Rhizome

Local Drug Name: Xiang-he(C), Sheung-hor(H), Yang-ha(K)
Processing: Dry under the sun(C, K), or use in fresh(C)
Method of Administration: Oral(decoction, C, H, K), Topical(paste or decoction: C)
Folk Medicinal Uses:

     1) Dysmenorrhea(H, K)
     2) Senile tussis(K)
     3) Red eyes(K)
     4) Inflammation(H, K)
     5) Cough(C)
     6) Bronchitis(C)
     7) Asthma(C)
     8) Toothache(C)
     9) Lumbago(C)
     10) Scrofula(C)
     11) Menstrual disorder(C)
     12) Leukorrhea(C)
     13) Rubella(C)

Scientific Research:

Chemistry

1) Monoterpene: iso-propyl *p*-benzaldehyde, borneol, borneol acetate, camphene, camphor, trans-carveol, carvone, 1,8-cineol, citral, trans-cymen-8-ol, *p*-cymene, fenchol, fenchone, geranic acid methyl ester, geranyl-acetone, limonene, limone-1,2-oxide, linalool, linalool acetate, 3-*p*-menthan-7-ol, neoisomenthol, mycene, mycene epoxide, myritenal, myritenol, myritenol acetate, cis-ocimene, trans-ocimene, perillaldehyde, α-phellandrene, β-phellandrene, α-pinene, β-pinene, pinocarveol, piperitone, sabinene, cis-sabinene hydrate, trans-sabinene hydrate, terpinene, 1-terpineol, α-terpineol, β-terpineol, thymol [1]

2) Diterpene: geranyl linalool[1]

3) Sulfur compound: benzothiazole[1]

4) Sesquiterpene: bicycloelemene, bicyclegermacrene, α-cardinol, caryophyllene formate, β-caryophyllene, β-, δ-, γ-elemene, α-farnensene, germacrene D, α-humulene, β-ionone, nerolidol [1]

5) Alkene: butyl-2-methyl-2-buteonate 3-methyl, dec-trans-2-en-1-al, dodecen-1-ol, dodecen-1-al, hept-5-en-ol 2-6-dimethyl, hep-5-en-2-one 6-methyl, hex-2-en-1-al 2-vinyl, hex-4-en-1-al 2-5-dimethyl-2-vinyl, hex-cis-3-en-1-al, hex-cis-3-en-1-ol, hex-cis-3-en-1-ol-2-methyl-2-butenoate, hex-trans-2-en-1-al, hex-trans-2-en-1-ol, oct-1-en-ol, oct-cis-2-en-1-ol, oct-trans-2-en-1-al, pentadecen-1-al, tridecen-1-al, undec-10-en-2-one [1], pent-1-en-3-ol, propyl-2-methyl-2-butenoate 2-methyl [4]

6) Alkane: decan-1-al, decan-2-one, dodecan-1-al, dodecan-2-one, heptan-1-al, heptane-2-one, heptan-2-one hydroxy, heptane-2-5-dione 6-methyl, hexan-1-al, hexan-1-ol, hexan-1-ol 2-methyl, nonan-1-al, nonan-2-ol, nonan-2-one, octan-1-ol, octan-3-ol, octan-3-one, pentan-1-ol, pentan-2-one 4-methyl, pentan-3-ol, pentan-3-one, tetradecan-1-al, tetradecan-2-one, tridecan-1-al, tridecan-2-oltridecan-2-one, undecan-1-al, undecan-2-ol, undecan-2-one [1]

7) Alicyclic: 4-iso-propyl cyclo-hex-2-enone, 4-iso-propyl cyclohexanol, cyclohexanone

8) Lipid: dodecanoic acid ethyl ester [1], lauric acid, myristic acid, oleic acid, palmitic acid, stearic acid [2]

9) Steroid: ergosterol, β-sitosterol, stigmasterol [2]

10) Phenylpropanoid: eugenol, isoeuenol methyl ether

11) Crbohydrate: glucose [2]

12) Proteid: glycine, serine, threonine, valine [2]

13) Indole alkaoid: indole [1]

14) Benzenoid: phenol, 2-phenylethanol, toluene, meta-xylene[1]

15) Alkaloid: 2-iso-butyl-3-methoxy pyrazine, 2-iso-propyl-3-methoxy pyrazine, 2-sec-butyl-3-

methoxy pyrazine[1]
16) Alicyclic: quinic acid, shikimic acid [4]
17) Miscellaneous: acetaldehyde, 3-methyl but-3-en-2-ol, but-3-en-2-one, 3-methyl but-trans-2-en-
1-al, butan-1-ol, 3-methyl butan-1-ol, butan-2-ol, butan-2-one, 3-methyl butyl acetate,ethanol,
ethyl acetate, ethyl formate, oxalic acid, propan-1-ol, 2-methyl propan-1-ol, propyl acetate [1]

Pharmacology
1) Tumor promotion inhibition effect [5]
2) Carcinogenic activity [6]
3) Antiedema activity [7]
4) Barbiturate potentiation effect, CNS depressant activity [8]
5) Desmutagenic activity[9]

Literiture:
[1] Kurobayashi, Y. et al.: Agr. Biol. Chem. **1991**, 55, 1655.
[2] Machida, K. et al.: Annu. Rep. Tohoku. Coll. Pharm. **1985**, 32, 129.
[3] Nakahara, K.: Eiyo. To. Shokuryo. **1974**, 27, 33.
[4] Yoshida, S. et al.: Phytochemistry. **1975**, 14, 195.
[5] Koshimizu, K. et al.: Cancer Lett. **1988**, 39, 247.
[6] Hirono, I. et al.: Cancer Lett. **1982**, 15, 203.
[7] Yasukawa, Y. et al. : Phytother Res. **1993**, 7, 185.
[8] Suzuki, Y. et al.: Folia Pharmacol. Japan. **1979**, 75, 731.
[9] Morita, K. et al.: Agr. Biol. Chem. **1978**, 42, 1235.

[C. K. Sung]

596.　　　　　*Cremastra variabilis* **Nakai**　　(Orchidaceae)
[= *C.appendiculata* Makino]

Du-juan-lan(C), Saihairan(J), Yak-nan-cho(K)

Bulb
Local Drug Name: Mao-ci-gu(C), Sanjiko(J), San-ja-go(K)
Processing: Dry under the sun(C, K)
Method of Administration: Oral(decoction, C, K), topical(paste, C)
Folk Medicinal Uses:
1) Snake bite(C, J, K)
2) Tuberculosis(C, K)
3) Carbuncle(C)
4) Abscess(J)
5) Frost bite(K)

Scientific Research:
Phamacology
1) Antitumor activity[1]

Literature:
[1] Chen, L. C.: Jhejiang J. Trad. Chin. Med. **1988**, 23(8), 365.

[C. K. Sung]

597.　　　　*Pleione bulbocodioides* **(Franch.) Rolfe**　　(Orchidaceae)

Du-shuan-lan (C), Sanjiko (J)

Related Plants: *P. yannanensis* Rolfe: Yun-nan-du-shuan-lan (C); *Cremastra appendiculata* (D. Don) Makino: Du-juan-lan (C).

Pseadobulb (CP)
  Local Drug Name: Shan-ci-gu (C), Sanjiko (J).
  Processing: Eliminate foreign matter, soak for about 1 hour, soften thoroughly, cut into thin slices, and dry, or dry after washing, pound to pieces before use (C).
  Method of Administration: Oral (decoction: C); Topical (decoction: C).
  Folk Medicinal Uses:
  > 1) Carbuncles (C, J).
  > 2) Boils (C, J).
  > 3) Tuberculosis of cervical lymph nodes (C).
  > 4) Snake and insect bite (C).

Scientific Research:
  Chemistry
  1) Dihydrophenanthropyran: Shanciol, bletilol B[1], bletilols A, C[5]
  2) Stilbenoids: Shancidin, shancinlin, shanciguol[2], shanciols C, D[5]
  3) Lignans: Sanjidins A, B[3]
  4) Bichromans: Pleionin A[3]
  5) Bibenzyl glycosides: 3'-Hydroxy-5-methoxybibenzyl-3-O-β-D-glucopyranoside, 3',5'-dimethoxybibenzyl-3-O-β-D-glucopyranoside, batatasin III, 3'-O-methylbatatasin III[4]
  6) Flavonoids: Shanciols A, B[5]

Literature:
  [1] Bai, L. et al.: *Phytochemistry* **1996**, 41(2), 625.
  [2] Bai, L. et al.: *Phytochemistry* **1996**, 42(3), 853.
  [3] Bai, L. et al.: *Phytochemistry* **1997**, 44(2), 341.
  [4] Bai, L. et al.: *Phytochemistry* **1997**, 44(8), 1565.
  [5] Bai, L. et al.: *Phytochemistry* **1998**, 47(6), 1125.

[J.X. Guo]

598.　　　　　*Spiranthes sinensis* **(Pers.) Ames**　　(Orchidaceae)

Shou-cao (C), Sau-cho (H), Ta-rae-nan-cho (K)

Root or Whole Plant
  Local Drug Name: Pan-long-shen (C), Poon-lung-sum (H), Bam-ryong-sam (K).
  Processing: Dry under the sun (C, H, K).
  Method of Administration: Oral (decoction: C, H, K); Topical (macerated fresh herb: C, H, K).
  Folk Medicinal Uses:
  > 1) Tuberculosis (C, H, K).
  > 2) Hemoptysis (C, H, K).
  > 3) Debility (C, H, K).
  > 4) Snake bites (C, H).
  > 5) Sore throat (C, H).
  > 6) Summer fever in children (C, H).
  > 7) Neurasthenia (C, H).
  > 8) Cough (H, K).
  > 9) Leukorrhea (C).
  > 10) Diabetes (C).
  > 11) Pyodermas (H).

12) Tonsillitis (H).

Scientific Research:
Chemistry
1) Spiranthols A and B, spirasineol A, orchinol, *p*-hydroxybenzaldehyde, *p*-hydroxybenzyl alcohol, hydrocarbons, sterols, ferulates [1].

Literature:
[1] Tezuka, Y. *et al.*: *Chem. Pharm. Bull.* **1989,** 37, 3195.

[P.P.H. But]

599. *Pegasus laternarius* **(Cuvier)**   (Pegasidae)

Hai-e (C), Hai-jerk (H)

Related animals: *P. volitans* Cuvier: Hai-e(C), Hai-jerk(H)

Whole fish
Local Drug Name: Hai-e (C), Hai-jerk (H)
Processing: Remove the visceral organs and dry under the sun (C).
Method of Administration: Oral (soup: C, H)
Folk Medicinal Uses:
  1) Cough and sputum (C, H).
  2) Bronchitis (C, H).
  3) Measles (C, H).
  4) Diarrhea (C).
  5) Thyroid tumor (C).

Scientific Research:
Chemistry
1) Proteins, peptides, amino acids, lipids, ceramid octasaccharide, mannose-6-phosphate [1].
Pharmacology
1) Anti-lipoperoxidation effect [2, 3].
2) Antitumor effect [2].
3) Anti-inflammatory effect [3].
4) Immunostimulatory effect [3].

Literature:
[1] Anonymous: *Medicinal Fauna of China (Zhongguo Yaoyong Dongwuzhi)* **1983,** 2, 271.
[2] Xu, S.P. *et al.*: *Acta Scientiarum Naturalium Universitatis Sunyatseni* **1990,** 29 (Suppl.), 101.
[3] Xu, S.P. *et al.*: *Acta Scientiarum Naturalium Universitatis Sunyatseni* **1990,** 29 (Suppl.), 105.

[P.P.H. But]

600. *Selenarctos thibetanus* **G. Cuvier**   (Ursidae)

Hei-xiong (C), Hark-hung(H), Tsukinowaguma(J), Heuk-gom(K)

Related animals: *Ursus arctos* L.: Zong-xiong(C), Chung-hung(H), Higuma(J), Gom(K)

Gall bladder or bile
Local Drug Name: Xiong-dan. (C), Hung-darm (H), Yutan(J), Ung-dam(K)

177

Processing: Dry in shade (C, H, J, K).
Method of Administration: Oral (powder: C, H, J, K)
Folk Medicinal Uses:

        1) Convulsion (C, H, J, K).
        2) Conjunctivitis (C, H, J, K).
        3) Pharyngolaryngitis (C, H, J, K).
        4) Jaundice (C, J, K).
        5) Febrile diseases (C, J, K).
        6) Furuncle (C, K).
        7) Chronic summer diarrhea (C).
        8) Ascariasis pain (C).
        9) Hyperemia (C).
        10) Nebula (C).
        11) Hemorrhoid (C).
        12) Carbuncle (C).

Note: Both *Selenarctos thibetanus* and *Ursus arctos* are listed on CITES Appendix I. Poaching and trading are prohibited[10].

Scientific Research:

Chemistry
    1) Ursodeoxycholic acid, chenodeoxycholic acid, cholic acid [1, 7].
Pharmacology
    1) Anti-inflammatory effect [2–4].
    2) Anticonvulsion effect [2–4].
    3) Analgesic effect [2].
    4) Prolong survival in hypoxic conditions [2].
    5) Gall stone dissolving effects [9, 11].
    6) Choleretic effects [4].
    7) Anti-arrhythmic effect [5].
    8) Vasodilatory effect. [6].
    9) Antibacterial effect [8].
    10) LD_{50} of bear bile: 1071.7 mg/kg s.c. [4].

Literature:

[1] Taguchi, H. *et al.*: *Chem. Pharm. Bull.* **1976,** 24, 1668.
[2] Li, Y. W. *et al.*: *J. Ethnopharm.* **1995,** 47, 27.
[3] Li, X. P. *et al.*: *J. Yanbian Medical College* **1976,** 14, 235.
[4] Li, W. J. *et al.*: *J. Chin. Mat. Med.* **1990** 13(2), 12.
[5] Ye, D. *et al.*: *Chin. J. Internal Med.* **1992,** 31, 241.
[6] Wang, Y. P. *et al.*: *J. China Med. Univ.* **1991,** 20, 297.
[7] Song, Z. J. *et al.*: *Chin. J. Patent Med.* **1991,** 13(7), 32.
[8] Liu, X. Y. *et al.*: *Chin. Trad. Patent Med.* **1991,** 13(4), 43.
[9] Leuschner, U. *et al.*: *Gasteroenterology* **1989,** 97, 1268.
[10] But, P. P. H.: *1995 AZA Annual Conference Proceedings* **1995,** 68.
[11] Sano, M.: *Proc. Int. Symp. on Trade of Bear Parts for Medicinal Use* **1995,** 43.

[P.P.H. But]

INDEX TO SCIENTIFIC NAMES

中文索引（繁體字、简体字、日字） (in Plant No.)

183

INDEX TO LOCAL HERB NAMES

Feng-dou-cai 571
Feng-ji-sheng 428
Feng-teng 453
Feng-xiang-shu 467
Feng-xiang-zhi 467
Foo-gui-choi 574
Foon-gun-teng 452
Fu-peng-zi 478
Fuk-poon-gee 478
Fukoushi 467
Fukubonshi 478
Fun-fong-gay 451
Funboi 451
Fung-shu 467
Futokazura 453
Fuu 467

Ga-che 548
Ga-geun 548
Ga-go-gwa 493
Ga-hwa 548
Ga-ja 504
Ga-ji 548
Ga-neun-ip-hal-mi-ggot 445
Ga-ri-reuk 504
Ga-yeop 548
Gae-byul-ggot 433
Gae-da-rae 456
Gae-gu-ri-gat 447
Gae-ja 463
Gae-yang-gwi-bi 461
Gagaimo 530
Gaishi 463
Gam-da 470
Gam-song 557
Gam-song-hyang 557
Gan-gi 492
Gan-song 557
Gang-ban-gui 430
Gang-hwal 513
Gang-liu 531
Gang-pan-gwi 430
Ganto 571
Gao-ben 512
Gat 463
Gat-beo-seot 407
Ge-zao 456
Gee-gum-ngau 520
Gen-chi-a-na 527
Genchiana 527
Geon-chil 492
Geum-aeng-ja 476
Ggot-i-ggi 415
Ggu-ji-bbong-na-mu 427
Gie-choi 463

Gie-gee 463
Gil-cho-geun 559
Gim 405
Giso 562
Go-bon 511
Go-chae 574
Go-chu-na-mul 459
Gobaishi 491
Goh-boon 512
Gohishokon 529
Gon-chut 492
Gon-po 402
Gong-barn-gwai 430
Gong-lao-mu 449
Gorenshi 485
Gu-maek 432
Guang-zao 490
Gui-muk 432
Gum-chung 557
Gum-ying-far 476
Gum-ying-gee 476
Gum-ying-gee-yip 476
Gum-ying-gun 476
Gung-loh-muk 449
Guo-lu-huang 522
Gwan-yeop-gam-song 558
Gwang-du-geun 483
Gwang-na-mu 524
Gweon-sam 429

Hae-dae 403
Hae-dang-hwa 477
Hae-pung-deung 453
Hae-tae 405
Hagekiten 533
Hai-dai 402
Hai-e 599
Hai-er-shen 433
Hai-feng-teng 453
Hai-jerk 599
Hai-zhong-cao-zi 444
Hakkadazetsuso 534
Hakurakukai 460
Hakusen 489
Hakusenhi 489
Hakushinin 422
Hakuto-o 445
Hamajisha 431
Hark-min-sun 487
Hark-min-sun-yip 487
Hashiridokoro 547
Hau-tau-gwoo 410
Hay-shue 506
He-tao-ren 424
He-zi 504

Hei-mian-shu 487
Hei-mian-ye 487
Heui-su 506
Heung-gar-pay 531
Hibatsu 454
Hicchoka 443
Hihatsu 454
Hiiragi-nanten 449
Hijitsu 423
Hikai 585
Himawari 567
Himeaikyo 510
Hin-myeong-a-ju 434
Hinageshi 461
Hiroha-okinagusa 446
Hirugao 537
Hitotsuba 419
Ho-do-in 424
Ho-du-na-mu 424
Ho-hwang-ryeon 552
Ho-hwang-ryun 553
Ho-ro 498
Hoi-dai 402
Hoi-fung-tunk 453
Homika 526
Hon-shakunage 518
Honpakuso 473
Hook-gay-sung 428
Hor-gee 504
Hou-tou 410
Houkigi 435
Hu-chu 455
Hu-chu-deung 453
Hu-chu-na-mu 455
Hu-huang-lian 553
Hu-jiao 455
Hu-man-teng 525
Hu-tao 424
Hua-dong-fu-pen-zi 478
Hua-shan-shen 546
Huan-ye-liao 429
Huang-jing 540
Huang-niu-cha 457
Huang-niu-mu 457
Hung-darm 600
Hup-toh 424
Hup-top 424
Hwal-na-mul 481
Hwang-jeong 581
Hyang-ga-pi 531
Hyang-il-gyu-ja 567
Hyotan 498

Ibuki-toranoo 429
Ibukijakoso 544

189

Moe-die-ding-cho 572
Moe-sair-heung 549
Mok-cheon-ryo-ja 456
Mok-hwa 495
Mokuji 408
Mokutenryo 456
Monkei 417
Mour-jour-cho 447
Mu-er 408
Mu-jing 540
Mu-u 466
Mube 450
Mug-gar 588
Mui-gwai 477
Muk-yee 408
Mun-hyung 417
Murasaki-omoto 586
Mutianliao 456
Mutianliao-zi 456
Myeo-neu-ri-bae-ggop 430
Myeon-hwa-geun 495
Myeon-hwa-ja 495
Myo-jo-cho 447
Myrobalan 504

Na-ma-ja 530
Na-ma-yeop 530
Nae-bok 466
Nan-hyang-cho 538
Nan-suan-zao 490
Nang-tang-geun 547
Nang-tang-yeop 547
Naniwaibana 476
Nanto 453
Nasu 548
Nezumimochi 524
Ngai-gwar 548
Ngie-keung 418
Nikuzuku 440
Ninjinboku 540
Nong-ji-li 481
Nung-gut-lay 481
Nurude 491
Nyoteishi 524
Nyoteiyo 524

O-bae-ja 491
Okinagusa 445
Ot-na-mu 492
Otogiriso 459
Ousei 581

Pa-geuk-cheon 533
Pal-gak-geum-ban 507
Pal-gak-hoi-hyang 438

Pal-gak-hoi-hyang-yu 438
Pal-son-i 507
Pan-long-shen 598
Pan-ram-geun 464
Parng-kay-guk 576
Pay-gie 585
Peng-qi-ju 576
Pil-bal 454
Pong-far 586
Poon-lung-sum 598
Pung-seon-deong-gul 493

Qi-shu 492
Qiang-huo 513
Qie-yi 514
Qie-zi-gen 548
Qu-mai 432
Quan-shen 429
Qun-dai-cai 404

Raigan 409
Rakanka 499
Ramashi 530
Ramayo 530
Reishi 494
Reishunka 461
Renge-tsutsuji 517
Rishiri-konbu 403
Ritsu-ka 425
Ritsu-yo 425
Rorotsu 467
Rou-dou-kou 440
Routokon 547
Routoyo 547
Rui-he 474
Rui-ren 474
Ryudo-sogoko 468

Sa-in 594
Sa-sang-ja 514
Sa-weon-ja 479
Saan-jar 471
Sak-wai 419
Sam-chil 508
Sam-chil-in-sam 508
Sam-reung 592
San-du-geun 483
San-gi 508
San-ja-go 596
San-leng 592
San-sa-ja 471
Sanjiko 596
Sanshichi 566
Sanshichi-ninjin 508
Sanzashi 471

Sanzukon 483
Sar-yuan-gee 479
Sar-yun 594
Sarm-ling 592
Sarn-die-doe 535
Sarn-dou-gun 483
Sarn-garn-larn 578
Sarn-tsarng 528
Seini 561
Sekii 419
Sekisho 416
Sekishozu 484
Senka 537
Senkoku-kon 587
Senpukuka 568
Seo-jang-ho-hwang-ryun 553
Seok-ji-gap 469
Seok-wi 419
Seok-ye-cho 415
Seon-bok-hwa 568
Seon-hwa 537
Seon-hwang-gi 479
Seu-ko-po-ri-a 547
Sha-yuan-zi 479
Shajin 594
Shakunage-yo 518
Shan-cheng 528
Shan-ci-gu 597
Shan-da-yan 535
Shan-dou-gen 483
Shan-ji-jiao 443
Shan-jian-lan 578
Shan-zha 471
Shen-jin-cao 416
Shen-jue 420
Sheung-hor 595
Shi-luo 510
Shi-rui 415
Shi-song 416
Shi-wei 419
Shikingyu 520
Shima-hasunohi-kazura 451
Shiroza 434
Sho-rengyo 459
Shobeki 448
Shui-rong 500
Shui-rong-gen 500
Shui-rong-hua 500
Shui-rong-pi 500
Shui-rong-ye 500
Shui-yung 500
Shui-yung-far 500
Shui-yung-gun 500
Shui-yung-pay 500
Shui-yung-yip 500

INDEX TO DISEASES AND BIOACTIVITIES

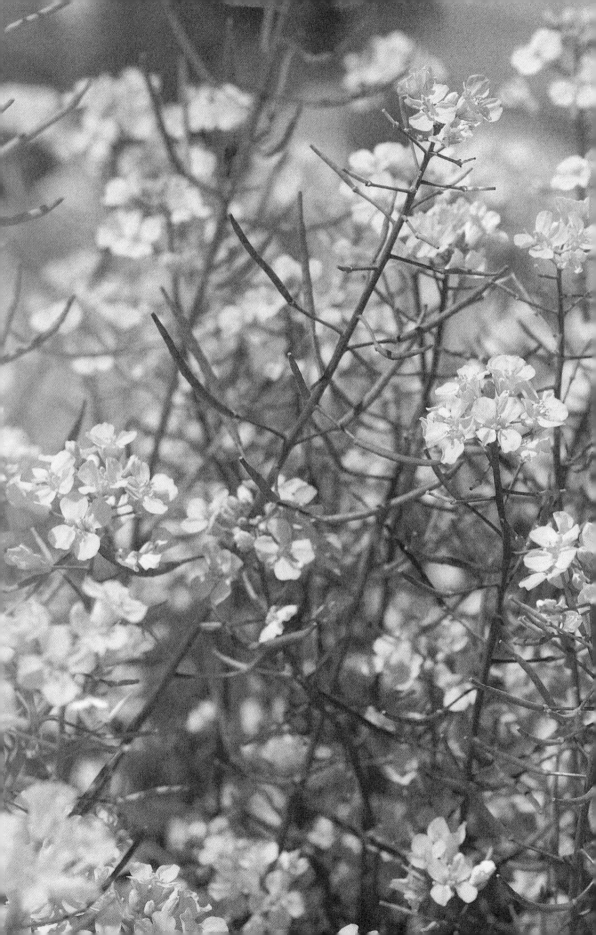